Neuronal Development

CURRENT TOPICS IN NEUROBIOLOGY

Series Editor

Samuel H. Barondes
Professor of Psychiatry
School of Medicine
University of California, San Diego
La Jolla, California

Tissue Culture of the Nervous System
Edited by Gordon Sato

Neuronal Recognition
Edited by Samuel H. Barondes

Peptides in Neurobiology
Edited by Harold Gainer

Neuronal Development
Edited by Nicholas C. Spitzer

Neuroimmunology
Edited by Jeremy Brockes

A continuation Order Plan is available for this series. A continuation order will bring delivery of each new volume immediatedly upon publication. Volumes are billed only upon actual shipment. For further information please contact the publisher.

Neuronal Development

Edited by
Nicholas C. Spitzer
University of California, San Diego
La Jolla, California

PLENUM PRESS • NEW YORK AND LONDON

Library of Congress Cataloging in Publication Data

Main entry under title:

Neuronal development.

(Current topics in neurobiology)
Includes bibliographical references and index.
1. Developmental neurology. I. Spitzer, Nicholas C. II. Series. [DNLM: 1. Nervous system—Embryology. 2. Nervous system—Growth and development. W1 CU82P v. 4/WL 0 101 N493]

QP363.5.N49 591.3′34 82-3693
ISBN 0-306-40956-9 AACR2

A Division of Plenum Publishing Corporation
233 Spring Street, New York, N.Y. 10013

Printed in the United States of America

Contributors

KATE F. BARALD — Department of Anatomy and Cell Biology
University of Michigan Medical School
Ann Arbor, Michigan

DARWIN K. BERG — Department of Biology
University of California, San Diego
La Jolla, California

SETH S. BLAIR — Department of Molecular Biology
University of California, Berkeley
Berkeley, California

W. MAXWELL COWAN — Salk Institute for Biological Studies
San Diego, California

JOHN S. EDWARDS — Department of Zoology
University of Washington
Seattle, Washington

THOMAS E. FINGER — Department of Anatomy
University of Colorado Medical Center
Denver, Colorado

MURRAY S. FLASTER — Department of Biological Sciences
Columbia University
New York, New York

COREY S. GOODMAN — Department of Biological Sciences
Stanford University
Stanford, California

MARCUS JACOBSON — Department of Anatomy
School of Medicine
University of Utah
Salt Lake City, Utah

PAUL C. LETOURNEAU — Department of Anatomy
University of Minnesota
Minneapolis, Minnesota

EDUARDO R. MACAGNO — Department of Biological Sciences
Columbia University
New York, New York

JOHN PALKA — Department of Zoology
University of Washington
Seattle, Washington

ROBERT S. SCHEHR — Department of Biological Sciences
Columbia University
New York, New York

GUNTHER S. STENT — Department of Molecular Biology
University of California, Berkeley
Berkeley, California

DAVID C. VAN ESSEN — Division of Biology
California Institute of Technology
Pasadena, California

DAVID A. WEISBLAT
Department of Molecular Biology
University of California, Berkeley
Berkeley, California

SAUL L. ZACKSON
Department of Molecular Biology
University of California, Berkeley
Berkeley, California

Foreword

Studies of simple and emerging systems have been undertaken to understand the processes by which a developing system unfolds, and to understand more completely the basis of the complexity of the fully formed structures. The nervous system has long been particularly intriguing for such studies, because of the early recognition of a multitude of distinctly differentiated states exhibited by nerve cells with different morphologies. Anatomical studies suggest that one liver cell may be very like another, but indicate that neurons come in a remarkable diversity of forms. This diversity at the anatomical level has parallels at the physiological and biochemical levels. It is becoming increasingly easy to characterize the different cellular phenotypes of neurons. The repeatability with which these phenotypes are expressed may account in part for the specificity and reliability with which neurons form connections, and it has allowed precise description of the first appearance and further development of the differentiated characteristics of individual neurons from relatively undifferentiated precursor cells. This represents a major advance over our knowledge of development at the level of tissues, and makes it feasible to define and address questions about the underlying molecular mechanisms involved.

Central to these advances has been the clear recognition that there is no single best preparation for the study of neuronal development. Furthermore, it has become evident that no single technique can tell us all we want to know. As this volume demonstrates, a multitude of techniques, many of them developed only recently, are being brought to bear on a wide variety of preparations. The breadth of the approaches has not only advanced our knowledge rapidly, but has simultaneously thrown into relief the similarities and divergences found among different nervous systems, potentially aiding in the recognition of general principles.

The fundamental question that the authors have addressed is "How does the nervous system acquire its differentiated state?" While each chapter approaches this from a different perspective, there are several common themes. The first of these is to ask, "What is the cell lineage or mitotic ancestry of particular neurons?" Several ingenious methods have been devised that permit the tracing of cell lineages. The answer to this question frames the next, which is "What is the role of cell lineage in the differentiation of particular cells? What are the relative contributions of the cytoplasm and its interaction with the genome, versus the contributions of the environment?" A second major theme is to ask, "What are the rules and the underlying molecular mechanisms that give rise to differentiated states, such as extended neurites or specific, stabilized synapses? What are the constraints on the normal outcome of development, and what macromolecules play roles in the expression of neuronal phenotypes?" Implicit throughout all of the authors' efforts is a concern with developing working hypotheses, or explicitly devising testable models, that shape the course of further experimentation.

The first five chapters are concerned with defining the lineage of the nervous system or of specific nerve cells in different organisms. Stent, Weisblat, Blair and Zackson have injected horseradish peroxidase or a fluorescently labeled D-amino acid peptide (not subject to digestion by intracellular proteases) into identified blastomeres of the leech, and examined the distribution of label to their progeny. In this system cell lineage appears to be a major determinant of cell fate, since ablation of specific blastomeres leads to the absence of their progeny; no replacement by progeny of other cells occurs. Jacobson has used the horseradish peroxidase tracer to evaluate the role of lineage in a vertebrate nervous system; his results indicate that ablation of small numbers of identified blastomeres causes no deficit in the development of neurons to which they normally give rise, and that some regulation occurs in the development of the frog embryo. He is led to conclude, however, that there are larger regions (that he terms compartments) in early embryos, which are committed from early stages to form whole regions of the nervous system; removal of all the cells in a compartment results in the absence of cellular structures they normally generate. A provocative theory is presented, supported by his experimental results, which directly challenges the organizer concept of Spemann and Mangold and explains the organization of the CNS by the early specification of compartments. Barald has used a different probe to study the development of chick ciliary ganglion neurons. Monoclonal antibodies recognizing cell surface components of the neurons have been found to recognize a small proportion of the neural crest cells from which they are derived, as well.

This finding raises the possibility of using immunological methods to map neuronal lineage; the role of lineage in development can then be assessed by complement-mediated ablations of cells at different stages in the early embryo. Goodman has focused on an invertebrate with a meroblastic cleavage that permits separation of the embryo from its associated yolk; it has been possible to make direct observations of mitotic ancestry in the grasshopper nervous system, by microscopic examination of living embryos of increasing age, comparable to the studies of developing nematodes. A role for lineage in development of this nervous system is suggested by the observation that all of the progeny of one neuroblast come to contain the same neurotransmitter. Palka has employed a genetic analysis of *Drosophila* to assess the role of the genome (and thus lineage) in directing neuronal development. Studies of pathways followed by outgrowing neurites in homeotic mutants suggest that some cuticular mutations do not affect the sensory axons, which develop normal projections in spite of the altered environment. Furthermore, sensory fibers ignore the classical compartment boundaries in the periphery, as they establish their paths, although the opposite result obtains in the CNS; the dominant guiding factors seem to be different for these two regions. These five chapters detail some of the most imaginative approaches to understanding the role of lineage in neuronal development. The work of these investigators, and others not included here, indicates that the relative contribution depends not only on the embryo studied but on the stage of development as well.

Five chapters are concerned with neurite extension and pathway formation. This typical feature of neuronal differentiation has received much attention because its characterization is straightforward, although its determinants may be complex. Three authors provide convergent evidence for a role of early developing pioneer fibers in directing subsequent neuronal outgrowth. Edwards' studies of development of the cercal nerve in the cricket are the most direct. Laser ablations of the peripheral pioneer cell bodies lead to disorganization of the ingrowing sensory axon bundles, when made at early stages; after pioneer tracts are established, the lesions are without effect. Goodman describes the earliest outgrowth of neurites in the grasshopper CNS, from midline precursor cells; since these are the first to lay down axonal pathways, which are followed by other outgrowing neurites, they appear to serve the role of pioneers. Palka is led to a similar conclusion for the development of peripheral sensory fiber pathways in *Drosophila*. Moreover, Flaster, Macagno and Schehr, in their investigations of the development of the visual system of the crustacean *Daphnia*, provide evidence for substrate guidance of axonal growth by a glial cell column; destruction of this column by UV radiation causes some photoreceptors to fail send axons to the lamina, their normal target. Finally, the possible mechanisms for neurite elongation and pathfinding are analyzed in tissue culture studies by Letourneau. A detailed model for nerve fiber growth is presented, involving a balance of protrusion, adhesion, and force generation by actomyosin. The power of this model is that the regulation of nerve fiber growth by environmental factors, including interactions with other cells and chemotaxis to agents such as NGF, can be understood in terms of the interaction of these extrinsic factors with the elements of the model.

The two chapters by Goodman and Letourneau illustrate the success with which specific membrane and cytoplasmic features of neuronal differentiation, respectively, are now being studied. The onset and further development of electrical excitability and chemosensitivity have been described for identified neurons of the grasshopper embryo. The cellular localization of actin and myosin in growth cones *in vitro* has been defined immunocytochemically. These immunological methods will allow determination of the time of appearance of characteristic neuronal proteins (such as transmitter receptors and ion channels); cDNA probes will allow determination of the time of appearance of specific mRNAs in particular cells, using the newly developed technique of hybridization histochemistry (not discussed in this volume).

The development of the nervous system includes formation of vast numbers of specific synaptic connections. The events involved in synaptogenesis have been extensively described elsewhere. Three chapters in this volume discuss aspects of synapse formation, maintenance and elimination; the findings are of particular interest since they go beyond the descriptive phase of investigation and present the results of perturbation analysis. Flaster, Macagno and Schehr propose that the specificity with which synapses are formed is a consequence of the spatiotemporal organization of axon growth in the visual system of *Daphnia*. Deletions of photoreceptors or delays in their differentiation produce defects that strongly support their model. Berg analyses the phenomenon of nerve cell death during development, an impressive event in which more than half of the cells generated typically disappear. Experimental manipulations indicate that the extent of cell death depends on the size of the normally innervated target tissue; additional targets reduce the extent of cell death. While some evidence indicates that functional synapses are necessary for neuronal survival, the findings are also compatible with the targets serving as sources of trophic factors, supplied to the neurites. In addition to NGF, critical for the development of sympathetic neurons, several recently discovered factors essential for parasympathetic neurons, and for other neuronal populations, are described. Van Essen discusses the phenomenon of initial polyneuronal innervation and subsequent synapse elimination at the mammalian neuromuscular junction, which occurs after the period of neuronal death. He develops a comprehensive model that accounts for both the processes of polyneuronal innervation and its subsequent elimination, on the basis of interactions already known to occur during synaptogenesis. A prominent element of this model is the role played by the synaptic scaffolding in stabilizing or relinquishing the contacts of motor neuron terminals upon the muscle, and attention is directed to further experimental efforts to identify its constituents.

The final chapter recapitulates a number of the themes previously developed. Cowan and Finger have observed a striking regenerative capacity in the chick, following unilateral ablations at early stages. New neurons are generated in the normal sequence, albeit somewhat delayed; the tectal cytoarchitecture is reconstituted normally; retinal projections to the regenerated tectum are normal in binocular chicks, but expand over the tectal surface in monocular embryos. Developmental regulation, precision of neurite outgrowth, and competition for target tissues are demonstrated here. That such processes can take place by regeneration at these stages of development emphasizes the remarkable degree of plasticity of the embryonic avian nervous system.

This is an exciting time for developmental neurobiologists. New technical advances and selective exploitation of a variety of preparations are yielding information about neuronal development at the cellular and molecular levels. It is a pleasure to thank the authors for their splendid contributions. The rapid recent expansion of knowledge suggests that the years ahead will be particularly productive ones.

Nicholas C. Spitzer
La Jolla

Contents

8. Mechanisms for the Formation of Synaptic Connections in the Isogenic Nervous System of *Daphnia Magna* 267

MURRAY S. FLASTER, EDUARDO R. MACAGNO, AND ROBERT S. SCHEHR

1

Cell Lineage in the Development of the Leech Nervous System

GUNTHER S. STENT, DAVID A. WEISBLAT, SETH S. BLAIR, and SAUL L. ZACKSON

1. INTRODUCTION

1.1. Developmental Cell Lineages

The intricate structure and function of the adult nervous system is the result of developmental interactions of factors both intrinsic and extrinsic to the embryonic neurons and their precursor cells. To fathom the mechanisms underlying these interactive processes, a detailed knowledge of the course of neurogenesis at the cellular level is essential. Once such knowledge is available, specific and well-focused questions can be formulated at the biophysical, biochemical, or genetic levels. One key aspect of the process of neurogenesis at the cellular level is *cell lineage*, i.e., the embryonic lines of descent of various types of neurons. The importance of cell lineage for understanding developmental processes was realized over a century ago by C. O. Whitman.[1] On the basis of his studies of the development of leeches, Whitman put forward the idea, then quite novel, that each identified cell of the early embryo, and the clone of its

GUNTHER S. STENT, DAVID A. WEISBLAT, SETH S. BLAIR, and SAUL L. ZACKSON · Department of Molecular Biology, University of California, Berkeley, CA 94720.

descendant cells, plays a specific role in later development. Cell lineage analyses were later extended to the embryos of other species, not only by direct observation but also by use of other techniques, such as selective ablation, application of extracellular marker particles, and, most importantly, production of chimera and genetic mosaics.[2–10] More recently, we have refined and extended Whitman's century-old cell lineage studies in leech embryos, with particular emphasis on the cellular origins of the leech nervous system. As will be seen in this chapter, leeches are well suited for cellular investigations of neuronal development because both their early embryos and their adult nervous systems comprise identifiable cells accessible to experimental manipulation.

Before giving an account of the results of our cell lineage studies, we provide a brief overview of the nervous system of the adult leech and of the general course of leech embryogenesis. We then present the novel techniques for cell lineage tracing that have allowed progress beyond the classical findings of Whitman and his followers. It should be noted that most investigations of the adult leech nervous system were carried out with species belonging to the family of Hirudinidae (order Gnathobdellidae).[11] By contrast, most investigations of leech embryology, including Whitman's and our own, were carried out with species belonging to the family of Glossiphoniidae (order Rhyncobdellidae).[12–15] Fortunately the nervous systems of leeches belonging to these two different orders are sufficiently similar that much of the neurophysiological and neuroanatomical knowledge available from the study of the Hirudinidae is applicable to the Glossiphoniidae.[16,17]

1.2. The Leech Nervous System

The leech CNS consists of a ventral chain of 32 segmentally iterated ganglia.[18] The first four and last seven segmental ganglia are fused, constituting a rostral and caudal ganglionic mass, respectively. The rostral ganglionic mass, or subesophageal ganglion, is connected at its anterior end to a dorsally situated supraesophageal ganglion. Each segmental ganglion contains about 400 bilaterally paired neurons,[19] as well as a few unpaired neurons (Fig. 1). Their somata form a cortex around the outer surface of the ganglion. The neurons are monopolar; their processes project into a central neuropil, where they make synaptic contacts. From there, the processes of some neurons project to other ganglia via a connective nerve. Sensory and effector neurons project their processes to targets outside the CNS via segmental nerves, whose roots emerge from the lateral edge of the ganglion. In each ganglion, the neuronal somata are distributed over six cell packets, of which two

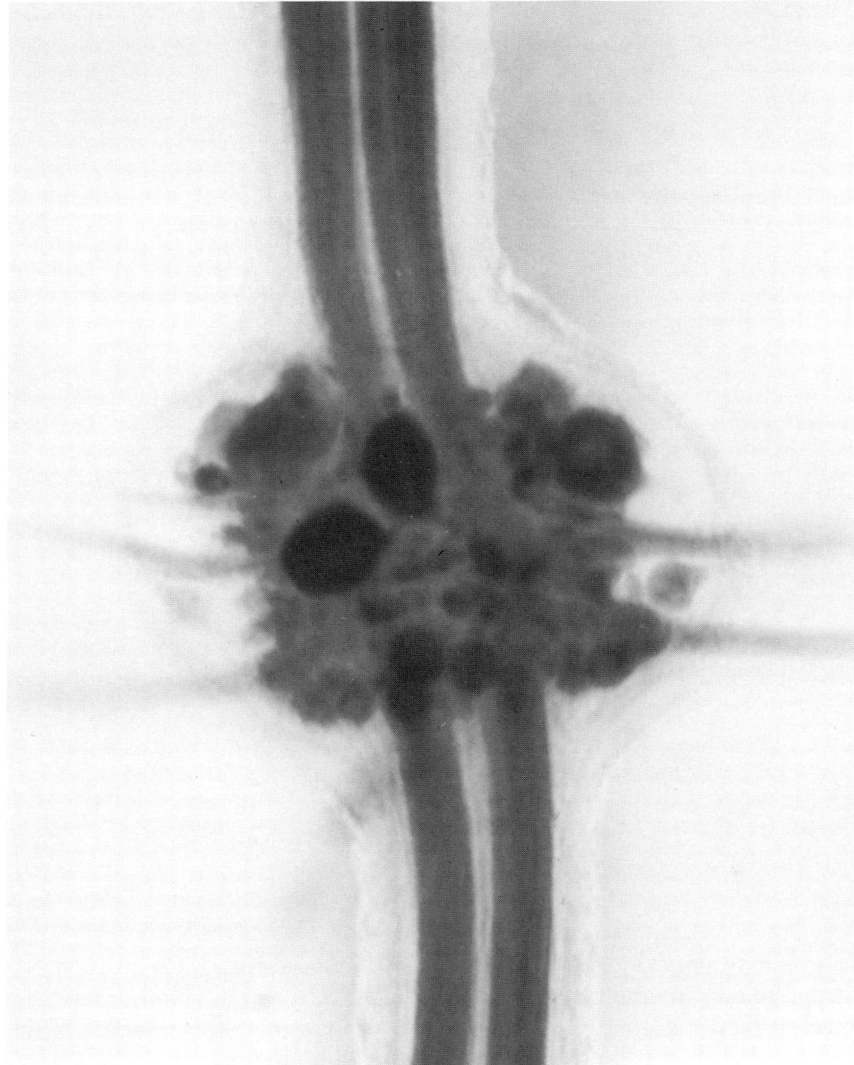

Figure 1. Segmental ganglion of the nerve cord of *Haementeria*, seen from the ventral aspect. The anterior edge is shown at the top. The diameter of the ganglion shown is about 700 μm.

form an anterior and two a posterior pair of lateral packets. The remaining two packets are unpaired, one lying anterior and the other posterior on the ventromedial aspect of all but the frontmost ganglia. (In the front, the two ventromedial cell packets lie nearly side by side across the ganglion midline). Each cell packet contains one giant glial cell, whereas two giant glial cells are associated with the ganglionic neuropil. Additional giant glia are present in the interganglionic connective nerves.[14,20]

The anatomy of the leech ganglion is sufficiently stereotyped that a large fraction of its neurons are identifiable. That is, after characterizing a particular neuron in a particular ganglion of a particular specimen according to such criteria as soma size and position, axonal and dendritic branching patterns, synaptic connectivity, or electrophysiological and histochemical properties, homologous neurons can usually be found on the other side of that same ganglion, in other ganglia of the same specimen, in the ganglia of other specimens of the same species, and even in other leech species, families, or orders. Despite this high degree of neural stereotypy, some systematic variations do occur in the number of cells among different segmental ganglia within the same nerve cord, and among corresponding ganglia in the nerve cords of different leech species. For instance, in the hirudinid leech *Hirudo medicinalis*, the ganglia in the two body segments containing the male and female copulatory organs of the hermaphrodite leech have nearly twice as many cells as the other ganglia.[19] Although the corresponding ganglia in the glossiphoniid leech *Haementeria ghilianii* also contain more cells than the other segmental ganglia, here the excess is only on the order of 5%. Moreover, there is even some slight variation in the exact number of neurons per ganglion between corresponding ganglia of different specimens of the same species. This "developmental noise" amounts to a variance of about 1% in the total number of neurons per corresponding ganglion.[19]

Roughly one-quarter of the neurons of the segmental ganglia of *H. medicinalis* have been identified according to various criteria, including function. Thus, many cells have been classified as sensory, motor, or interneurons, and their conectivity has been elucidated.[21–25] These surveys have culminated in the description of sensory pathways and of neuronal networks controlling various behaviors, such as body shortening, heartbeat, and swimming.[26–29] Thanks to this detailed knowledge of its functional elements, the leech nervous system presents developmental neurobiologists with a clearly defined conceptual end point in the search for understanding how a complex ensemble of specifically interconnected neurons develops from the fertilized egg.

2. LEECH EMBRYOGENESIS

2.1. *Two Experimentally Favorable Leech Species*

Glossiphoniid leeches are well suited for developmental studies because their eggs are large and undergo stereotyped cleavages that produce a blastula containing large identifiable cells, or blastomeres. The embryos can be observed, manipulated, and cultured to maturity in simple media. Moreover, development from egg to adult is direct, without passage through larval forms.[12] The developmental cell lineage studies summarized in this article were carried out with two glossiphoniid leech species, maintained as continuously breeding laboratory colonies since 1976. One of these is the dwarf species, *Helobdella triserialis*, which reaches an adult length of up to 4 cm and propagates with an egg-to-egg generation time of about 6 weeks. The other is the giant species *H. ghilianii*, native to French Guyana, which can reach an adult length of up to 50 cm and has an egg-to-egg generation time of about 10 months. Its short generation time and robust embryo make *Helobdella* a favorable material for developmental studies, but its small size renders it less favorable for neurophysiology. By contrast the enormous size of *Haementeria* makes its adult and embryonic nervous systems both accessible to intracellular electrical recording and other techniques that require penetration of single cells, but the long generation time, more demanding breeding conditions, and less hardy embryo also present drawbacks compared to *Helobdella*. Despite their disparate sizes, both species are sufficiently similar in adult body plan and embryonic development that they can be considered as interchangeable for many developmental studies, thus providing greater scope for experimentation than would either species alone.

Helobdella and *Haementeria* lay yolk-rich eggs about 0.5 mm and 2.5 mm in diameter, respectively. The eggs are laid in clutches, enclosed in transparent, fluid-filled cocoons that remain attached to the ventral body wall of the brooding parent. Embryonic development begins as soon as the eggs are laid, and, at a temperature of 25°C, two weeks later (*Helobdella*), or a month later (*Haementeria*), a juvenile leech has arisen whose form differs from the adult mainly by its smaller size. The eggs can be removed from the cocoon at any stage of development and cultured to maturity in a saline whose composition resembles that of the cocoon fluid. The egg yolk provides the nutrients needed for this development. Upon exhaustion of the yolk, the juvenile leech takes its first meal from a host animal. Subsequent, postembryonic growth and maturation of the juvenile leech represents both an increase in cell size and, to a lesser degree, cell number.

2.2. *A Developmental Staging System*

The following generalized staging system has recently been devised for the embryonic development of glossiphoniid leeches, based on studies carried out with *Helobdella*,[14] *Haementeria*,[30] and *Theromyzon rude*.[13]

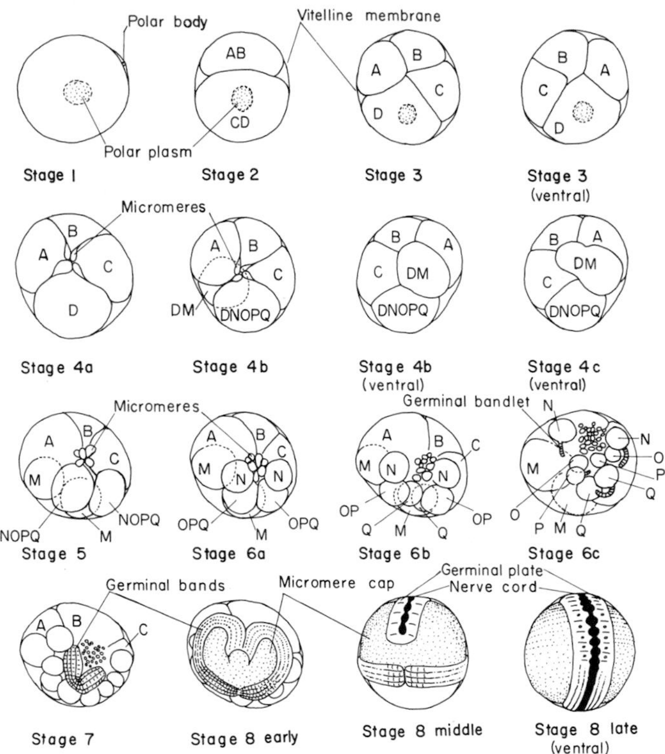

Figure 2. The 11 stages of development of glossiphoniid leeches, beginning with the uncleaved egg (stage 1). All drawings, unless otherwise noted, are views of the future dorsal aspect of the embryo.

The notation used here to designate various blastomeres and their descendants is simpler than that used in previous descriptions of cell lineage in annelid development[12,31] (Figs. 2 and 3).

Stage 1. Uncleaved egg. As the egg approaches its first cleavage there becomes visible at each of its two poles a region of colorless cytoplasm, or *polar plasm,* as distinct from the colored yolk that fills most of the egg. One of these poles marks the future dorsal and the other the future ventral surface of the embryo.

Stage 2. Two cells. The egg cleaves to yield a smaller cell AB and a larger cell CD. Cell CD receives the bulk of the polar plasm.

Stage 3. Four cells. Cell CD cleaves to produce a smaller cell C and a larger cell D. The bulk of the polar plasm goes to cell D. Cell AB cleaves soon thereafter to produce cells A and B.

Stage 4. This stage has been subdivided as follows: Stage 4a. Mi-

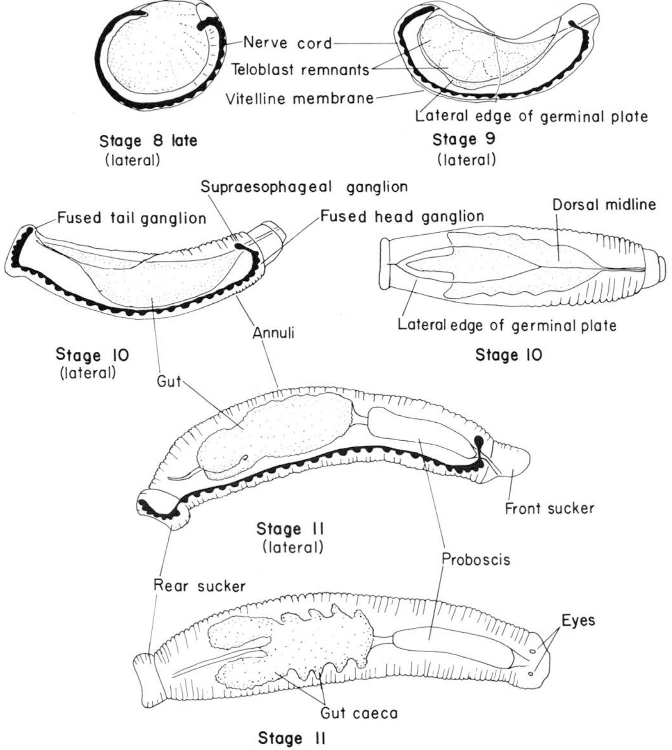

Figure 2 (*continued*).

cromere quartet. At the dorsal junction of the four cleavage furrows, each of the four cells A, B, C, and D cleaves unequally to produce a macromere (still designated by the capital letter of its parent cell) and a much smaller micromere (designated by the lower-case letter corresponding to its sister macromere), beginning with cell D. Stage 4b. Macromere quintet. The D macromere cleaves to produce cells DNOPQ and DM. Since Whitman, cell DNOPQ is regarded as the source of ectoderm, cell DM as the source of mesoderm, and the A, B, and C macromeres as the source of endoderm. Stage 4c. Mesoteloblast formation. The mesodermal precursor cell DM cleaves to yield the left and right mesoteloblast—M*l* and M*r*.

Stage 5. Ectoteloblast precursor. The ectodermal precursor cell DNOPQ cleaves symmetrically to yield the left and right ectoteloblast precursors NOPQ*l* and NOPQ*r*.

Stage 6. Teloblast completion. Bilaterally homologous cells cleave at about the same time. This stage has been subdivided as follows: Stage 6a. Cell NOPQ cleaves, yielding the smaller ectoteloblast N and the larger cell OPQ. Stage 6b. Cell OPQ cleaves, yielding the smaller ectoteloblast Q and the larger cell OP. Stage 6c. Cell OP cleaves, yielding the ectoteloblasts O and P. Thus at the conclusion of Stage 6, one bilateral pair of mesoteloblasts (M*l* and M*r*) and four bilateral pairs of ectoteloblasts (N*l* and N*r*, O*l* and O*r*, P*l* and P*r*, and Q*l* and Q*r*) have been formed. By the end of stage 6, the number of micromeres lying at the dorsal pole of the embryo has increased by processes that have not yet been fully elucidated. It has been reported for several glossiphoniid leech species that the A, B, and C macromeres undergo further rounds of micromere formation[12] and also that the ectoteloblasts and their precursors cleave to produce additional micromeres during stages 5 and 6.[13,32] Further proliferation of the micromeres, derived largely from progeny of the DM blastomere (S. S. Blair, D. A. Weisblat, and S. L. Zackson, unpublished observations), eventually gives rise to the *micromere cap*.

Stage 7. Germinal band formation. Each teloblast initiates a series of unequal divisions that produces a one-cell-wide column of small *stem cells*. Each column is called a *germinal bandlet*. The stem cells and the germinal bandlets are designated by a lower-case letter corresponding to the teloblast of origin. On each side the germinal bandlets merge to form the *germinal band*. The left and right germinal bands move rostrally on the future dorsal surface of the embryo, as more stem cells are added to the rear of each bandlet. In the germinal bands, the m bandlet (arising from the M mesoteloblast) lies under the n, o, p, and q bandlets (arising from the N, O, P, and Q ectoteloblasts). The ectodermal bandlets are arranged in alphabetical order, with the q bandlet lying most medially and the n bandlet most laterally. The germinal bands grow in crescent shape around the micromere cap. This growth entails a circumferential migration over the surface of the embryo, attended by an expansion of the micromere cap. Right and left germinal bands meet at the future head of the animal.

Stage 8. Coalescence of the germinal bands. The germinal bands elongate as the result of further stem cell production and division and continue their circumferential migration. The right and left germinal bands coalesce zipperlike at their former lateral edges in a rostrocaudal progression along the future ventral midline to form the *germinal plate*. As the germinal bands move circumferentially over the surface of the embryo, the area behind them is covered by a layer of cells. After migration and coalescence, the right and left n bandlets lie most medially in the germinal plate, directly apposed across the ventral midline. The o, p, and q bandlets lie progressively more laterally.

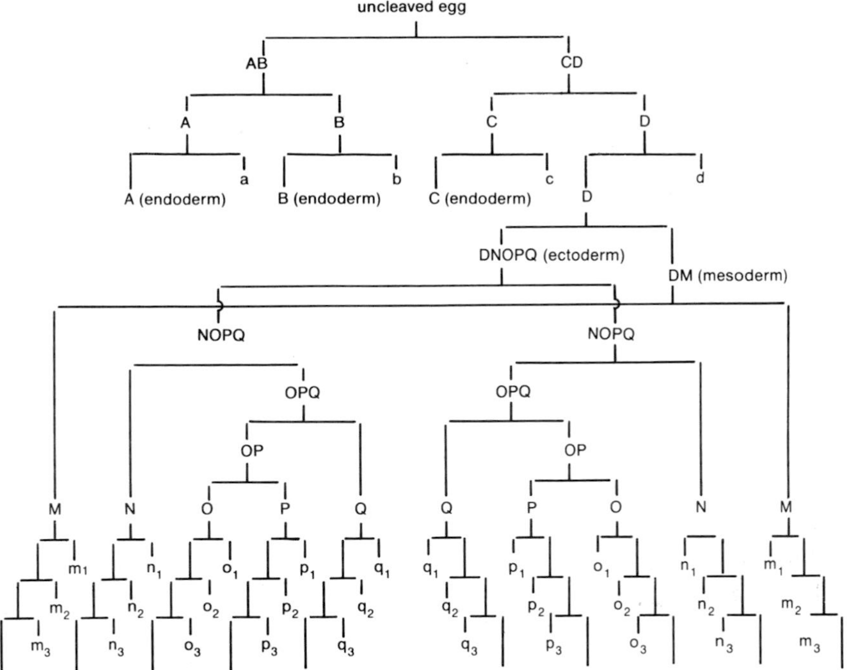

Figure 3. Cell pedigrees during the first seven stages of glossiphoniid leech development. (The divisions responsible for the proliferation of the micromere cap have been omitted.)

Stage 9. Segmentation. The first sign of incipient segmentation of the embryo is provided late in stage 7, when, in rostrocaudal progression, the mesodermal component of the germinal bands becomes fragmented into a column of hollow tissue blocks. Each of these blocks is a primordial half-somite. As coalescence of the germinal bands proceeds during stage 8, right and left primordial half-somites come to lie in register in the germinal plate and form successive somites separated by transverse septa. Late in stage 8, another sign of incipient segmentation is provided by the formation (also in rostrocaudal progression) of paired ectodermal cell masses on either side of the midline of the germinal plate. Upon its coalescence at the midline, each of these cell mass pairs becomes the primordium of a ganglion of the future nerve cord. By the end of stage 8, the frontmost 4 primordia, precursors of the subesophageal ganglion, have appeared. The next 21 primordia to appear are the precursors of the abdominal ganglia. By the end of stage 9, all 32 ganglionic primordia have appeared; the rearmost 7 eventually form the caudal ganglionic mass.

Stage 10. Body closure. The cells of the germinal plate divide to produce the precursors of the adult tissues. This cell proliferation results in a progressive thickening and circumferential expansion of the germinal plate over the surface of the embryo. By the end of stage 9, the expanding germinal plate covers only about half of the ventral surface. Later, right and left leading edges of the expanding germinal plate enter dorsal territory and finally meet and fuse on the dorsal midline. By the end of stage 10, closure of the leech body has taken place. During stage 10 gut formation also occurs. The gut first appears as a long cylinder (filled with yolk from the macromeres and spent teloblasts), and then becomes segmented as a result of annular constrictions of the yolk-filled cylinder, in register with the septa. This process gives rise to paired gut expansions, or caeca, in register with the abdominal body segments.

Stage 11. Yolk exhaustion. Body closure is followed by a morphological and functional maturation of the embryo. Maturation of the embryonic nervous system is reflected by the appearance of some adult behaviors, in particular of the locomotory routines of walking and swimming. During this final stage of embryogenesis the yolk stored within the gut is digested. Stage 11 ends when the yolk store has been exhausted and the juvenile leech is ready to take its first meal from a host animal.

3. A NOVEL CELL LINEAGE TRACING METHOD

Whitman and his followers established the lines of descent of cells A, B, and C, of the teloblasts, and the stem cell bandlets by direct microscopic observation of early embryos. But with the increase in cell number at later developmental stages the method of direct observation becomes too cumbersome for following the further fate of individual cells. Hence in order to make possible more detailed developmental cell pedigrees we devised a novel cell lineage tracer technique.[14,33,34] This technique consists of injecting a tracer substance into an identified cell of the early leech embryo. After tracer injection, embryonic development is allowed to progress to a later stage, whereupon the distribution pattern of the tracer within the tissues is visualized. The success of this tracer method requires that three conditions be satisfied: (1) after injection of the tracer substance, embryonic development must continue normally; (2) the injected tracer must remain intact and not be diluted too much in the developing embryo; and (3) the tracer must not pass through the gap junctions that link embryonic cells, so that it is passed on exclusively to lineal descendants of the injected cell.

3.1. *Horseradish Peroxidase Tracer*

The first substance which we used as a cell lineage tracer and which satisfies the three necessary conditions is horseradish peroxidase, or HRP. For cell lineage tracing, the embryo is placed in a well in the bottom of a dish filled with Sylgard or Epon, oriented with the target cell facing upward, and immobilized by gentle suction applied through a small hole in the bottom of the well. The target blastomere is penetrated with a micropipet filled with a 2–5% solution of HRP (Sigma Chemical Co., Type VI or IX) in 0.2 M KCl, and a small volume of the solution is forced into the cell by pressure. The injection process can be followed visually by including 0.1–1.0% Fast Green in the HRP solution. At some later developmental stage, the embryo is fixed and stained for HRP by standard histological techniques.[35] The stained embryos can be examined under the microscope either as wholemounts or, after embedding them in plastic (Epon or glycolmethacrylate resin), as serial thick sections. The examination of sections is aided by counterstaining them with toluidine blue, which causes the yellow HRP-stained cells (that do not take on toluidine blue) to stand out against the blue background of other cells.

As shown in Fig. 4, condition (3) for cell lineage tracers is satisfied by HRP, but not by the fluorescent dye lucifer yellow. In this experiment individual NOPQ cells of several embryos were injected at stage 6a with a mixture of HRP and lucifer yellow.[36] Without allowing further development, the injected embryos, as well as some uninjected embryos, were first photographed under fluorescent conditions, then fixed, stained for HRP, and rephotographed under standard illumination. As shown in Fig. 4a, injection of a single NOPQ cell with lucifer yellow caused the whole embryo to fluoresce. Thus, it can be inferred that all cells of the leech embryo at this stage are linked by junctions that permit intercellular passage of lucifer yellow (of molecular mass of 450 daltons). (We have also observed low-resistance electrical coupling between blastomeres using electrophysiological techniques.) By contrast, Fig. 4b shows that the larger HRP molecules (of molecular mass of about 40,000 daltons) remain confined to the injected cell. Hence, the HRP tracer does not move between blastomeres, despite an extensive network of intercellular junctions.

3.2. *Fluorescent Tracer*

The use of HRP as a cell lineage tracer has at least two limitations. First, since fixation and staining for HRP kills the tissue, the tracer

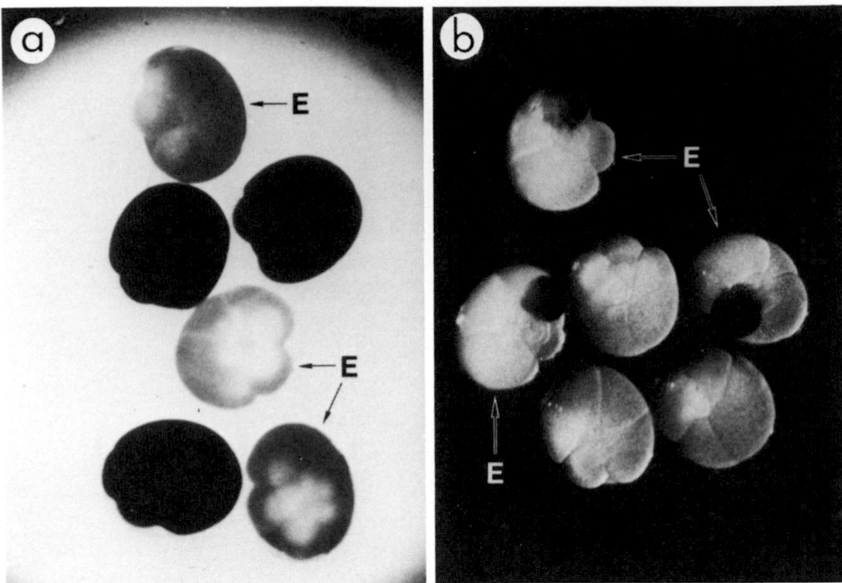

Figure 4. Differential mobility of HRP and lucifer yellow through junctions linking the cells of early embryos. (a) Fluorescence micrograph of 3 stage 6a *Helobdella* embryos (E) taken within 30 min after cell NOPQ had been injected with a mixture of HRP and lucifer yellow, and of three uninjected control embryos. (b) The same injected (E) and control embryos as in panel (a), after fixation and staining for HRP, photographed under white light.

cannot be observed in living cells. Second, since the histochemical HRP reaction product is opaque, this method is unsuitable for experiments in which intracellular features of the tracer-labeled cells, such as the mitotic state of the nucleus, are to be examined in wholemounts. Fluorescent dye tracers would overcome both of these limitations. But the molecular weight of most such dyes is too low to permit their direct use as cell lineage tracers because they diffuse throughout the entire embryo upon injection into a single blastomere (see Fig. 4). Nevertheless, a fluorescent dye can be confined to the injected cell and its lineal descendants if it is attached to a larger *carrier molecule*. For instance it has been reported that the molecular mass limit for the permeation of insect salivary gland gap junctions by oligopeptide–fluorescent-dye complexes lies between 1200 and 1900 daltons.[37]

One fluorescent-dye–carrier complex that we examined for its suitability as a cell lineage tracer is fluorescein linked to dextran of molecular mass about 3000 daltons (FITC dextran). FITC dextran is intensely fluorescent, highly soluble, can be readily pressure injected intracellularly from a micropipet, and appears to be nontoxic to the embryonic cells. However, FITC dextran has the drawbacks that the maximum of its emission spectrum is near that of tissue autofluorescence (which reduces the sensitivity of its detection) and that it does not react with aldehydes, so that upon tissue fixation it leaks from the labeled cells. For these reasons, our use of FITC dextran as a cell lineage tracer has been limited to short-term observations on living embryos. For example, FITC dextran has been injected into teloblasts to monitor their cessation of stem cell production after later injection of cytotoxic agents.

In view of these drawbacks of FITC dextran as a cell lineage tracer, we sought a carrier that offers flexibility in the choice of fluorophore and also reacts with formaldehyde fixative. For that purpose the dodecapeptide (glu-ala)$_2$-lys-ala-(glu-ala)$_2$-lys-gly, of molecular mass about 1200 daltons and composed of amino acids in the unnatural D configuration, was synthesized by the Merrifield solid phase method.[34,38] The synthetic peptide was coupled to rhodamine isothiocyanate, and the product, rhodamine-D-peptide (RDP), was isolated by column chromatography and lyophilized.[39]

4. DEVELOPMENT OF GERMINAL BANDS

The utility of RDP as a cell lineage tracer was demonstrated in studies of the development of the germinal bands.[34] For this purpose, a teloblast (or teloblast precursor) was injected with RDP. After formation of the germinal bands was underway (i.e., at stage 7 or 8), the embryo was fixed, cleared of yolk by the acid method of Fernandez,[13] and treated with the blue-fluorescing, DNA-specific stain Hoechst 33258.[40] The blue fluorescence of the nuclei and the red fluorescence of the RDP-labeled cytoplasm were then viewed separately through appropriate filters. By focusing through the cleared embryo, the labeled bandlet could be traced from its point of origin at the teloblast to its anterior end within the germinal band.

4.1. *Ectodermal Stem Cell Bandlets*

Figure 5a shows an embryo whose left N teloblast had been injected with RDP at stage 6a. The embryo was fixed, cleared,and Hoechst-stained at early stage 8. The numerous fluorescent dots visible in this photograph represent nuclei of diverse embryonic cells, but the nuclei belonging to the n bandlet can be distinguished because they lie within

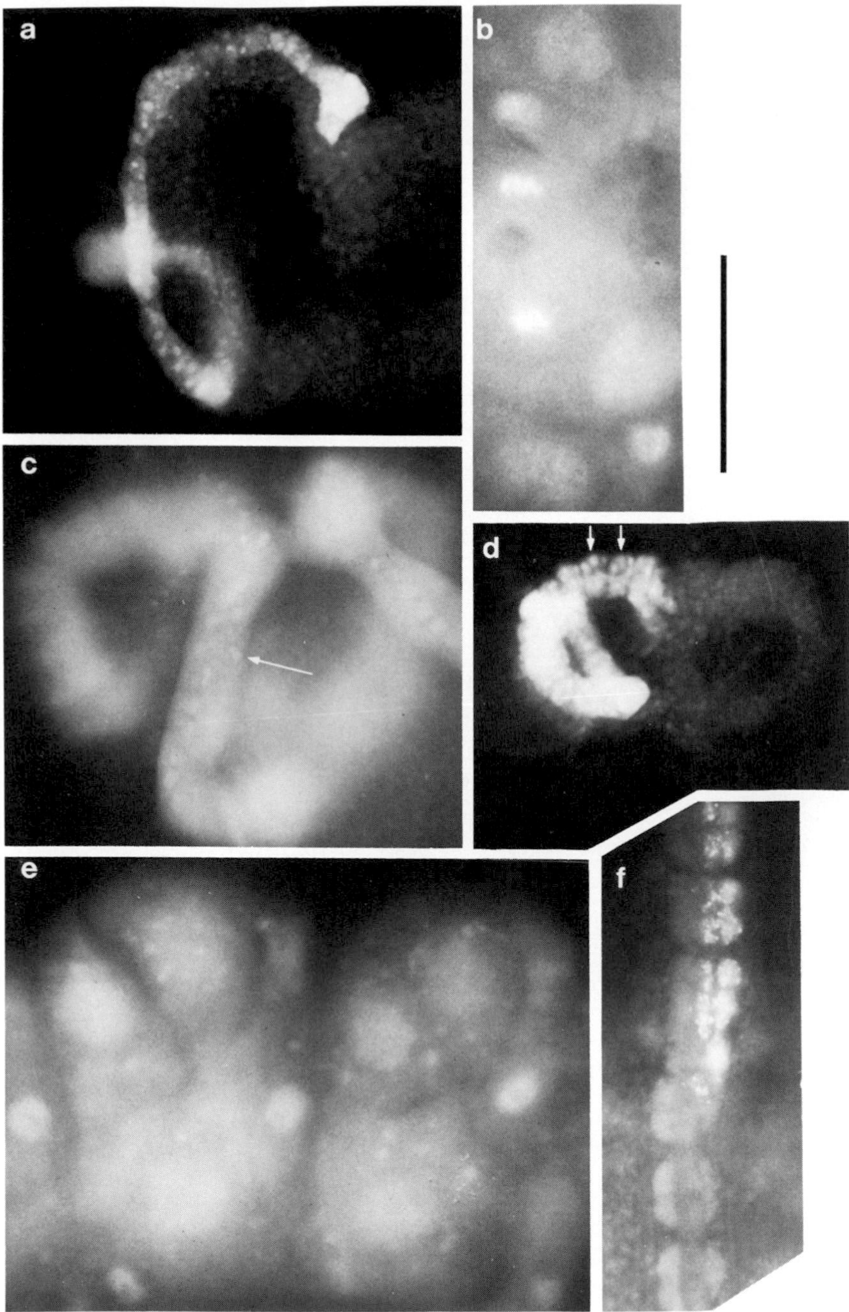
a
b
c
d
e
f

RDP-labeled N teloblast progeny. Closer inspection of bandlet nuclei reveals them to be of two types: interphase nuclei with diffuse fluorescence, and mitotic nuclei showing brightly fluorescent, condensed chromosomes[40] (Fig. 5b). The alignment of condensed chromosomes on the metaphase plate indicates the orientation of the spindle axis of cell division. Upon examination of 26 stage 7 embryos in which an N teloblast had been injected with RDP at stage 6, no mitotic n stem cells were found at a separation of less than 20 stem cells from the parent teloblast. At that point the bandlet cells are already within the germinal band. Hence it takes about 20 times as long for the newly born n stem cell to make its first division as it did for the N teloblast to cleave off that stem cell. The spindle axis of all observed early n stem cell divisions was nearly parallel to the long axis of the bandlet, as shown in Fig. 5b.

Figure 5. Photomicrographs of RDP-injected, Hoechst 33258-stained *Helobdella* embryos. (a) Early stage 8 embryo whose cell N*l* had been injected with RDP at stage 6a. The labeled n bandlet extends caudally from its origin at the N teloblast (left) to its point of entry into the left germinal band (bottom), then rostrally along the lateral edge of the germinal band to the future head (top right). The numerous dots are nuclei of cells of the germinal bands and micromere cap. (b) Enlarged view of the n bandlet of an embryo treated similarly to that shown in (a). In the middle of this picture is a telophase cell with the spindle axis parallel to the longitudinal axis of the bandlet. Above and below the dividing cell, interphase nuclei are visible. (c) Early stage 8 embryo whose cell DM had been injected with RDP at stage 4b. The left m bandlet extends from the left M teloblast (out of focus at bottom center). Part of the right m bandlet can be seen in the upper right hand portion. Interphase nuclei are visible as pale dots within the m bandlet. The arrow points to the daughter cells of an m stem cell cleavage which took place prior to the entry of the bandlet into the germinal band. The position of the daughter cell nuclei indicates that the spindle axis was perpendicular to the longitudinal axis of the bandlet. Rows of nuclei of unlabeled ectodermal bandlets converge at the point of origin of the germinal band. (d) Late stage 7 embryo whose cell M*l* had been injected with RDP at stage 5. The labeled m bandlet extends from its origin at the M teloblast (left) to its point of entry into the germinal band (center), then arcs beneath the ectodermal bandlet to the future head (top center). The arrows indicate two adjacent clusters of m stem cell progeny. (e) Enlarged view of the cell clusters marked by arrows in (d), showing some of the cells in each cluster. Topographically and morphologically corresponding cells can be seen within these clusters. (f) Ventral view of a portion of the nerve cord of a 9-day-old embryo whose cell N*l* had been injected with RDP at stage 6a and with pronase at stage 7. Anterior is at the top; seven ganglia are shown. Ganglia 1, 2, and 3 (from the top) are normal; RDP-labeled cells can be seen in the left (apparent right) sides of these ganglia. Ganglia 6 and 7 are abnormal, in that they contain fewer cells on the left (apparent right) side; the remaining cells are not RDP-labeled. Ganglion 4 (tilted and only partially visible) and ganglion 5 are at the border between the normal, anterior and the abnormal, posterior parts of the nerve cord; ganglion 4 contains some RDP-labeled cells at its left lateral edge, and ganglion 5 at its left anterior midline. The labeled background beneath ganglia 6 and 7 results from the fluorescence of RDP and of the dye Fast Green (coinjected with pronase) in teloblast remnants in the gut. Scale bar: 160 μm in (a), (c), and (f); 25 μm in (b) and (e); 250 μm in (d).

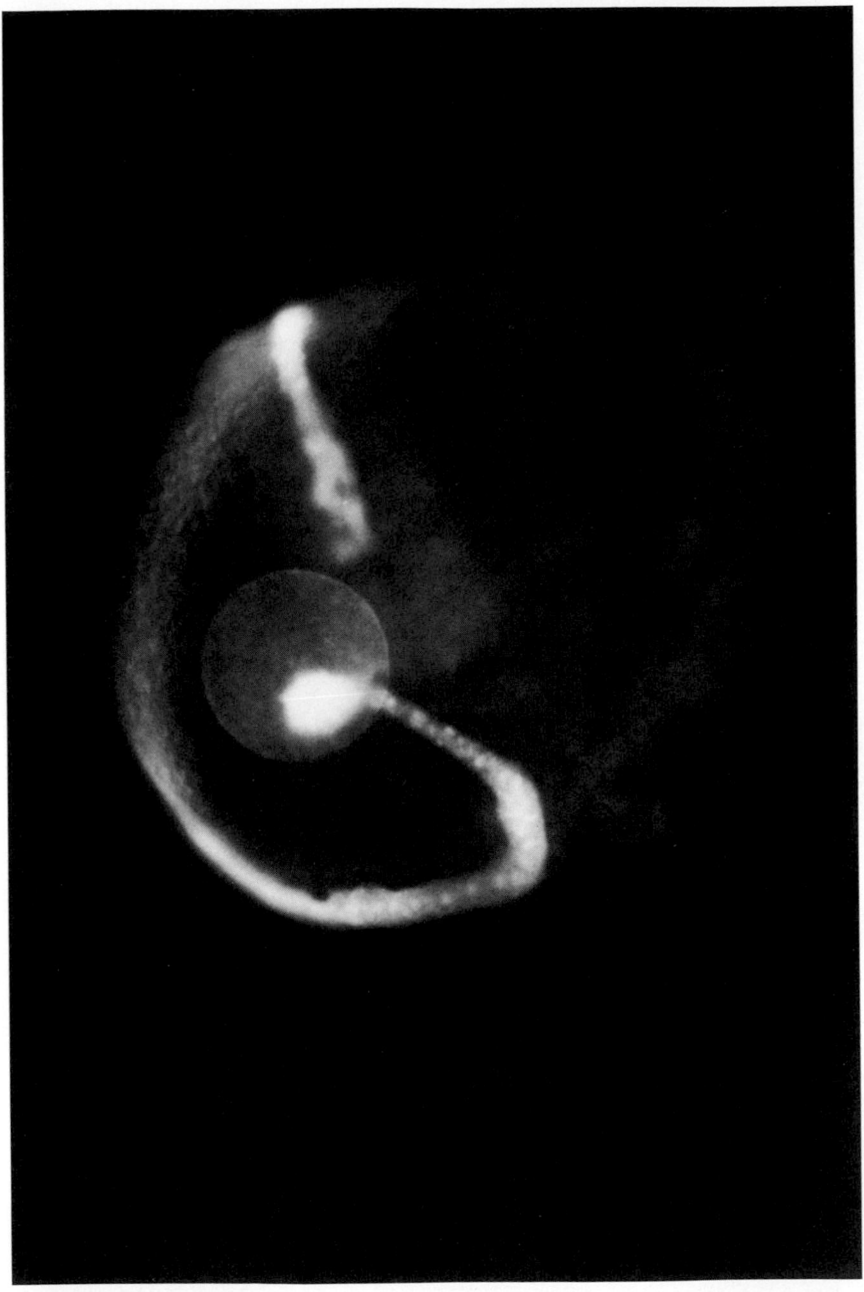

After that first division, therefore, the bandlet still remains one cell wide. Figure 6 presents an embryo whose left N cell had been similarly injected at stage 6a, but whose development had been allowed to progress to mid-stage 8 prior to fixation, clearing, and Hoechst staining. Here formation of the germinal plate is well under way, and the column of fluorescent N-derived cells, which previously lined the lateral edge of the crescent-shaped germinal bands, now borders the ventral midline of the germinal plate. Analogous experiments (whose results are not presented here), in which the O, P, or Q teloblasts were RDP-labeled prior to onset of stem cell production, have similarly revealed that the o, p, and q bandlets follow the n bandlet in their alphabetic sequence in lateromedial order within the germinal bands, and in mediolateral order within the germinal plate.

4.2. Mesodermal Stem Cell Bandlets

Figure 5c shows an embryo whose M teloblasts had been labeled with RDP by injecting their precursor, cell DM, at stage 4b. In this preparation, progeny of m stem cell mitoses are visible at a distance of about 10 cells from the M teloblast, before that bandlet has joined the ectodermal, n, o, p, and q bandlets in the germinal band. Thus it takes about 10 times as long for the newly born m stem cell to make its first division as it did for M teloblast to cleave off that stem cell. The spindle axis of the initial stem cell division in the m bandlet is perpendicular to the long axis of the bandlet, so that the m bandlet becomes two cells wide after the first stem cell division. Similar observations were made in 17 RDP-labeled m bandlets. Thus, combined use of RDP and Hoechst stain reveals that the mesodermal, m stem cells differ from the ectodermal, n stem cells in both the timing and the orientation of their first cleavage: whereas the n stem cells cleave only after entering the germinal band, and with spindle axes parallel to the long axis of the bandlet, the m stem cells cleave prior to entering the germinal band, and with spindle axes perpendicular to the long axis of the bandlet.

Figure 5d presents an embryo in which the left M teloblast had been injected with RDP at stage 5. Here the large fluorescent M teloblast is lying deep and out of focus. From it a bandlet of fluorescent stem cells projects upwards, makes a sharp left turn on reaching the surface of the embryo, and joins the crescent-shaped left germinal band. At its

Figure 6. *Helobdella* embryo whose left N teloblast had been injected with RDP at stage 6a and which was fixed and stained with Hoechst 33258 at mid-stage 8, when formation of the germinal plate was well under way.

front end, the m bandlet is evidently subdivided into iterated clusters of labeled cells. This subdivision is the first overt sign of segmentation of the mesodermal tissue, which occurs even before the coalescence of right and left germinal bands. The enlarged photograph of the front end of the germinal band of this embryo (Fig. 5e) shows that adjacent clusters are isomorphic, in that their cells are in topographical and morphological correspondence. This isomorphism suggests that the early development of the mesoderm of each body segment proceeds, as does cleavage and teloblast formation in the whole embryo, by a sequence of stereotyped cell divisions.

5. ORIGIN OF THE SEGMENTAL GANGLIA

Because of the medial disposition of the n bandlets within the germinal plate, Whitman[1,41] and later workers[42] inferred that the leech nerve cord derives from the N teloblast pair. However, this inference could not be certain: after stage 6 it is difficult to follow the fate of the stem cells because they and their descendant cells are small, numerous, and form multiply-layered arrays. Use of the HRP cell lineage tracer method has now shown that the origin of the nerve cord is more complex than was previously supposed. In order to ascertain the lines of descent of the neurons of the segmental ganglion, various blastomeres of early embryos were injected with HRP and the resulting distribution of HRP label was examined in early-stage 10 embryos, when expansion of the germinal plate covers nearly all of the ventral surface and all 32 segmental ganglia of the nerve cord are present.

5.1. *Ectoteloblast Contribution*

Figure 7 presents the result of one such experiment, in which an N, O, P, or Q teloblast in each embryo had been injected during stage 7. Evidently, the HRP-labeled descendants of a given teloblast form a characteristic pattern within the germinal plate that is repeated from segment to segment. Moreover, in replicate injections of different embryos, this distinct pattern is the same from specimen to specimen. (About 30–50% of such HRP injections are successful. Of the remainder, some injected embryos die before the time of fixation, others show an irregular, irreproducible staining pattern indicative of abnormal development or leakage of HRP tracer from the injected teloblast, and yet others fail to stain at all upon histochemical processing.) In each case, the stained cells lie on only one side of the ventral midline, namely, on the same

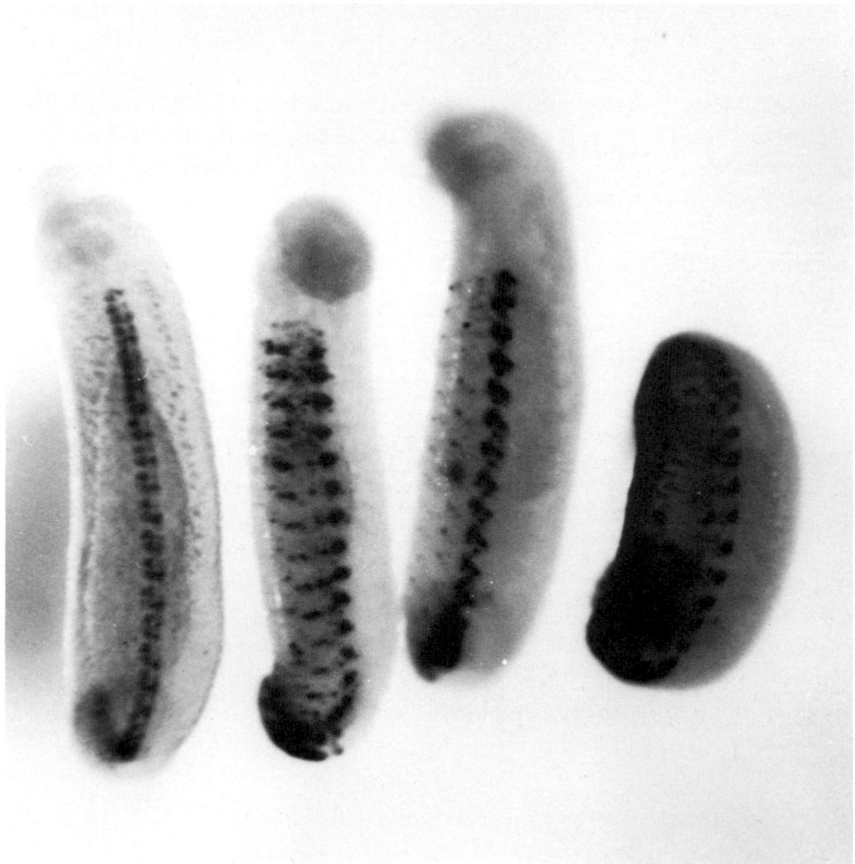

Figure 7. Ventral views of 4 *Helobdella* embryos at early stage 10, when expansion of the germinal plate covers nearly all of the ventral surface. In each embryo, a different teloblast (in left to right sequence N, O, P, and Q) had been injected with HRP at stage 7.

side as the injected teloblast. (Injection of the other member of the teloblast pair on the opposite side results in a mirror image pattern.) Apparently there is little or no cell migration of teloblast descendants across the ventral midline. The size, shape, and location of the segmentally repeated stain pattern following injection of the N teloblast indicate that the HRP-labeled cells lie mainly within the half-ganglia of the ventral nerve cord. However, the ganglia are not stained uniformly; within each half-ganglion the HRP stain appears as a longitudinal strip next to the ventral midline and two transverse strips extending laterally from it. The presence of unstained tissue between the two transverse strips in each ganglion indicates that some of the neurons of the segmental ganglion have an origin other than the N teloblast. The stain pattern following injection of the O, P, and Q teloblasts suggests that these teloblasts are that other origin. Although the HRP-labeled descendants of the O, P, and Q teloblasts are located mainly in ectodermal tissues outside the CNS, there also appear in each case some segmentally repeated patches of stain whose position indicates that they are located within the segmental ganglia. Comparison of all four staining patterns suggests that the cells labeled with HRP following injection of the O, P, and Q teloblasts are just those left unlabeled following injection of the N teloblast.

The cellular distribution of HRP stain was seen in more detail in serial histological sections of the HRP-injected embryos. Examination of such sections confirms, first of all, that all four ectoteloblasts do contribute cells to the ventral nerve cord and that in the case of the N teloblast, its progeny lie almost exclusively within the segmental ganglia. The sections confirm also that the descendants of the O, P, and Q teloblasts each give rise to a characteristic pattern of cell clusters both within the segmental ganglia and in ectoderm outside the CNS. Even at this higher level of resolution the size and position of these clusters is seen to be quite invariant from segment to segment and from specimen to specimen. Indeed the cluster pattern is sufficiently characteristic that the identity of the injected teloblast can be inferred from the stain distribution in the embryo.

5.2. *Distribution Pattern of Four Neuronal Kinship Groups*

Reconstructions of the total neuronal staining pattern from the ensemble of serial sections indicates that, with the few exceptions to be discussed later, between them the N, O, P, and Q teloblasts supply all of the cells (including glia) of the segmental ganglion. As for the major ganglionic subpopulations arising from each of four ectoteloblasts, they are distributed as follows: the progeny of N form two transverse slabs of cells in the anterior and posterior regions of the hemiganglion and a longitudinal band of cells near the midline of the ventral part of the ganglion, including the morphologically distinct neuropil glia; those of O, an oblique column of cells extending from the midportion of the ventral aspect to the anterior portion of the dorsal aspect of the ganglion; those of P, a thin transverse band of cells near the center of the ventral aspect of the ganglion; and those of Q, two small patches of cells near the midline at the anterior and posterior edges of the ganglion (Fig. 8). N and O each contribute many more cells to the ganglion than do P or Q. These findings suggest that the developmental cell lineages repre-

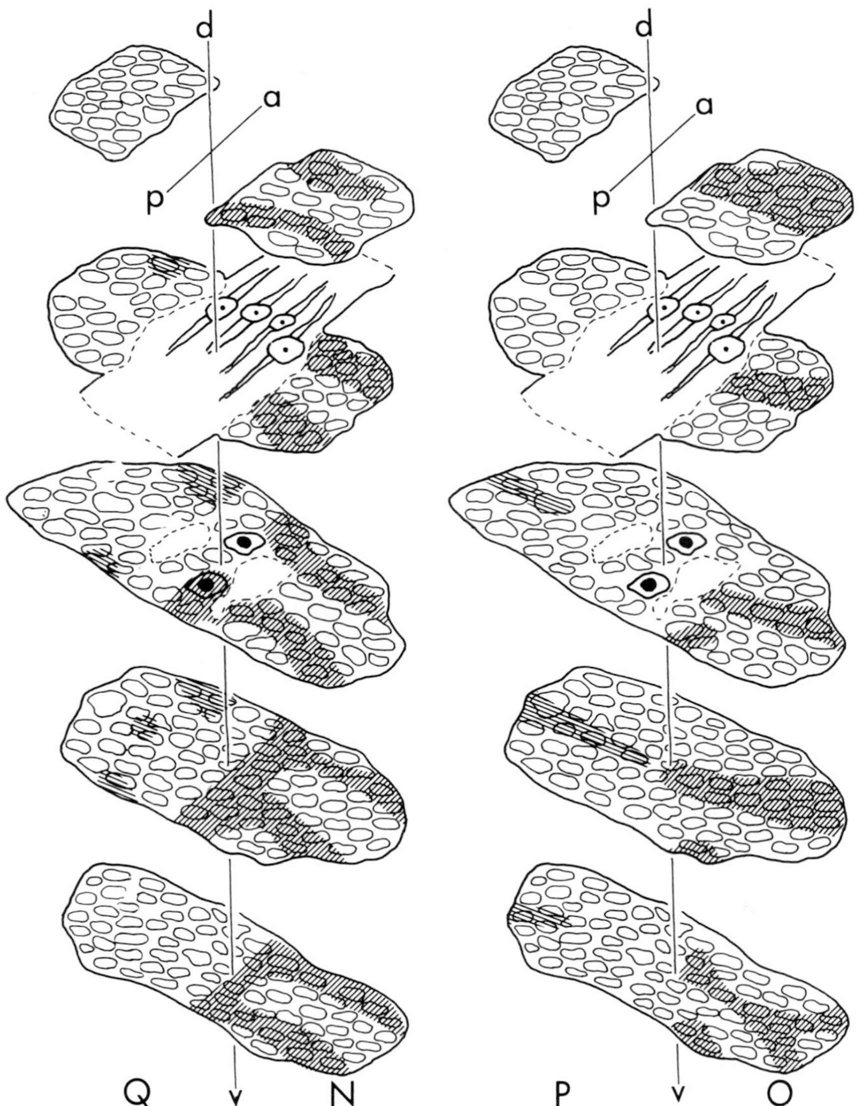

Figure 8. Embryonic origins of the cells of the *Helobdella* segmental ganglion. The drawing shows five horizontal sections through a midbody segmental ganglion of the embryo at mid-stage 10. (Dorsal aspect at the top; front edge facing away from the viewer.) The two pairs of dark, elongated contours in the center of the second section from the top represent identifiable muscle cells in the longitudinal nerve tract. They are descendants of the M teloblast pair. The two dark, circular contours in the center of the middle section represent two identifiable glial cells, each a descendant of one N teloblast. The faint contours do not correspond to actual cells but are shown to indicate the approximate size, disposition, and number of neurons in the ganglion. In each half-ganglion, domains are shown cross-hatched that contain descendants of the teloblast, designated at the bottom of the figure.

sented by the descendants of each of the four teloblast pairs correspond to four distinct, identifiable neuronal kinship groups. In view of the positional invariance of identified neurons in the segmental ganglia, it would appear that each identified neuron is the lineal descendant of a particular teloblast. The observation that neuropil glia regularly derive from the N teloblast pair supports the inference of a fixed line of descent of identified cells.

5.3. *Number of Ganglion Founder Cells*

If we now ask how many ectodermal stem cells found each segmental ganglion, the data of Fig. 8 already provide a preliminary answer. Since some of the neuronal cell bodies of the ganglion arise from stem cells of the n bandlet and others from stem cells of the o and p and q bandlets, it follows that at least four stem cells must contribute to the founding of each half-ganglion. The following experiment was carried out to ascertain whether within a single bandlet, only one or more than one stem cell contributes to the founding of each half-ganglion.[14]

This experiment is made possible by a feature of the embryos shown in Fig. 7, whose teloblasts had been injected with HRP after their stem cell production had begun. Careful examination of the staining pattern in the germinal plates of these embryos shows that there is a sharp anterior boundary of the HRP-staining pattern. This boundary separates the progeny of two successive stem cells, one produced just prior to and the other just after the HRP injection of the parent teloblast. The sharpness of this boundary suggests that there is little or no longitudinal migration of cell bodies within the germinal plate. Thus an examination of the position of the stain boundary relative to the ganglion in a series of embryos allows an indirect determination of the number of stem cells from a given teloblast that found a single half-ganglion.

If a single stem cell founded one half-ganglion, the stain boundary seen in embryos injected after the initiation of stem cell production should always coincide with a ganglion border. If, however, more than one stem cell contributed its progeny to a single half-ganglion, it will sometimes be the case that a half-ganglion at the stain boundary received progeny from labeled and unlabeled stem cells. In this case the stain boundary should sometimes fall within a ganglion. Moreover, the greater the number of stem cells contributing to a single ganglion, the greater should be the proportion of intrasegmental stain boundaries observed in a series of labeled embryos. Upon examining, both in wholemount and in serial sections, a number of embryos whose N teloblast had been HRP-injected after its stem cell production was underway, we found that in about half the cases the stain boundary coincided with a ganglion border and that in the other half the boundary ran midway through a ganglion.[14] Hence it can be concluded that in the n bandlet more than one, and probably two, stem cells contribute their progeny to each half-ganglion. Of these, the elder (i.e., firstborn) stem cell contributes its progeny to the anterior part and the younger (i.e., last-born) stem cell to the posterior part of the ganglion.

5.4. *Mesoteloblast Contribution*

In confirmation of the previous inference that between them the N, O, P, and Q teloblasts account for nearly the whole CNS, it was found that HRP injection of the ectodermal precursor cell NOPQ at stage 5 results in labeling of almost all of the cells of the half-ganglion. However, two readily identifiable (paired) cells in each embryonic half-ganglion remain unlabeled. These two cell pairs, located in the anterior dorsal aspect of the ganglionic nerve tract, are precursors to the muscle cells of the interganglionic connective nerve. In addition, a very few other cells within the ganglion also remain unlabeled. To trace the developmental source of these unlabeled cells, one of the pair of M teloblasts of stage 5 embryos was injected with HRP and subsequent development was allowed to proceed to early stage 10. Serial sections through the ganglia of such preparations show that the precursor of the connective nerve muscle cells and a very small number of other cells within the ganglion are now stained on one side.[14] Although these stained intraganglionic cell bodies have not been positively identified, it is likely that some of them are precursors of the connective tissue sheaths that envelop the ganglion and delimit the cell packets. Thus some (nonneural) cells of the ganglion are evidently derived from the M teloblast. In accord with the M teloblast pair being the source of the leech mesoderm, wholemounts of M-teloblast-labeled embryos show extensive HRP staining of germinal plate tissues outside the ventral nerve cord (Fig. 9). Moreover, stain is also manifest beyond the lateral edge of the germinal plate. There the stain appears in the form of circumferential fibers extending from the germinal plate to the dorsal midline. Thus the cells composing these fibers seem to have been left behind by the m bandlets during the circumferential migration of the germinal bands at stage 8. Moreover, if such M-teloblast-labeled embryos are fixed early in stage 8 (rather than early in stage 10), most of the cells of the micromere cap are stained. This indicates that the M teloblast pair is the main source of the micromere cap, rather than the proliferation of the initial micromeres formed at stage 4 from the A, B, C, and D blastomeres.

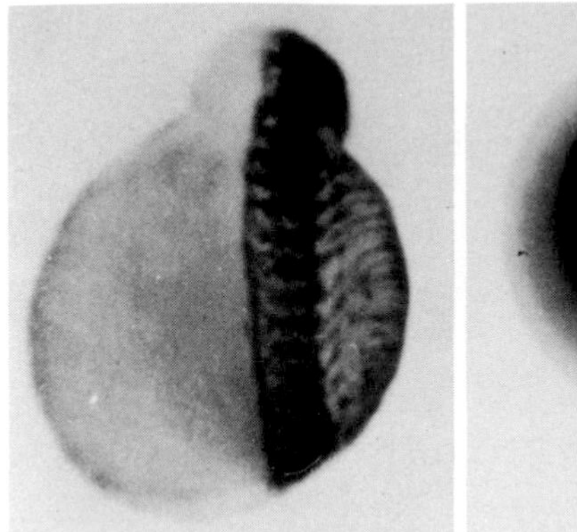
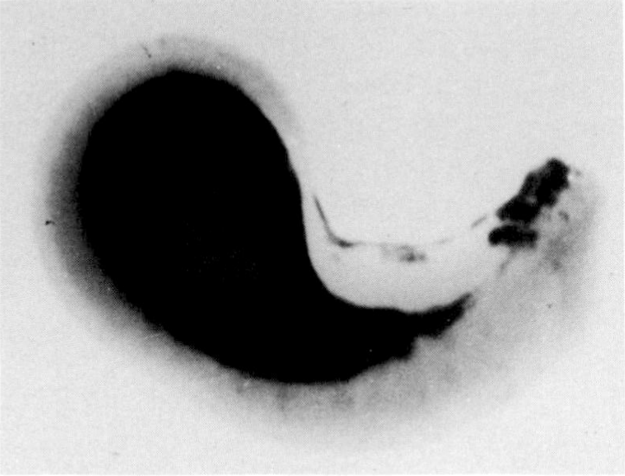

Figure 9. *Helobdella* embryos fixed and stained for HRP at early stage 10. In the embryo shown on the left (from the ventral aspect), cell M*l* had been injected with HRP at stage 5c. In the embryo shown on the right (from the lateral aspect) the A, B, or C macromere had been injected with HRP at stage 3. (The exact identity of the injected macromere was not determined.) Parts of the supraesophageal ganglion and body wall are stained. The large area of intense staining in the center of the embryo derives from the incorporation of the injected macromere into the primordial gut.

5.5. *Origin of the Supraesophageal Ganglion*

There is one component of the leech CNS that remains unlabeled after HRP injection of either the NOPQ ectodermal precursor cell *or* the mesodermal M teloblast: the supraesophageal ganglion at the front of, and dorsal to, the ventral nerve cord. If the failure of the supraesophageal ganglion to stain following injection of HRP into any of the teloblasts or teloblast precursors is not artifactual, these results support Whitman's contention, later contradicted by Mueller,[32] that the frontmost part of the leech nerve cord is derived from a source other than the germinal bands. To test this possibility HRP was injected into an A, B, or C blastomere of stage 3 embryos, i.e., prior to micromere formation. After allowing development of the embryos to early stage 10, they were fixed and stained. Wholemounts of such preparations show HRP stain in the frontmost end of the embryo as well as in the gut, which contains the remnants of the injected blastomere (Fig. 9). Sections of the embryos show that the rostral stain is confined to the supraesophageal ganglion and the frontmost body wall. Thus, in accord with Whitman's original inference, the supraesophageal ganglion does have a different embryological origin from the remainder of the nerve cord, namely, the A, B, or C blastomere, and, presumably therefore, the micromeres to which they give rise at stage 4.

6. CELL-SPECIFIC ABLATION

These cell lineage analyses, or fate maps, thus show that leech neurogenesis is highly determinate, in the sense that a particular blastomere or teloblast regularly gives rise to a given part of the nervous system during normal development. Another aspect of this determinacy is that upon death or malfunction of a blastomere, its normal developmental role is not taken over fully by any other cell. Thus killing or ablating a particular blastomere of the early embryo leads to characteristic developmental aberrations.[43] In this section we summarize the results of a set of experiments in which the consequences of killing identified blastomeres by injecting them with deoxyribonuclease, or DNase I, were examined. The lethal effect of DNase I is thought to devolve either from its hydrolytic action on DNA or from its destruction of actin filaments.[44,45] In some experiments blastomeres were ablated by injecting them with the proteolytic enzyme pronase.[46] In order to be able to visualize more clearly the morphogenetic effects of cell ablation, the embryonic cells were injected also with RDP or HRP cell lineage tracer before or after ablation.

Study of the development of oligochaete embryos had previously suggested that the formation of body segments in annelids has its origin in the mesoderm.[47–50] According to this view, the mesodermal embryonic tissue is first partitioned into segmental blocks, which then induce the organization of segments within ectodermal tissues, including the formation of segmental ganglia. The early appearance of protosegmental clusters of mesodermal tissue in the germinal bands in leech embryos prior to formation of the germinal plate, and hence long before there is any sign of ectodermal segmentation or ganglionic primordia, is thus fully consonant with this view. Nevertheless, despite the lack of overt ectodermal segmentation in the germinal bands, their ectodermal component bandlets might contain some covert segmental cues. In order to elucidate the relative roles played by mesoderm and ectoderm in the segmentation of leech embryos, the morphogenetic effects of ablation of specific precursors of either of these germinal tissue layers were investigated.

6.1. *Role of Mesoderm in Ectodermal Development*

The role of mesoderm in the segmental organization of ectodermal tissue was ascertained by a series of experiments in which one of the M teloblasts was ablated.[51] In one of these experiments cell DM, precursor of the M teloblast pair, was injected with RDP lineage tracer at stage 4b and the left M teloblast was later ablated by DNase I injection at stage 6b. At this stage the M teloblast pair has already produced a substantial fraction of its m stem cells. Development was allowed to proceed until early or middle stage 8, at which time the embryos were fixed and counterstained with Hoechst dye. The right germinal band and right half of the germinal plate of such embryos were completely normal in appearance, containing the RDP-labeled tissue clusters (Fig. 10). By contrast, only the anterior sector of the left germinal band and the left half of the germinal plate consisted of normally segmented mesodermal tissue clusters. The posterior sector was devoid of RDP-labeled cells and showed a lower density of total cell nuclei, owing to the absence of cells ordinarily derived from the ablated M teloblast. Those nuclei that *were* present in the posterior sector of the left side reflected the presence of cells derived from the ectodermal teloblasts. This finding indicates that the earliest stem cells produced by the M teloblast prior to its ablation continue their normal development and give rise to the mesodermal segments of the anterior body. Furthermore, the mesodermal stem cells eliminated by the ablation of the M teloblast are not replaced by any other descendants of the mesodermal precursor blastomere DM. However, after ablation of the M teloblast, the ipsilateral ectodermal teloblasts still continue to produce their stem cells, and these stem cells are still capable of division, despite the absence of underlying mesodermal tissue.

In order to reveal more clearly the effect on ectodermal development of ablating the left M teloblast at stage 6b, the left N teloblast was injected with RDP tracer at stage 6a prior to such ablation.[51] These embryos were allowed to develop until stage 10. Here the distribution of RDP label in the anterior, normal sector of the left germinal plate corresponded to the segmentally iterated pattern typical of tissue normally derived from the N teloblast (Fig. 11). However, within the posterior, abnormal sector of the germinal plate the RDP label showed no sign of segmental organization; rather, RDP-labeled progeny of the N teloblast formed an irregular bandlet along the midline of the germinal plate. Indeed, in this posterior sector some of the RDP-labeled progeny of the left N teloblast were found in the right half of the germinal plate, having evidently migrated across the ventral midline after germinal band coalescence. Since the absence of mesodermal tissue from the posterior sector of the left germinal plate resulted in a profound disorganization of ectodermal tissue derived from the ipsilateral N teloblast, it can be inferred that the underlying mesoderm is necessary for normal morphogenesis of the overlying ectoderm, including the nervous system. However, the absence of mesodermal tissue on one side does not impair segmentation

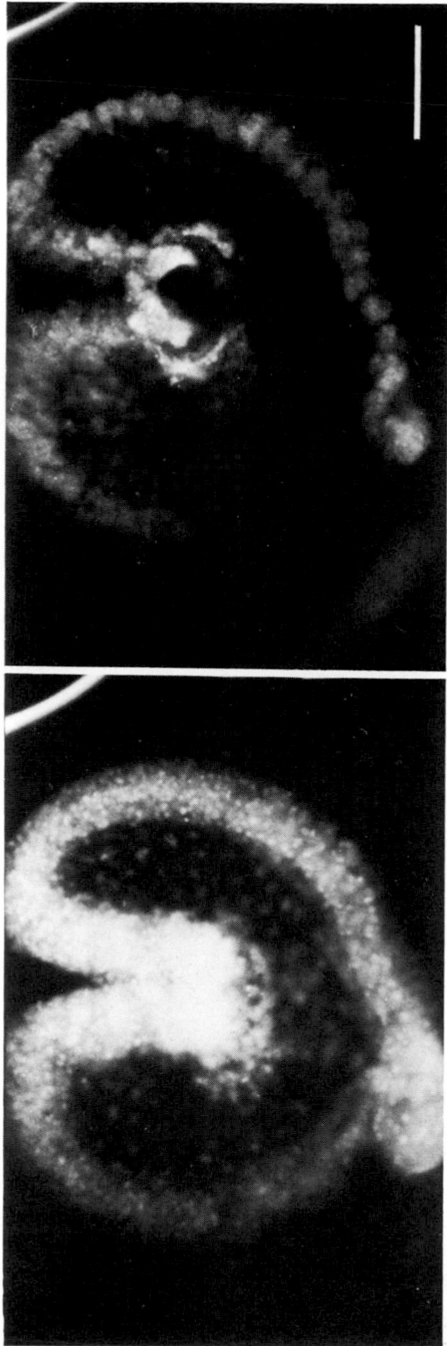

Figure 10. Early stage 8 *Helobdella* embryo whose DM cell had been injected with RDP at stage 4b and whose left M teloblast had been ablated at stage 6b. (In this figure, and in Fig. 11 and 12, the left-hand photographs show the pattern of blue-fluorescing cell nuclei stained with Hoechst 33258, whereas the right-hand photographs show the pattern of red-fluorescing cells containing RDP.) The two germinal bands both appear almost normal, though slightly asymmetric, the left band being somewhat shorter. Red-fluorescing cells form the normal pattern following injection of cell DM, appearing in the micromere cap as segmental blocks in the two germinal bands. However, because of ablation of the left M teloblast, no red-fluorescing cells are seen in the posterior zone of the left germinal band, which is formed by ectodermal bandlets only. Scale bar: 100 μm.

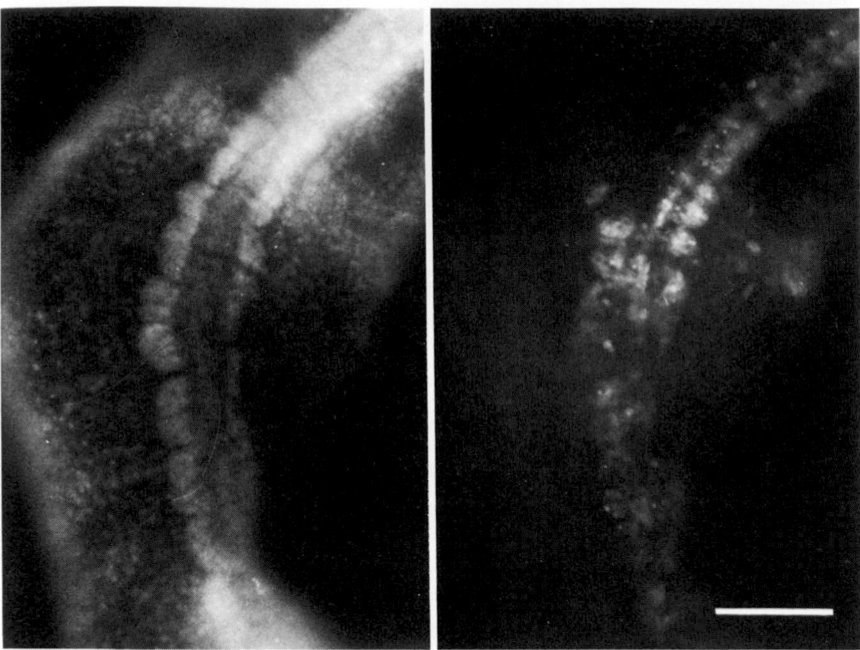

Figure 11. Ventral aspect of a stage 10 embryo whose left N teloblast had been injected with RDP at stage 6a and whose left M teloblast had been ablated at stage 6b. The anterior zone of this embryo is of normal morphology. Normal segmental ganglia are seen as paired clusters of nuclei along the ventral midline. The posterior zone is abnormal on the left (apparent right) side; the body wall is deformed and the segmental hemiganglia are completely absent. The right (apparent left) hemiganglia lying opposite the abnormal zone are well formed, though they appear abnormally large. Red-fluorescing cells in the normal zone form the segmental pattern typical of the progeny of the left N teloblast. In the posterior zone this pattern is totally disrupted, and red-fluorescing cells are seen within the right hemiganglia. Scale bar: 100 μm.

on the other side of the germinal plate that still has its mesodermal component.

6.2. *Role of Ectoderm in Mesodermal Development*

That the ectoderm plays a converse role in the segmental organization of the mesoderm was shown by experiments in which the left NOPQ teloblast precursor cell was ablated at stage 5 and development was allowed to proceed to early or middle stage 8.[51] In line with the cell pedigree of Fig. 3, ablation of the left NOPQ teloblast precursor resulted in the loss of all four ectodermal teloblasts and hence of ectodermal tissue on the left side of the embryos. On the nonablated right side of the embryos the cells continued to cleave normally and gave rise to intact germinal bands. In one set of these embryos, the fate of mesodermal tissue in the ablated embryos was visualized by injecting RDP tracer into cell DM at stage 4b. On the basis of the subsequent distribution pattern of RDP label the ablated stage 8 embryos fell into two classes, *switched* and *unswitched*. In the unswitched class (24 out of 79 embryos), the m stem cell bandlet derived from the left M teloblast remained on the left, ablated, ectoderm-deficient side, where it formed disorganized cell clumps rather than the full set of regular mesodermal segmental structures (Fig. 12a). On the right, nonablated side of these embryos, however, normal mesodermal segmental structures were formed. Thus the disorganization of the left mesodermal bandlet cannot be attributed to a global effect of ablation of the left NOPQ cell on the general health of the early embryo. Rather the disorganization of the mesoderm is due to the absence of overlying ectodermal tissue on the ablated side. In the switched class (55 out of 79 embryos), part or all of the left m stem cell bandlet had deviated from its normal path around the left side of the micromere cap and been incorporated into the right germinal band. That is to say, the right germinal band now contained *both* right and left m stem cell bandlets lying side by side under the right ectodermal bandlets (Fig. 12b,c). In the switched embryos, both mesodermal bandlets formed segmental blocks of tissue of normal appearance, except that the blocks were somewhat compressed in the transverse direction. It should be noted, however, that the segmental boundaries in the two adjacent mesodermal bandlets are not necessarily in register. Even though the mesodermal bandlets would be subject to the same ectodermal cues, they laid down their segmental boundaries independently of each other and of the overlying ectoderm. These consequences of NOPQ cell ablation indicate that the ectoderm is necessary for formation of mesodermal segments but does not appear to determine the position of their boundaries.

In another set of embryos with ablated left NOPQ ectodermal precursor cells the fate of mesodermal tissue was followed by injecting the left M teloblast with RDP tracer at stage 5. The embryos were allowed to develop to early stage 10, at which time expansion of the germinal plate would normally have covered nearly all of the ventral embryonic surface. As expected, in some of these ablated embryos no switching had occurred. Here the RDP-labeled tissue derived from the left M teloblast lay wholly to the left of the intact half-plate, being disorganized and lacking normal segmental organization. In other embryos, instances of switching were found. Here the RDP-labeled tissue derived from the

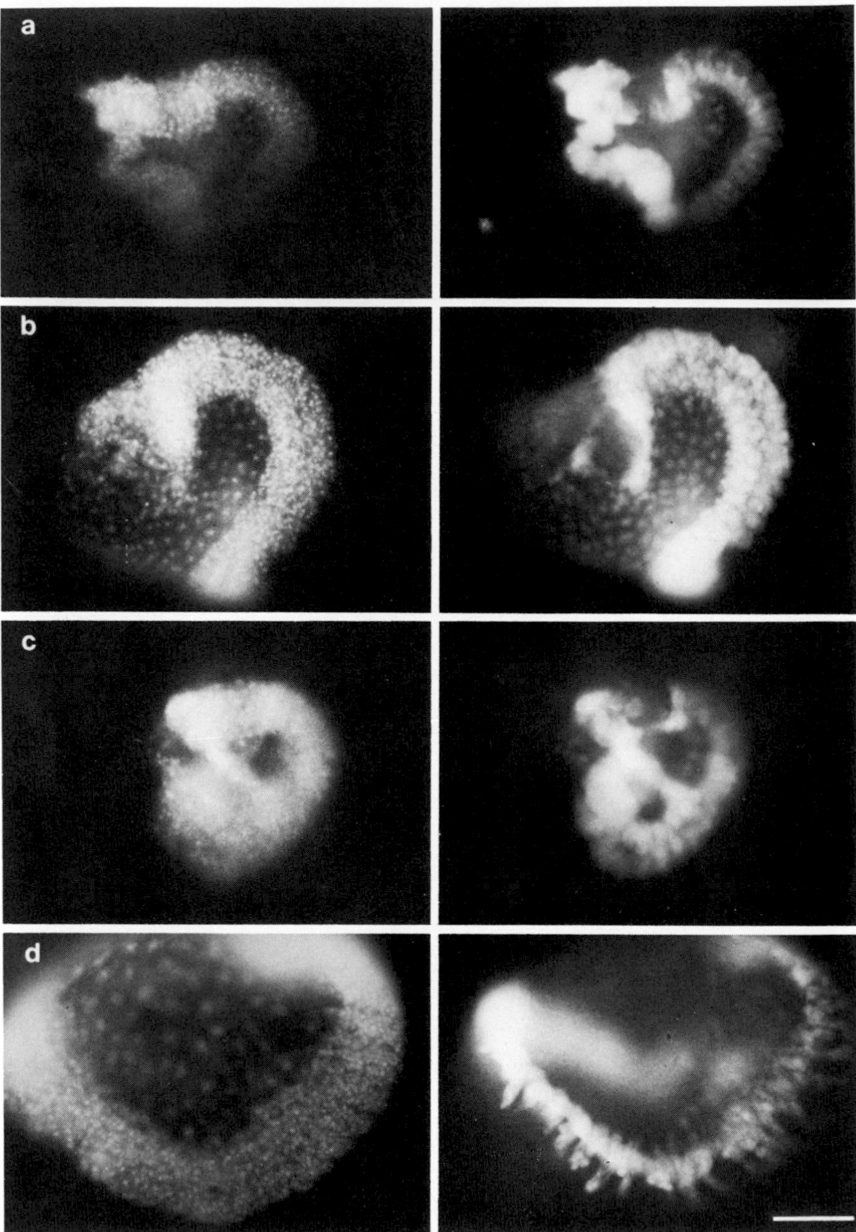

Figure 12. Embryos whose left NOPQ cell had been ablated at stage 5. Panels a, b, and c show early stage 8 embryos whose DM cell had been injected with RDP at stage 4b, prior to ablation of the left NOPQ cell. Panel a shows an unswitched embryo whose right

left M teloblast was present in the right half-germinal plate. Moreover, the mesodermal cells derived from the switched m bandlet were spread across the entire width of the right half-plate, apparently dispersed among the (nonlabeled) mesodermal cells derived from the right M teloblast (Fig. 12d). This dispersion indicates that when right and left m bandlets happen to come into precocious contact by switching during germinal band formation at stage 7 (and come to share a common overlying hemilateral ectoderm), their progeny cells comingle in later mesodermal histogenesis of the germinal plate. This behavior is to be contrasted with the complete lack of left–right intermingling in the normal situation, where the cells derived from either m bandlet (each provided with its own overlying ectoderm) come into contact at the ventral midline during germinal band coalescence at stage 8.

In both switched and unswitched embryos of this experiment, formation of a hemilateral nerve cord, consisting of a chain of half-ganglia linked by a connective, had occurred on the nonablated side. Thus, following ablation of one NOPQ ectodermal precursor cell, neither the presence of a double set of mesodermal cells in the one surviving germinal band nor the absence of a structured contralateral germinal band prevents the morphogenesis of hemilateral ectodermal structures on the nonablated side.

The results of these ablation experiments thus show that in leech embryogenesis *both* mesoderm and ectoderm are necessary for segmentation of the germinal plate; neither is capable of segmentation in the absence of the other. As far as segmentation of the mesoderm is concerned, it would appear that the necessary role of the ectoderm in this process is of a general mechanical or trophic nature. However, in the switched embryos resulting from unilateral NOPQ ablation, segments

---

germinal band appears normal and whose left, ectoderm-deficient germinal band is profoundly disorganized. The left, unswitched mesodermal bandlet shows no signs of segmental organization. Panel b shows a switched embryo whose left germinal band is completely absent. The right germinal band contains both right and left mesodermal bandlets, lying side by side and having segmented slightly out of register. Panel c shows a half-switched embryo. In the anterior portion of the embryo the left mesodermal bandlet has not switched into the right germinal band, and shows no segmental structure. In the posterior portion, the left mesodermal bandlet has merged with the right germinal band, lying side by side with the right mesodermal bandlet. These two bandlets segment out of register in the posterior portion of the right germinal band. Panel d shows the right germinal band of a mid-stage 8, switched embryo whose left M teloblast had been injected with RDP at stage 5 prior to the ablation of the left NOPQ cell. The switched left mesodermal bandlet is confined to the left edge of the germinal band in its posterior region (apparent left); more anteriorly (apparent right) the cells from the left M-bandlet have spread across the whole band. Scale bar: 100 μm.

in the two adjacent mesodermal bandlets are out of register; this indicates that the mesodermal segment boundaries are set autonomously, rather than being determined by positional cues from the overlying ectoderm. This inference is fully consonant with the conclusion reached earlier in this article on other grounds, that each of the 32 mesodermal body segments arises from the stereotyped cleavages of m stem cells (Section 4.2). By contrast, as far as the segmentation of the ectoderm is concerned, it would appear that the one-bilateral-founder-cell-pair-one-segment hypothesis cannot account for the mechanism of formation of ectodermal segments. As was also shown earlier in this article, the progeny of stem cells from all the ectodermal bandlets, including two from the n bandlet, coalesce to form the segmental half-ganglion (Sections 5.1–5.3). And since mesodermal and ectodermal segmental structures are phase-locked, there must occur some boundary-aligning interaction between mesodermal and ectodermal segments. Thus it seems plausible that at least one necessary role of the mesoderm in the formation of ectodermal segments is to provide positional cues for the location of segmental boundaries, although additional mechanical or trophic influences upon the ectoderm are not, of course, excluded.

6.3. *Morphogenetic Interactions within the Ectoderm*

In addition to the morphogenetic interactions between mesodermal and ectodermal tissues revealed by the foregoing experiments, interactions within the ectoderm also appear to play a role in the normal development of the segmental ganglia. Such interactions were revealed by ablation of the N teloblast, or of the OPQ teloblast precursor cell, on one side of an early embryo. As before, the fates of particular cells in ablated embryos were visualized using cell lineage tracers.

In initial experiments, an N teloblast was labeled by RDP injection at stage 6a (prior to the onset of n bandlet stem cell production), and then ablated at stage 7 (after n stem cell production was underway) by a second injection with pronase.[34] The morphology of the resulting embryo was visualized at stage 10 using Hoechst 33258 as a counterstain. As expected on the basis of the previous cell lineage analyses, the nerve cord of these embryos consisted of morphologically normal (bilaterally symmetric) ganglia anteriorly, whereas the posterior part consisted of abnormal (bilaterally asymmetric) ganglia reduced in size on the side of the ablated N teloblast. The pattern of these abnormalities was not regular; the abnormal half-ganglia on the ablated side varied greatly in size within the same specimen, ranging from nearly normal to a total absence of neurons. Moreover, some ganglia showed morphological abnormalities on the other, nonablated side. The distribution of RDP stain in these embryos showed that the variability in anatomical deficits is not attributable to a variable residual production of stem cells by the N teloblast after the ablation procedure (Fig. 5f). RDP label was present only in the morphologically normal anterior ganglia; all posterior ganglia lacked RDP label. Thus the morphologically normal anterior ganglia contain progeny of n stem cells produced prior to ablation of the N teloblast, and the posterior ganglia, are abnormal because they received no contribution from the ablated N teloblast.

The following set of experiments revealed the source of the morphological variability of ganglia following N teloblast ablation.[52] Here one N teloblast was injected with HRP tracer at stage 6a, the other N teloblast was ablated at stage 7, and the embryos were fixed and stained for HRP at stage 10 (Fig. 13). In these embryos, the anterior ganglia (derived from the normal stem cell complement produced prior to N teloblast ablation) contain HRP-labeled progeny of the surviving N teloblast in the normal, exclusively ipsilateral distribution pattern. By contrast, the posterior ganglia (derived from the n-deficient stem cell complement produced after N teloblast ablation) show an abnormal distribution of HRP-labeled progeny of the surviving N teloblast: here the clones of HRP-stained cells extend across the ventral midline. Moreover, that distribution pattern varies considerably from ganglion to ganglion. In some ganglia, the stained cells lie mostly ipsilaterally to the injected N teloblast, resembling the normal pattern, whereas in other ganglia they lie mainly contralaterally, forming a mirror image of the normal pattern. In most ganglia the distribution is intermediate between these extremes, in that stained cells are present on both sides of the ventral midline. The total number of stained cells per ganglion appears to be constant, however, as if only the position within the ganglion, but not the number of neurons produced by the stem cells of the surviving N teloblast, is altered by ablation of its contralateral homolog. The variability of the pattern suggests that random factors determine whether or not an N teloblast derived neuron crosses the midline under these conditions. This is to be contrasted with the normal situation where, in the presence of the progeny of the contralateral N teloblast, the neurons do not cross over at all. But having crossed over in the absence of their contralateral homologs, the N-teloblast progeny appear to take an appropriate place among the O-, P- and Q-teloblast-derived progeny on the inappropriate side. This suggests that on crossing over, the progeny of the surviving N teloblast select specific sites left vacant by their missing homologs on the ablated side.

That vacant, teloblast-specific sites play a role in crossing over is

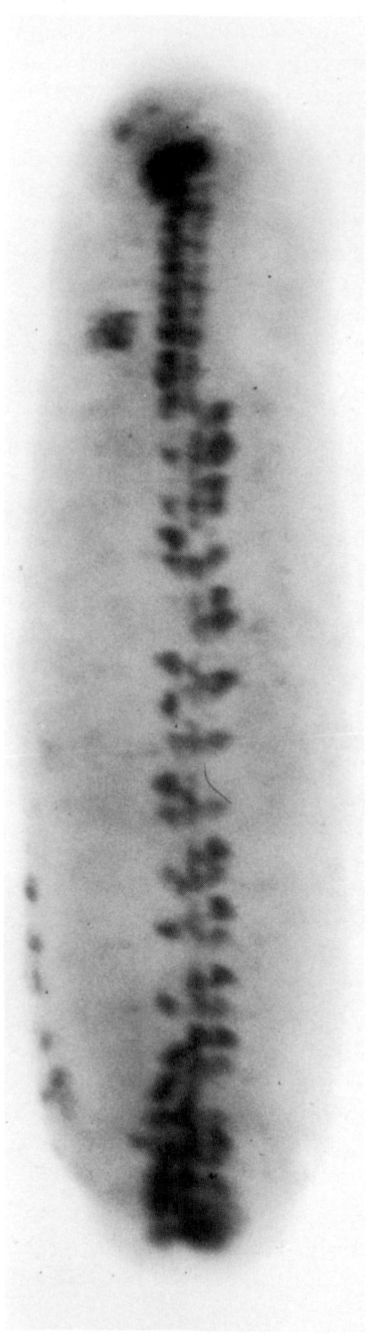

Figure 13. Stage 10 embryo whose left N teloblast had been HRP-injected at stage 6a and whose right N teloblast had been ablated at stage 7.

supported by the findings that the progeny of an HRP-labeled N teloblast do not cross over upon ablation of the contralateral OPQ teloblast precursor cell, and that the progeny of an HRP-labeled OPQ teloblast precursor do not cross over upon ablation of the contralateral N teloblast.

An unexpected result was obtained, however, when this inference was tested further. One OPQ-teloblast precursor cell was injected with HRP tracer at stage 6a, the other OPQ-teloblast precursor cell was ablated at stage 7, and the embryos were fixed and stained for HRP at stage 10.[52] If the inference of midline crossover for occupation of contralateral vacant specific sites were generally applicable to all neurons, this experiment should have yielded results analogous to those obtained for N-teloblast progeny following ablation of the other N teloblast. Contrary to that expectation, a fully normal distribution of O-, P-, and Q-teloblast-derived progeny was found on the nonablated side in the anterior sector of the nerve cord. In the posterior sector of the nerve cord, however, a segmentally repeated distribution pattern of stained cells appeared on the ablated side, attended by a constant reduction in stained cells on the nonablated side. The stain seen on the ablated side formed the pattern characteristic of the contribution of the Q teloblast. The boundary between the anterior sector in which all stained cells were lying on the ipsilateral side and the posterior sector in which a segmentally iterated pattern of stained cells was present also on the contralateral side was quite sharp, as if to the rear of that boundary all progeny of one or more of the labeled O, P, and Q teloblasts had switched from the normal to the ablated side.

The differences between the midline violations by N-derived and OPQ-derived cells under conditions of ablation suggest that two different mechanisms are at work. This notion is reinforced by consideration of the topography of the germinal bandlets within the germinal band and of the formation of the germinal plate. At the initial formation of the germinal bands, the left and right q stem cell bandlets lie at the medial edges of the nascent bands and are very near to each other. Thus when one q bandlet is missing due to ablation of the OPQ teloblast precursor cell, the opportunity exists for the surviving q bandlet to switch to the ablated side and take the vacant place of its absent contralateral homolog at the point of germinal band formation. In that case, posterior to the point of the q bandlet switch, all Q-teloblast-derived cells will be in contralateral tissues. By contrast, the n bandlets lying at the lateral edges of the nascent bands are separated by three pairs of intervening o, p, and q bandlets. Thus upon ablation of the N teloblast, the surviving n bandlet has no access to the vacant place of its absent contralateral homolog at the point of germinal band formation and cannot switch to the other side there. After the bands have migrated circumferentially and coalesced to form the germinal plate at stage 8, the mediolateral bandlet order is reversed, however. Now the cells of the n bandlet pair are in direct apposition across the ventral midline, and individual neuroblasts in that bandlet can cross the midline to fill sites in the contralateral half-ganglion left vacant by ablation of the N teloblast.

To test the idea that the two different modes of abnormal midline violation arise by distinct mechanisms, one blastomere was injected with RDP tracer, its contralateral homolog was ablated, and the embryos were fixed and examined late in stage 8, *prior* to the completion of germinal band coalescence.[52] When this experiment was carried out with the N teloblast pair, the crossover of n bandlet cells was observed in the anterior, developmentally most advanced sector of the embryo where formation of the germinal plate was already complete. But in the midsector of the embryo, where the germinal bands had just coalesced, no crossover of n bandlet cells was found: all stain was confined to the half-germinal plate ipsilateral to the labeled, nonablated teloblast. Similarly, in the rear, least advanced sector of the embryo, where the germinal bands were still separate, all stain was confined to the germinal band ipsilateral to the labeled teloblast. This result shows that, in agreement with the preceding explanation, abnormal crossover by n bandlet cells occurs only after germinal band coalescence, when under normal conditions the two n bandlets would have met along the ventral midline. Each cell of the surviving n bandlet approaches the midline from its side of origin and appears to have the choice of crossing or not crossing the midline, independently of the choice of other n bandlet cells. This freedom of choice would account for the segment by segment variability of the extent of crossover.

By contrast, when this experiment was carried out with the OPQ teloblast precursor pair, all stain was found ipsilateral to the labeled OPQ cell in the anterior sector of the germinal plate, and the stain switched abruptly from the nonablated to the ablated side of the germinal plate in the midsector of the germinal plate. In the rearmost sector of the embryo, where the germinal bands were still separate, the switched, stained bandlets extended into the germinal band on the *ablated* side. Thus, upon ablation of the OPQ teloblast precursor, the surviving q bandlet (and occasionally the o or p bandlet as well) appears to break at the point at which the two q bandlets would normally come into close proximity, at the origins of their germinal bands. The stem cells in the anterior sector of the broken bandlet remain with, and continue their development within, the original germinal band, while cells posterior to the break switch to join the germinal band on the ablated side.

7. CONCLUSION

7.1. Governance of Cell Fate by Cell Lineage

The findings presented here imply that cell lineage largely governs cell fate in the development of the leech. Evidently, the determinate cleavage pattern of the leech egg entails an irrevocable commitment of blastomeres as precursors of distinct tissue types at the earliest stages of development. Thus by the end of stage 4, the main lines of descent have been established. Early during stage 4, formation of micromeres provides the precursors of the frontmost tissues, including the supraesophageal ganglion, which are not derived from the germinal plate. Of the macromeres then present, A, B, and C will form the endoderm of the embryo, whereas D (recipient of the egg polar plasm) will give rise to the germinal plate, comprising the segmental tissues. Late in stage 4, cleavage of D into blastomeres DM and DNOPQ segregates the germinal plate cell lineage into mesodermal and ectodermal sublines. This segregation appears to be irrevocable, since upon ablation of the precursor cell of either mesodermal or ectodermal subline, no other blastomere can furnish a replacement for the missing germinal layer. In that cleavage, it should be noted, the polar plasms derived from the ventral and dorsal poles of the egg pass on to the DM and DNOPQ, respectively.

Next, upon cleavage of cells DM and DNOPQ into the M and NOPQ cell pairs, the two germinal sublines are separated into their left and right components. In the course of normal embryogenesis, the left and right components respect the body midline and give rise to tissues strictly ipsilateral to their blastomere of origin. However, under the abnormal conditions caused by unilateral blastomere ablation, stem cell bandlets may switch from one germinal band to the other at the point of germinal band formation, and neuroblasts may cross the midline of the germinal plate after germinal band coalescence. Hence we infer that its lineage does not irrevocably commit a cell to a given side of the embryo. Instead, the normally strict right–left cell compartmentalization is the consequence of the initial blastomere positioning by the determinate cleavage pattern. Upon subsequent cell proliferation and migration, this lateralization is preserved by some exclusionary interaction between homologous cell populations on opposite sides. In this connection it should be noted that many of the motor neurons on the dorsal aspect of the leech segmental ganglion innervate the *contralateral* musculature.[21,53] This contralateral motor neuron innervation pattern is therefore attributable to a developmental decussation of motor neuron axons, rather than to an initially uncrossed projection followed by a reciprocal migration of homologous cell bodies across the midline. In fact, in exceptionally favorable preparations, stained neuronal processes can be seen in the segmental nerves contralateral to an HRP-injected teloblast.

7.2. *Neuronal Kinship Groups*

Further cleavage of the NOPQ cell pair gives rise to the four ectodermal N, O, P, and Q teloblast pairs, of which N, Q, and O or P are one, two, and three cleavages removed from NOPQ, respectively. The orientation of these cleavages is also sufficiently stereotyped that every teloblast comes to lie in a characteristic position. Once in that position, each ectodermal teloblast cleaves many times to generate its bandlet clone of progeny stem cells. These progeny stem cells, in turn, appear to divide in a determinate manner, in that the plane and timing of the first division are highly stereotyped. After subsequent circumferential migration and proliferation of the bandlets, the stem cell progeny of each make a characteristic, segmentally iterated contribution to the future ectoderm. As for the n bandlet pair (which lies next to the ventral midline of the germinal plate), its progeny cells are almost wholly destined for the segmental ganglia of the ventral nerve cord; the o, p, and q bandlets (which are more lateral in the germinal plate) contribute progeny both to the segmental ganglia and to ectodermal tissues outside the CNS. Within each segmental ganglion, moreover, the progeny of each teloblast form a characteristic, invariant pattern of cell clusters. The known descent of the neuropil glia from the N teloblast, along with preliminary neuroanatomical and neurophysiological characterization of other neurons within these clusters (J. Kuwada, A. P. Kramer, and D. A. Weisblat, unpublished observations), suggests that these cluster patterns arise because particular identified and positionally invariant neurons of the segmental ganglion are the lineal descendants of a particular teloblast.

This conclusion is consonant with findings made on the development of the segmental ganglia of locusts[54] (see Chapter 5). Here a particular neuronal precursor cell has been identified with each of several ganglionic primordia. This precursor cell undergoes a series of iterated, highly asymmetric divisions to form a chain of progeny cells whose neuronal developmental fates appear to be governed by their lines of descent.

The mere fact that cell lineage governs cell fate in neurogenesis does not necessarily mean that the differential character of various cell types, or indeed the unique character of each identified neuron, is due to the orderly segregation of a set of intracellular determinants in successive cell divisions. Instead, cell differentiation and cell pattern formation could still be the result of intercellular interactions, in which the fate of each cell would depend on its position in a morphogenetic field, rather than on having inherited a particular set of determinants from its progenitor blastomere. In that event, cell lineage would govern cell fate simply because, in view of the highly regular cleavage pattern, it determines cell position. A few hints are available that would suggest some role for segregation of intracellular determinants in leech development, however. First, it would seem likely that the mesodermal or ectodermal character of the descendants of the DM or DNOPQ blastomere devolves from the passage of the ventral polar plasm to DM and of the dorsal polar plasm to DNOPQ. Second, the finding that the descendants of one N teloblast may cross the midline of the germinal plate and fill in sites left vacant by their absent homologs suggests that the neuroblasts of each kinship group carry some kind of differential characters that identify them as members of the group in the course of ganglion morphogenesis. All the same, this finding shows also that under normal conditions cell lineage governs the sidedness of a neuron by placing its precursor cell on one side of the midline, rather than by marking it with a right- or left-hand determinant.

Do the members of each of the four pairs of neuronal kindship groups have any overt properties in common, other than common descent, that set them apart from the members of the other groups? That is to say, do they share some distinctive functional, biochemical, or morphological neuronal traits? No clear-cut answers are as yet available to that question (however, see Chapter 3). In any case, the fact that the N-teloblast-derived kinship group also includes the neuropil glial cells indicates that this group is unlikely to be exclusively constituted of some particular functional neuronal type, such as motor-, sensory-, or interneurons. However, in the case of the development of the locust nerve cord, some evidence exists that cell lineage governs eventual neurotransmitter synthesis[54] (see Chapter 5). Here it has been found that all the neuronal progeny of an identified, segmentally iterated precursor cell are octopaminergic.

7.3. *Segmentation*

The present findings lead to the conclusion that cell lineage governs also the formation of the metameric body segments. First, individual mesodermal segments, or somites, seem to arise on either side via a stereotyped division pattern of an m stem cell in the germinal band. The mesodermal segments are, therefore, clonal ensembles descended from individual founder cells, with the rostrocaudal sequence of segments reflecting the order in which the founder cells arose from the M teloblast pair. Second, the neural segments, or segmental ganglia, arise on either side from the coalescence of progeny of (probably) two n stem cells, and of at least one o, p, and q stem cell each. As shown by the specific blastomere ablation experiments, the mesodermal segmental tissues appear to play a necessary organizing role in this coalescence process.

Since coalescence of the ganglia occurs on the ventral midline of the germinal plate, the n-stem-cell-derived neuroblasts are already in place. By contrast (as can be shown by appropriate cell-labeling experiments) the o-, p-, and q-stem-cell-derived neuroblasts migrate towards the midline from their more lateral positions of origin. In the case of the neural segment, however, not all of the progeny of the founder stem cells necessarily have the ganglion as their destination, since some of these progeny will form nonneural ectoderm of the same segment. Thus the lineage relation between the cells of the ganglion and their founder stem cells is more properly referred to as kinship rather than clone. As with the mesodermal segment, the rostrocaudal sequence of segmental ganglia reflects the order in which their founder stem cells were produced by the teloblast pairs.

The conclusion that the cells making up individual body segments of the leech are clonally related corresponds to the view of students of the development of *Drosophila*, that the body segments of flies are tissue "compartments" composed of "polyclones," i.e., containing all of and only the descendants of a small number of founder cells[55] (see Chapter 4). Although the body segments of annelids and arthropods are undoubtedly phylogenetically homologous structures, this concordance in the role of cell lineage in the segmentation process seems nevertheless surprising, in view of the radically different early development of leeches and flies. In flies, the segmental boundaries appear to be imposed on a two-dimensional sheet composed of thousands of cells, the blastoderm, in which the nuclei of neighboring cells do not appear to bear any fixed clonal relation to each other. It is only after formation of the segmental pattern in the blastoderm that clonal relations are established in subsequent development. In the leech, by contrast, where the segmentation pattern of the germinal plate is already implicit in the ordered linear array of teloblast-derived stem cells, the segmental founder cells do bear a fixed lineage relation to each other that can be traced back to the uncleaved egg. Thus it would appear that in the evolution of higher insects from some putative annelid-like ancestor the determination of cell fate has been postponed to a later developmental stage.

Although the concept of the annelid and arthropod segment as a lineage-related ensemble, or "compartment," of cells gives some insight into the developmental origin of the segment, it does not provide an obvious explanation of how a given number of segments arises in the embryo. In the leech that number is 32, since there arise 32 readily countable ganglionic primordia in the germinal plate. (The supraesophageal ganglion, not being derived from the germinal plate, is not to be included in the number of neural segments into which the germinal plate is subdivided.) As was suggested by Turing,[56] the fragmentation of an initially homogeneous band of tissue into a discrete number of segmental subcompartments could be accounted for by a system of "morphogens" that react with each other and diffuse through the tissue. However, Maynard-Smith[57] recognized that this mechanism cannot account for the formation of an invariant number of more than 30 segments. As he showed, mechanisms such as that proposed by Turing would lead to fluctuations, so that many embryos should arise which have more, or fewer, than the average number of segments. Since in the case of the leech, individuals having other than the standard number of 32 segments arise very rarely, if at all, it seems more likely that this invariant number is generated by some iterative geometric process based on a smaller number of discrete steps, in each of which the number of elements present is doubled by reduplicating them or halving their size. Accordingly, five such steps would generate 2^5, or 32 segments. In this connection it might be noted that the embryos of some insects are initially subdivided into 16, or 2^4 segments. For instance, the *Bombyx* embryo comprises 1 cephalic, 1 gnathal, 3 thoracic and 11 abdominal segments.[58] Uncovering the nature of the segmental counting mechanism appears to be a challenging problem whose solution would constitute a major advance in the understanding of developmental processes.

Acknowledgments

The authors' work summarized in this article was supported by NIH research grant NS12818, by NIH training grants GM-07232 and

GM-07048, by NSF grant BN577-19181, and by a research grant from the March of Dimes Birth Defects Foundation.

8. REFERENCES

1. Whitman, C. O., 1878, The embryology of Clepsine, *Q. J. Micros. Sci.* **18:**215.
2. Wilson, E. B., 1892, The cell lineage of *Nereis, J. Morphol.* **6:**361.
3. Sturtevant, A. H., 1929, The claret mutant type of *Drosophila simulans*: A study of chromosome elimination and cell lineage, *Z. Wiss. Zool. Abt. A* **135:**325.
4. Tarkowski, A. K., 1961, Mouse chimera developed from fused eggs, *Nature* (*London*) **190:**857.
5. Mintz, B., 1965, Genetic mosaicism in adult mice of quadriparental lineage, Science **148:**1232.
6. Stern, C., 1968, *Genetic Mosaics and Other Essays*, Harvard University Press, Cambridge, MA.
7. Garcia-Bellido, A., and Merriam, J. R., 1969, Cell lineage of the imaginal discs in *Drosophila* gynandromorphs, *J. Exp. Zool.* **170:**61.
8. Le Douarin, N., 1973, A biological cell labeling technique and its use in experimental embryology, *Dev. Biol.* **30:**217.
9. Sulston, J. E., and Horvitz, H. R., 1977, Post-embryonic lineages of the nematode *Caenorhabditis elegans, Dev. Biol.* **56:**110.
10. Deppe, V., Schierenberg, E., Cole, T., Krieg, C., Schmitt, D., Yoder, B., and von Ehrenstein, G., 1978, Cell lineages of the embryo of the nematode *Caenorhabditis elegans, Proc. Natl. Acad. Sci. U.S.A.* **75:**376.
11. Nicholls, J. G., and Van Essen, D., 1974, The nervous system of the leech, *Sci. Am.* **230:**38.
12. Schleip, W., 1936, Ontogenie der Hirudineen, in: *Klassen und Ordnungen des Tierreichs*, vol. 4, div. III, book 4, (H. G. Bronn, ed.), Part 2, pp. 1–121, Akad. Verlagsgesellschaft, Leipzig.
13. Fernandez, J. 1980. Embryonic development of the glossiphoniid leech *Theromyzon rude*: Characterization of developmental stages, *Dev. Biol.* **76:**245.
14. Weisblat, D. A., Harper, G., Stent, G. S., and Sawyer, R. T., 1980, Embryonic cell lineages in the nervous system of the glossiphoniid leech *Helobdella triserialis, Dev. Biol.* **76:**58.
15. Fernandez, J., and Stent, G. S., 1980, Embryonic development of the glossiphoniid leech *Theromyzon rude*: Structure and development of the germinal bands, *Dev. Biol.* **78:**407.
16. Kramer, A. P., and Goldman, J. R., 1981, The nervous system of the glossiphoniid leech, *Haementeria ghilianii*. I. Identification of neurons, *J. Comp. Physiol.* **144:**435.
17. Kramer, A. P., 1981, The nervous system of the glossiphoniid leech *Haementeria ghilianii*. II. Synaptic pathways controlling body wall shortening. *J. Comp. Physiol.* **144:**449.
18. Mann, K. H., 1962, *Leeches* (*Hirudinea*). Pergamon, Oxford.
19. Macagno, E. R., 1980, The number and distribution of neurons in leech segmental ganglia, *J. Comp. Neurol.* **190:**283.
20. Coggeshall, R. E., and Fawcett, D. W., 1964, The fine structure of the central nervous system of the leech, *Hirudo medicinalis, J. Neurophysiol.* **27:**229.

21. Stuart, A. E., 1970, Physiological and morphological properties of motoneurones in the central nervous system of the leech, *J Physiol.* **209:**627.
22. Nicholls, J. G., and Baylor, D. A., 1968, Specific modalities and receptive fields of sensory neurons in CNS of the leech, *J. Neurophysiol* **31:**740.
23. Nicholls, J. G., and Purves, D., 1972, A comparison of chemical and electrical synaptic transmission between single sensory cells and a motorneuron in the central nervous system of the leech, *J. Physiol. (London)* **225:**637.
24. Lent, C. M., 1973, Retzius cells: Neuronal effectors controlling mucus release by the leech, *Science* **179:**693.
25. Muller, K. J., 1979, Synapses between neurones in the central nervous system of the leech, *Biol. Rev.* **54:**99.
26. Kretz, J. R., Stent, G. S., and Kristan, W. B., Jr., 1976, Photosensory input pathways in the medicinal leech, *J. Comp. Physiol.* **106:**1.
27. Nicholls, J. G., and Purves, D., 1970, Monosynaptic chemical and electrical connexions between sensory and motor cells in the central nervous system of the leech, *J. Physiol.* **209:**647.
28. Stent, G. S., Thompson, W. J., and Calabrese, R. L., 1979, Neural control of heartbeat in the leech and in some other invertebrates, *Physiol. Rev.* **59:**101.
29. Stent, G. S., Kristan, W. B., Jr., Friesen, W. O., Ort, C. A., Poon, M., and Calabrese, R. L., 1978, Neuronal generation of the leech swimming movement, *Science* **200:**1348.
30. Sawyer, R. T., Kramer, A. P., Stuart, D. K., and Weisblat, D. A., in preparation.
31. Anderson, D. T., 1973, *Embryology and Phylogeny in Annelids and Arthropods,* Pergamon, Oxford.
32. Mueller, K. J., 1932, Ueber normale Entwicklung, inverse Asymmetrie und Doppelbildungen bei Clepsine sexoculata, *Z. Wiss. Zool. Abt. A* **142:**425.
33. Weisblat, D. A., Sawyer, R. T., Stent, G. S., 1978, Cell lineage analysis by intracellular injection of tracer, *Science* **202:**1295.
34. Weisblat, D. A., Zackson, S. L., Blair, S. S., and Young, J. D., 1980, Cell lineage analysis by intracellular injection of fluorescent tracers, *Science* **209:**1538.
35. Muller, K. J., and McMahan, U. J., 1975, The arrangement and structure of synapses formed by specific sensory and motor neurons in segmental ganglia of the leech, *Anat. Rec.* **181**:432.
36. Stewart, W. W., 1978, Junctional connections between cells as revealed by dye-coupling with a highly fluorescent naphthalimide tracer, *Cell* **14:**741.
37. Simpson, I., Rose, B., and Lowenstein, W. R., 1977, Size limit of molecules permeating junctional membrane channels, *Science* **195:**294.
38. Stewart, J. M., and Young, J. D., 1969, *Solid Phase Peptide Synthesis,* W. H. Freeman, San Francisco.
39. Nairn, R. C., 1969, *Fluorescent Protein Tracing,* Williams and Wilkins, Baltimore, MD.
40. Sedat, S., and Manuelides, M., 1977, A direct approach to the structure of eukaryotic chromosomes, *Cold Spring Harbor Symp. Quant. Biol.* **42:**331.
41. Whitman, C. O., 1887, A contribution to the history of germ layers in Clepsine, *J. Morphol.* **1:**105.
42. Bergh, R. S., 1891, Neue Beitraege zur Embryologie der Anneliden, II. Die Schichtenbildung im Keimstreifen der Hirudineen, *Z. Wiss. Zool. Abt. A* **52:**1.
43. Mori, Y., 1932, Entwicklung isolierter Blastomeren und teilweise abgetoeteter aelterer Keime von *Clepine sexoculata, Z. Wiss. Zool. Abt. A* **141:**399.
44. Mannherz, H. G., Barrington-Leigh, J., Leberman, R., and Pfrang, H., 1975, A specific 1:1 G-actin:DNase I complex formed by the action of DNase I on F-actin, *FEBS Lett.* **60:**34.

45. Hitchcock, S. E., Carlsson, L., and Lindberg, U., 1976, Depolymerization of F-actin by deoxyribonuclease I, *Cell* **7**:531.
46. Parnas, I., and Bowling, D., 1977, Killing of single neurones by intracellular injection of proteolytic enzymes, *Nature (London)* **270**:626.
47. Penners, A., 1934, Experimentelle Untersuchungen zum Determinationsproblem am Keim von Tubifex rivulorum Lam. III. Abtoetung der Teloblasten auf verschiedenen Entwicklungsstadien des Keimstreifs, *Z. Wiss. Zool. Abt. A* **127**:1.
48. Devriès, J., 1969, Le développement des embryons d'*Eisenia foetida* après la destruction unilatérale des mesotéloblastes, *Bull. Soc. Zool. France* **94**:663.
49. Devriès, J., 1974*a*, Le mesoderme, feuillet directeur de l'embryogenèse chez le lombricien *Eisenia foetida*. II. La différenciation du tube digestif et des dérivés ectodermiques, *Acta Embryol. Exp.* **2**:156.
50. Devriès, J., 1974*b*, Le mesoderme, feuillet directeur de l'embryogenèse chez le lombricien *Eisenia foetida*. III. La détermination des ectotéloblastes, *Acta Embryol. Exp.* **2**:181.
51. Blair, S. S., 1982, Interactions between mesoderm and ectoderm in segment formation in the embryo of a glossiphoniid leech, *Dev. Biol.*, in press.
52. Blair, S. S., and Weisblat, D. A., 1982, Ectodermal interactions during neurogenesis in the glossiphoniid leech *Helobdella triserialis*, *Dev. Biol.*, in press.
53. Ort, C. A., Kristan, W. B., and Stent, G. S., 1974, Neuronal control of swimming in the medicinal leech. II. Identification and connections of motor neurons, *J. Comp. Physiol.* **94**:121.
54. Goodman, C. S., and Spitzer, N. C., 1979, Embryonic development of identified neurones: Differentiation from neuroblast to neurone, *Nature (London)* **280**:208.
55. Crick, F. H. C., and Lawrence, P. A., 1975, Compartments and polyclones in insect development, *Science* **189**:340.
56. Turing, A. M., 1952, The chemical basis of morphogenesis, *Philos. Trans. R. Soc. London Ser. B* **237**:37.
57. Maynard-Smith, J., 1960, Continuous, quantized and modal variation, *Proc. R. Soc. Ser. B***152**:397.
58. Tazima, Y., 1964, *The Genetics of the Silkworm*, Logos Press, London.

2

Origins of the Nervous System in Amphibians

MARCUS JACOBSON

Our doubt is our passion and our passion is our task.
Henry James, *The Middle Years* (1893)

1. INTRODUCTION

The embryonic origins of the central nervous system (CNS) can be traced back to the fertilized egg, in which the information for establishing the basic pattern of the nervous system is encoded not only in the nucleus but also in the cytoplasm, as Wilhelm His[1,2] first proposed in his book *Unsere Körperform*. His modified the 18th-century preformationism[3] and proposed a more advanced theory of prelocalization of "organ-forming germ regions" in the egg cytoplasm and hence under control of the maternal genome. The problem of how much control of development is exerted by maternally derived determinants in the egg cytoplasm and how much the embryo's own genome contributes to its development are central themes of books by Wilson[4] and Davidson.[5] These books, written 90 years apart, show how little progress had been made in that

MARCUS JACOBSON · Department of Anatomy, School of Medicine, University of Utah, Salt Lake City, UT 84132.

time in understanding the control of development of morphological patterns.

Regardless of the amounts of information encoded in the chromosomes and cytoplasmic determinants, a qualitative difference between them appears to be important for developing morphological patterns: the information in the chromosomes is programmed linearly as a temporal order, but the egg cytoplasm could contain two- or three-dimensional positional information in the form of prelocalized determinants that could be segregated into separate lineages and thus into spatial patterns of differentiation.[4,5]

In seeking the origins in development of the basic morphological pattern, one is inevitably forced to consider progressively earlier stages until one has to seek the origin of the pattern in the egg. In amphibians the constituents of the egg cytoplasm are unequally distributed before fertilization; five or six cytoplasmic regions can be seen by means of light microscopy,[6,7] and further differential distribution of cytoplasmic materials occurs after fertilization in relationship to the point of sperm entry (reviewed in reference 8). Some of these differences in localization of materials are visible to the naked eye or can be seen at low magnification, while others are invisible but can be inferred. For example, inversion of the egg for some time extending from fertilization until after the first cleavage results in development of a second neural axis on the ventral side. From this result one may infer the presence of bouyant materials, freely mobile under the influence of gravity, that act as determinants of the development of a neural axis[9–11] (Fig. 1). I have observed that duplication of the longitudinal axis starts in the first few cleavages (Fig. 2) so that the formation of a second CNS is not primarily due to the formation of a second blastopore, which always occurs in such cases. The fact that the numbers or amounts of cytoplasmic determinants are sufficient to specify the position of two neural axes shows that there is considerable redundancy in the system. However, the physicochemical nature of the cytoplasmic determinants and their modes of action are not known. Experiments to demonstrate cytoplasmic determinants by showing that transposition of cytoplasm from one position to another in the egg results in the expected transfer of positional information have given positive results.[12–14] But the experiments are subject to criticism for lack of controls and the possibility that during the operation of transfer of cytoplasm inversion of the egg itself may result in formation of a second axis.[15]

The essential questions have remained the same for more than a century: how do materials for making cells originate; how do cells multiply, grow, and interact to form organized multicellular tissues; how

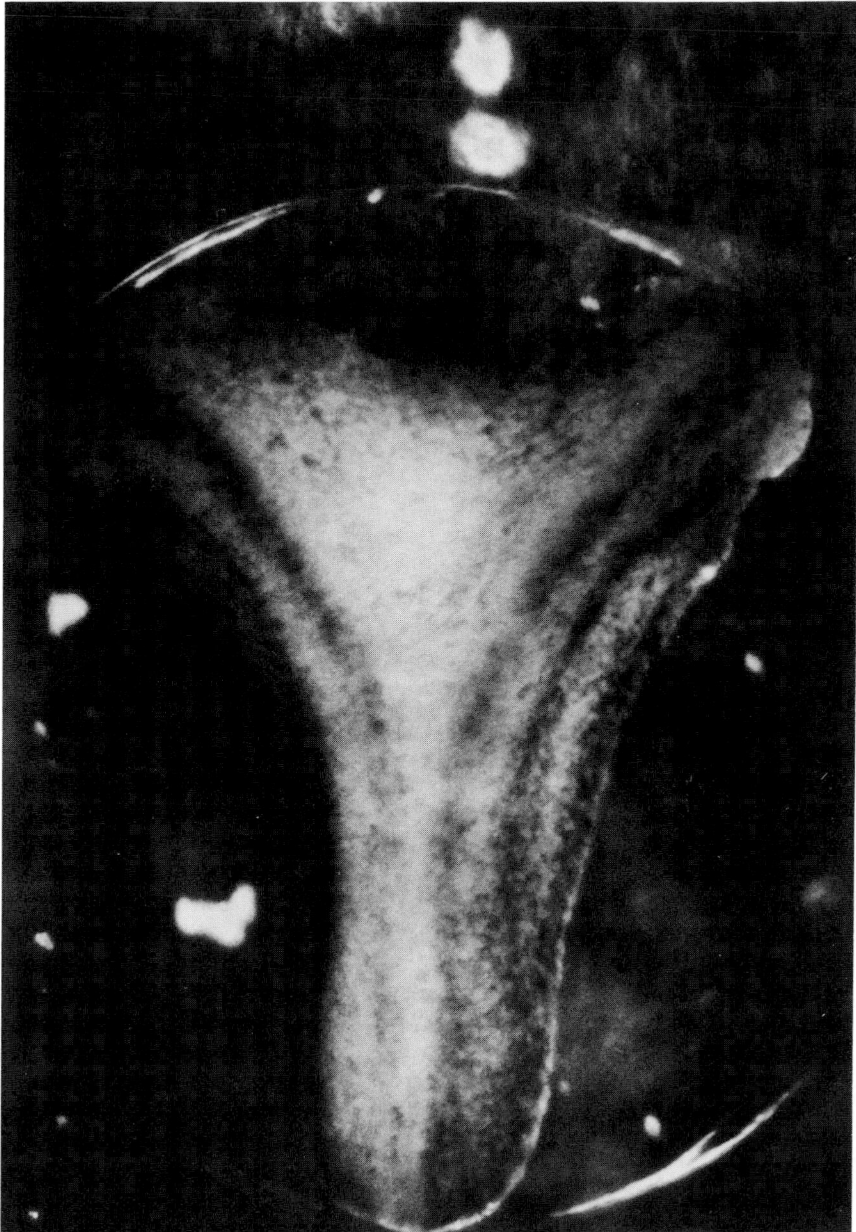

Figure 1. Twin Embryo of *Xenopus laevis* at larval stage 26 produced by turning the fertilized egg ventral side up for 1 hr until the second cleavage, using the method of Penners and Schleip.[10]

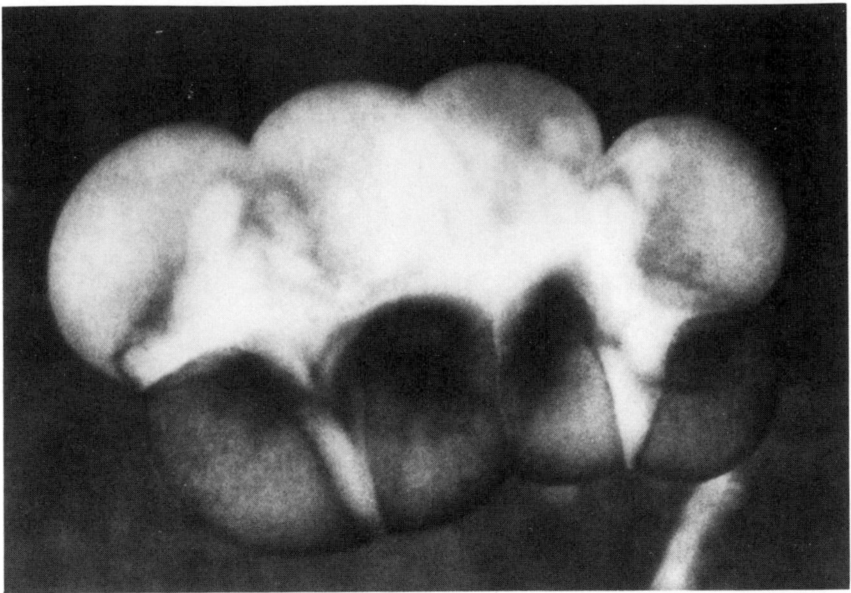

Figure 2. Twin embryo of *Xenopus laevis* at the eight-cell stage, showing duplication of the pattern of cleavage. The twin was produced by removing the vitelline membrane shortly after fertilization and turning the egg ventral side up for 1 hr until after the first cleavage.

do the tissues become harmoniously organized to form an organism? It is to Wilhelm His that we owe the revitalization of the preformationist concept that a kind of blueprint of the morphological pattern of the whole structure is already present in the egg and cleavage stages, and that cell proliferation, differentiation, and assembly are constrained by that blueprint.

In this article I shall show that the basic morphological plan of the central nervous system can be identified in mid-blastula stages and that the developmental programming of that pattern starts before any of the programs that control cell proliferation and differentiation of various types of nerve cells.[16] The keys to understanding these earliest stages of development of the CNS are to recognize that (1) the basic morphological pattern arises in small populations of ancestral or founder cells, (2) developmental programming of this basic morphological pattern results from interaction between the chromosomes and constituents of the egg which are regionally localized and are therefore distributed differentially into various cell lineages,[17] and (3) differentiation of sets of founder cells that compose the basic morphological pattern promotes further interactions at later stages that result in commitment of cells to restricted programs leading to development of many different types of nerve cells. The global primary pattern develops first as a "promorphology," and the subpatterns of regional differentiation develop later, within the primary pattern; the global pattern is not assembled gradually, bit by bit, as is commonly believed.

The early origin of the basic morphological pattern of CNS development, for which I shall give evidence, is under control of the egg cytoplasm. It has been shown, for example, by species hybrid experiments,[18] that early embryonic development is under maternal control (i.e., egg cytoplasmic control) until early gastrula stages and that the embryo's genome does not take over control in amphibians until neural plate stages (Davidson,[5] pp. 34–58, 83). Although transcription is not necessary for the egg to develop to gastrula stages, it may be very significant that in amphibian embryos the establishment of the primordial morphological pattern at stage 8, the 512-cell stage, is followed by a sudden increase in transcription of new RNA, resulting in "at least a twenty-fold relative increase in the amount of labeled RNA per nucleus . . . as the embryos progress from stage 8 to stage 8½, i.e., within a period of about one hour" (Davidson,[5] p. 148). During cleavage stages there are changes in RNA and protein synthesis,[19–21] great increases in cell adhesiveness[22,23] and the appearance of intercellular materials,[24–30] and I suggest that some of these changes are related to the development of compartment-specific cell recognition.

Whereas most of this chapter will be devoted to my theory of compartmentation in the blastula, it is worth noting that the primordial pattern of organization of the CNS of the frog deduced from my experimental results is essentially in agreement with the results of earlier workers who deduced the primordial pattern from comparative anatomical studies on brains of various species at different stages of development.[31–39] The history of research on that problem has been surveyed by Kuhlenbeck.[40] All workers agree on the basic morphological plan of the rhombencephalon and spinal cord, but some disagree on the plan of organization of more rostral parts of the brain (Fig. 3). My contribution has been to confirm Kingsbury's discovery of a continuity of the pattern across the ventral midline of the brain ahead of the rostral end of the floor plate[37–39] and also to show that the sulcus limitans of His extends rostrally as a boundary between dorsal and ventral parts of the mesencephalon, diencephalon, and telencephalon. It is especially satisfying to have found such a large measure of consistency between the classical concepts of primordial morphological pattern in the CNS and my theory of compartmentation in the early embryo.

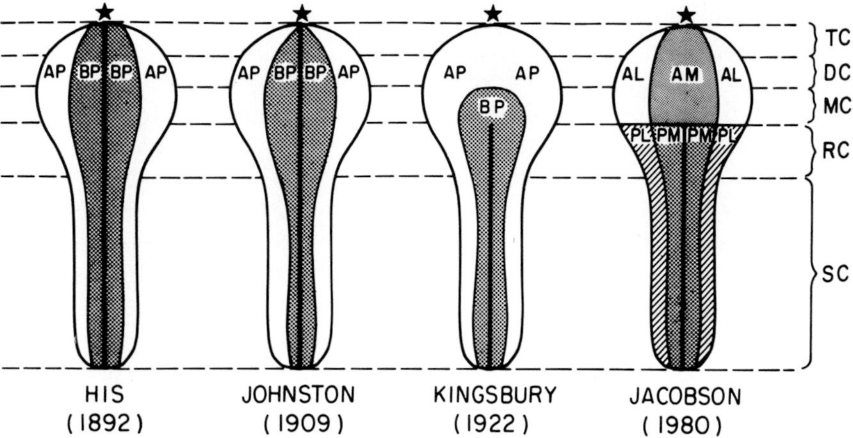

Figure 3. The basic morphological pattern of the vertebrate CNS as proposed by various authors. The star is at the lamina terminalis. The CNS is shown as if slit open along the dorsal midline and opened out like a book with the ventral midline as the hinge. The central heavy line shows the extent of the floor plate. The compartments are named as if they belong to the neural plate. AM, anterior medial compartment; AL, anterior lateral compartment; AP, alar plate; BP, basal plate; DC, diencephalon; MC, mesencephalon; PL, posterior-lateral compartment; PM, posterior-medial compartment; RC, rhombencephalon; SC, spinal cord; TC, telencephalon.

2. THE THEORY OF COMPARTMENTATION

The theory is that the primary morphological pattern of the CNS arises in the mid-blastula, probably at the 512-cell stage, in the form of groups of founder cells; the descendants of each group exclusively populate a region of the CNS, called a compartment, which is not shared with the descendants of any other founder cell group. The spatial arrangement of the seven founder cell groups (Fig. 4) persists as a pattern of compartmentation at later stages of development and in the mature system. Mingling of cells between compartments is prohibited but is permitted within each compartment. Descendants of each founder cell group are committed, from the time of foundation of the groups, to associate selectively with other descendants of their own groups. As a result the arrangement of the original seven groups is preserved, although topologically transformed as a consequence of different rates of cell proliferation, migration, growth, and differentiation of many types of cells in each compartment. Neither the differentiation of specific cellular phenotypes nor the paths of outgrowth of axons and dendrites are determined or limited by compartmentation.

From its inception,[16] this theory has been stimulated and informed by the work on the development of compartments in imaginal discs of *Drosophila*[41] (see Chapter 4). Accordingly there are a number of similarities between my theory of compartmentation in the frog's central nervous system and the theory of compartmentation in imaginal discs. But there are such great differences between the development of frogs and of insects, especially those in which organs develop from imaginal discs, that it is better, at present, to regard any similarities as fortuitous. Therefore, no further reference shall be made to the extensive literature on compartments in *Drosophila*.

This theory is based mainly on the results of clonal analysis, using a heritable cell tracer, horseradish peroxidase (HRP), which can be injected into individual ancestral cells and can later be used as a means of mapping the spatial distribution of labeled descendants[42–46] (see

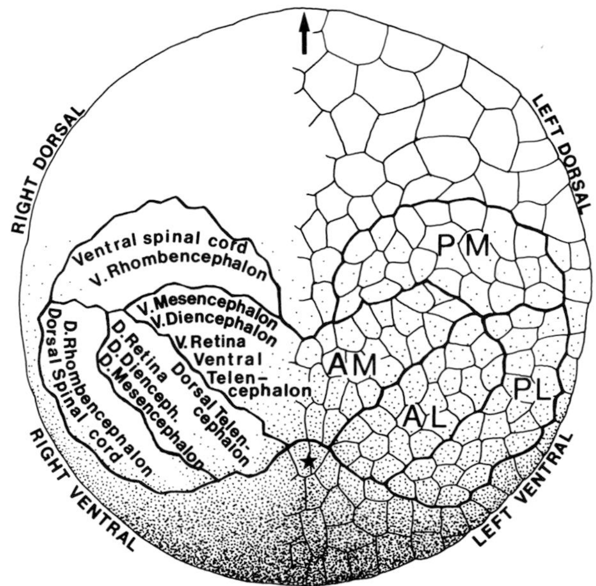

Figure 4. Diagram of the 512-cell embryo of *Xenopus* to show the locations and relative positions of the founder cell groups on the left that give rise to compartments in the CNS as shown on the right side of the embryo. The star is at the animal pole, and the arrow point is at the vegetal pole. AM, anterior-medial founder cell group (which gives rise to ventral retina, telencephalon, diencephalon, and mesencephalon); AL, anterior-lateral founder cell group (which gives rise to dorsal retina, telencephalon, diencephalon, and mesencephalon); PM, posterior-medial founder cell group (which gives rise to ventral rhombencephalon and spinal cord); PL, posterior-lateral founder cell group (which gives rise to dorsal rhombencephalon and spinal cord). (From Jacobson, 1980.[16])

Chapter 1; see also Chapters 3 and 5 for other approaches to the analysis of neuronal lineage). The theory is also supported by my experiments in which specific ancestral cells or their labeled descendants, which are known to contribute to parts of compartments or to form entire compartments, were removed or grafted to new positions.[47] The theory allows certain predictions to be made about the behavior of clones that arise from particular ancestral cells and the consistency between those predictions and the experimental evidence will be discussed in Section 3. The new theory is also somewhat at variance with Spemann's theory of the organizer,[48] making it necessary to give a critique of the orthodox theory and to show how parts of the old theory can be assimilated in the new theory (Sections 4 and 5).

3. PREDICTIONS MADE FROM THE THEORY AND THEIR EXPERIMENTAL VERIFICATION

The strength of the theory of compartmentation is that it enables one to predict the outcome of a number of different kinds of experiments. Some of these have already been done and provide support for the theory; others are feasible and will be done soon: their results could either support the theory or falsify it. There are three main predictions of the theory of compartmentation, and failure to validate any of these would falsify the theory or require major changes in it. If these three predictions are shown to be true, then others can be made and tested experimentally, which will open the way to understanding the mechanisms of patterning of differentiation in the early stages of development of the CNS of vertebrates. The three principal parts of the theory and the predictions that can be made from them are as follows.

1. The theory states that a compartment is a region of the central nervous system which is populated, from a particular time in mid-blastula stages known as the foundation time, exclusively by all the descendants of a small group of founder cells. The theory predicts that labeling any prospective neural cell after the foundation time will result in restriction of all the labeled descendants to one compartment. Conversely, the result of labeling any prospective neural cell before foundation time will depend on the position of that cell in relation to future compartment boundaries and on the amount of cell dispersal and mingling that occurs between the time of labeling and the foundation time. Therefore, in order to determine whether the experimental results are consistent with the theory, the amount and time of onset of cell dispersal and mingling must be known.

2. The theory states that compartment-specific properties develop which result in selective affinity between all cells of the same compartment and selective disaffinity between cells of different compartments. The theory predicts that those compartment-specific properties can be demonstrated biochemically or by tests of affinities between cells.

3. The theory states that all founder cells of the same group have an equal probability of giving rise to any of the many types of nerve cells that differentiate in the compartment that stems from that founder cell group. From this it can be predicted that removal of part of a founder cell group may reduce the final number of descendants but will not change the types of cells that differentiate in a compartment. However, removal of the entire founder cell group or removal of the whole compartment at any time will result in a corresponding permanent deficit in the structure. The effects of removal of part of a compartment will depend on the time of the operation in relation to times of commitment to differentiation of specific types of cells in that compartment.

3.1. *Deployment of Labeled Clones after HRP Injection into Ancestral Cells at Various Stages*

We have shown that HRP injected into single blastomeres of *Xenopus laevis* does not alter normal development, does not leak out of the injected cells, is transmitted to all its descendants, can be recognized in them up to several days later by means of a histochemical procedure applied to serial sections through the entire embryo.[42–46]. Maps were made of the distribution of the labeled cells in the well-differentiated CNS and in other tissues (Figs. 5–10). In all cases the labeled cells were mingled with unlabeled cells and were dispersed throughout a region which we call a *clonal domain*. The clonal domain of any cell labeled at or after the 512-cell stage is located entirely inside one of the compartments, but the clonal domain of any cell labeled before the 512-cell stage may be in more than one compartment. We could correlate the position of the clonal domain in the differentiated nervous system with the position of the originally labeled ancestral cell in the early embryo. This is fate mapping at the level of resolution of single ancestral cells and of every one of its descendants (Fig. 11 and Table I). Because the label persists in the descendants beyond the time of their differentiation, and because the label enters the outgrowing axons and dendrites (Figs. 12 and 13), specific types of labeled nerve cells can be identified and the clonal relationships between specific types of cells and identified ancestral cells can be determined (Table I).

We have completed a clonal analysis, by labeling individual cells

Table I. Lineage Diagram of Xenopus from the Zygote to the 64-Cell Blastula Stage[a]

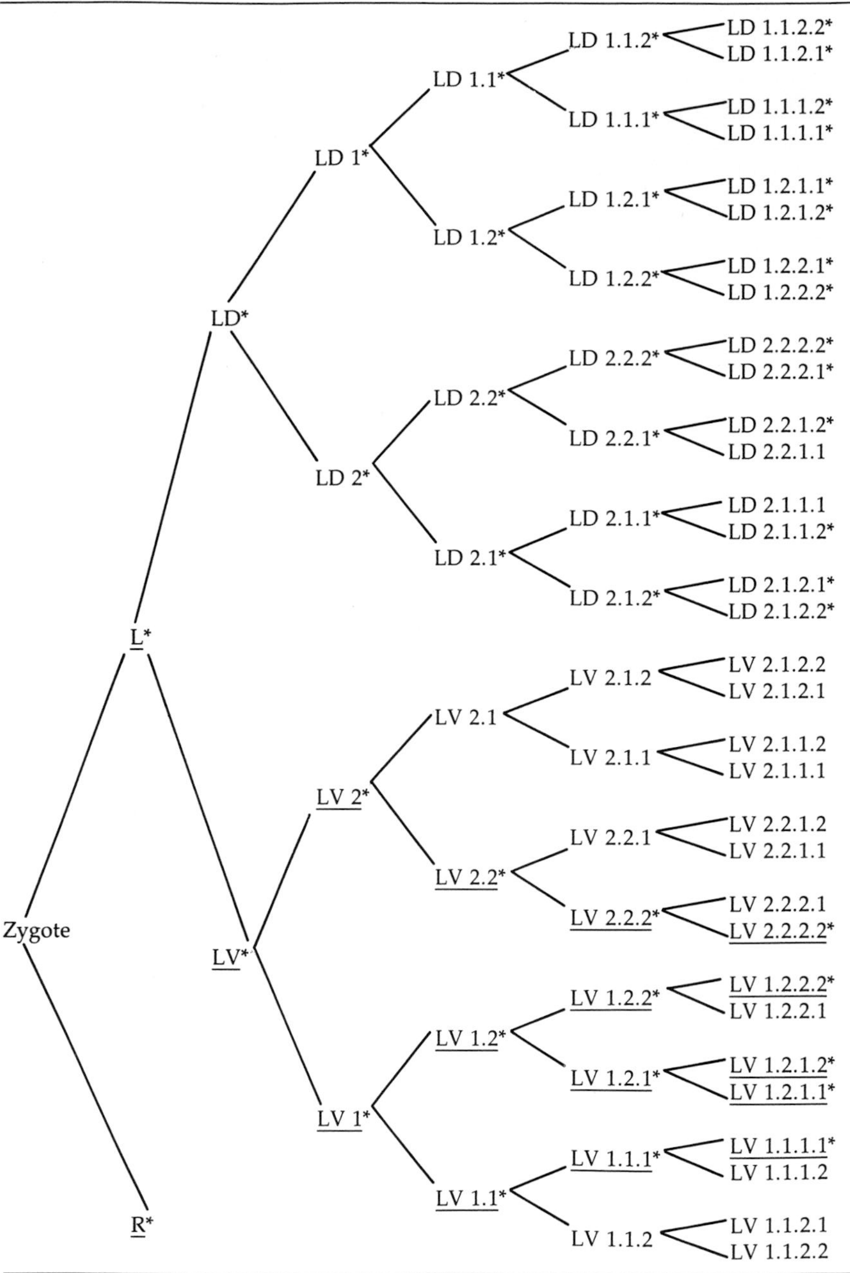

[a] Only the left side is shown: the right is identical. Blastomeres contributing descendants to the CNS are indicated by an asterisk. Underlined blastomeres give rise to Rohon-Beard neurons in type X embryos.[46] L, left; R, right; D, dorsal; V, ventral. Cells designated .1 are closer to, and those designated .2 are farther from, the mid-sagittal plane or the animal pole.

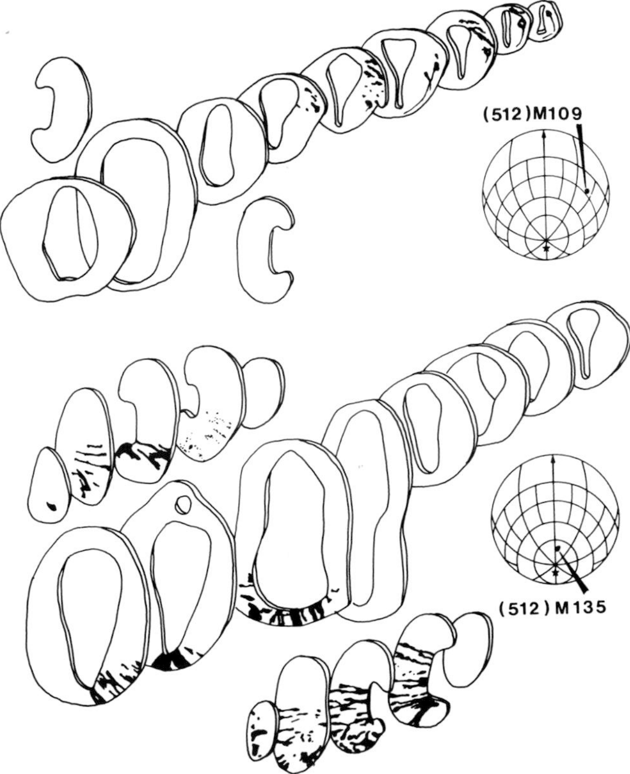

Figure 5. Serial section reconstructions of the CNS and retinae of larval *Xenopus* that had received an injection into a single ancestral cell at the 512-cell stage at the positions indicated on the diagrams of the embryos shown at the right. In the upper specimen the injected cell was in the posterior-lateral ancestral cell group and all the labeled descendants, shown in black, are located in the posterior-lateral compartment of the CNS. In the lower specimen the injected cell was located in the anterior-medial ancestral cell group and all the labeled descendants, shown in black, were located in the anterior-medial compartment of the CNS. (From Jacobson, 1982.[45])

at progressively later cleavage stages, beginning with the egg and progressing systematically to the 512-cell stage.[42–47] The results of this analysis show the spatial and phenotypic relationships between clones that arise from individual ancestral cells injected at progressively later stages. In particular, the results show how the clonal domain of a maternal cell is shared or partitioned by the clones arising from the daughter cells, and if partitioning occurs, where the boundaries are located.[44] The main results of these experiments can be summarized as follows.

1. Dispersal of labeled cells and mingling of labeled and unlabeled

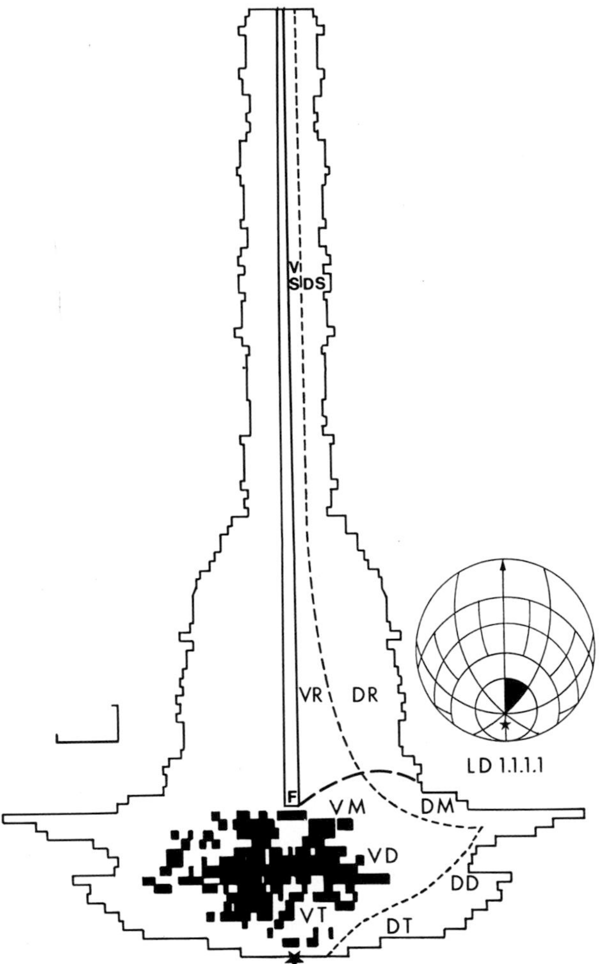

Figure 6. Topological map of the CNS of larval *Xenopus* at stage 37 that had received an injection of HRP into blastomere LD1.1.1.1 at the 64-cell stage. The labeled regions (black) and unlabeled regions (white) are shown in 113 consecutive serial sections extending from the lamina terminalis (star) to near the caudal end of the spinal cord. The CNS is shown as if opened along the dorsal midline and folded out with the ventral midline forming the axis of symmetry. Labeled cells were projected onto the ventricular surface, resulting in considerable superimposition in the regions shown in black. The light dashed line shows the approximate position of the boundary between dorsal and ventral compartments, while the heavy dashed line shows the approximate position of the boundary between anterior and posterior compartments in the CNS. DD, dorsal diencephalon; DM, dorsal mesencephalon; DR, dorsal rhombencephalon; DS, dorsal mesencephalon; DT, dorsal telencephalon; F, floor plate; VD, ventral diencephalon; VM, ventral mesencephalon; VR, ventral rhombencephalon; VS, ventral spinal cord; VT, ventral telencephalon. Scale, 100μm.

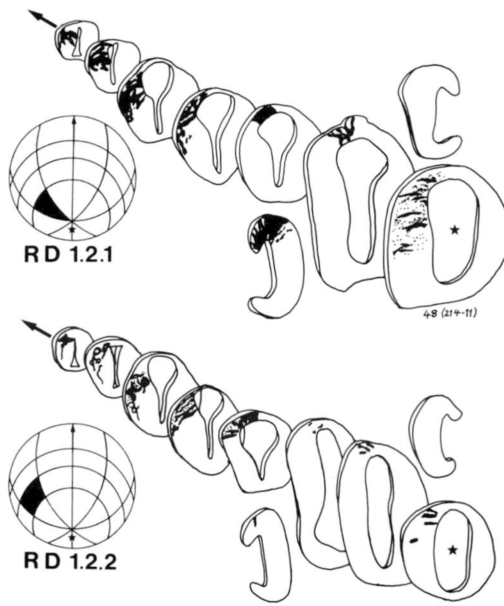

Figure 7. Serial section reconstructions of the CNS and retina of *Xenopus* in two specimens at early larval stages after injection of HRP into single blastomeres (RD1.2.1 and RD1.2.2) at the 32-cell stage. Labeled cells are black, unlabeled regions white. The star is at the lamina terminalis. The arrow points to the caudal end of the spinal cord.

cells occurred in all cases. I have observed that clones of ancestral cells labeled at early cleavage stages (2- to 16-cell stages) and fixed before the 1024-cell stage showed coherent clonal growth[49] (see also reference 50). Dispersal and mingling of cells started after the 1024-cell stage and were well advanced by the beginning of gastrulation (Figs. 14 and 15). The significance of this will be discussed later (Section 4.3.1).

2. Ancestral cells of the 2- to 512-cell stages are polyvalent, that is, each ancestral cell that contributed descendants to the CNS also contributed to other organs and tissues. Each ancestral cell gave rise to many types of cells in the CNS as well as in other tissues. There were one-to-many and many-to-many relationships between ancestral cells and cellular phenotypes to which they give rise. It is not yet known how lineages may become restricted after the 512-cell stage.

3. Boundaries, across which cells did not disperse or mingle, were found at invariant places in the CNS (and preliminary analysis indicated such boundaries in other systems also). The boundaries were seen in the CNS at the following positions: (1) A *dorsal midline boundary* separated left and right sides in the dorsal midline along its entire length. (2) A *ventral midline boundary* between left and right sides was located in the ventral midline of the rhombencephalon and spinal cord. This boundary was absent in the ventral midline of more rostral parts of the brain with

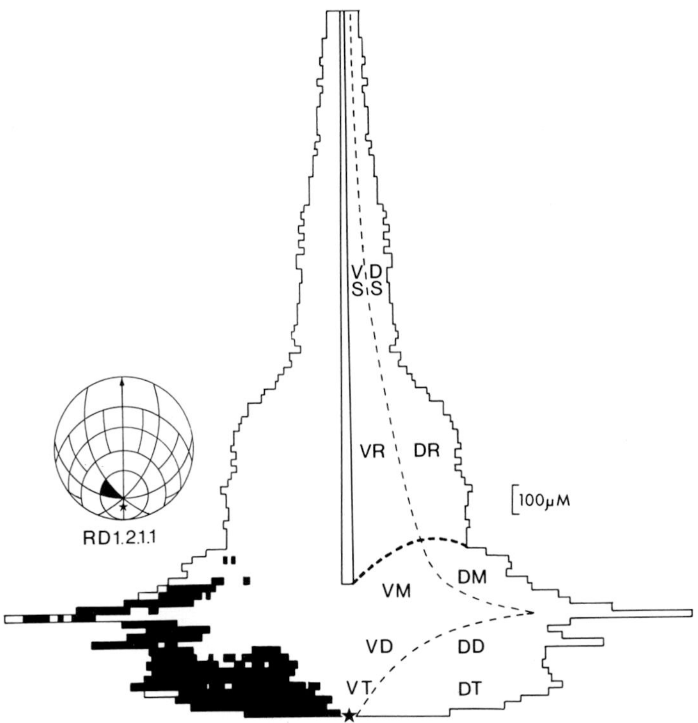

Figure 8. Topological map of the CNS of larval *Xenopus* at stage 39 that had received an injection of HRP into blastomere RD1.2.1.1 at the 64-cell stage. Labeled cells are shown in black, unlabeled regions in white. Other conventions are given in the legend to Fig. 6. (From Jacobson and Hirose, 1981.[44])

the result that cells mingled and dispersed across the ventral midline of the presumptive telencephalon, diencephalon, and mesencephalon and mingled cells from both sides contributed to the ventral parts of both retinae[42] (Figs. 5, 6, and 16). Their dispersal into the dorsal parts of the CNS was restricted by the boundary to be mentioned next. (3) A *dorsal–ventral boundary* occurred between dorsal and ventral parts of the CNS throughout its entire length and between dorsal and ventral parts of the retina (Figs. 17 and 18). In its caudal part this boundary was coincident with the sulcus limitans and extended rostrally to the lamina terminalis. (4) An *anterior–posterior boundary* extended transversely in the coronal plane at the level of the isthmus, separating the rhombencephalon caudally from more rostral regions of the brain (Figs. 5, 6, 9, and 10).

Note that these boundaries are named according to their positions in the neural tube and well-differentiated CNS, and their names do not reflect their positions at stages before the neural plate rolls up to form a tube. The positions of these boundaries at earlier stages, as shown by fixing labeled embryos at late blastula, gastrula, and neurula stages, are given in Table II.

These boundaries were respected in many cases by descendants of cells initially labeled before the 512-cell stage.[44] Whenever the clonal domain of a maternal cell was partitioned between the clones of the daughter cells, the partitioning occurred at one of those boundaries. Those boundaries were always respected by clones arising from every cell labeled at the 512-cell stage.[45]

The positions of compartment boundaries have been determined in a series of several hundred embryos in which a single cell has been labeled by intracellular injection of HRP at 2- to 512-cell stages and the positions of all the labeled descendants have been mapped at later

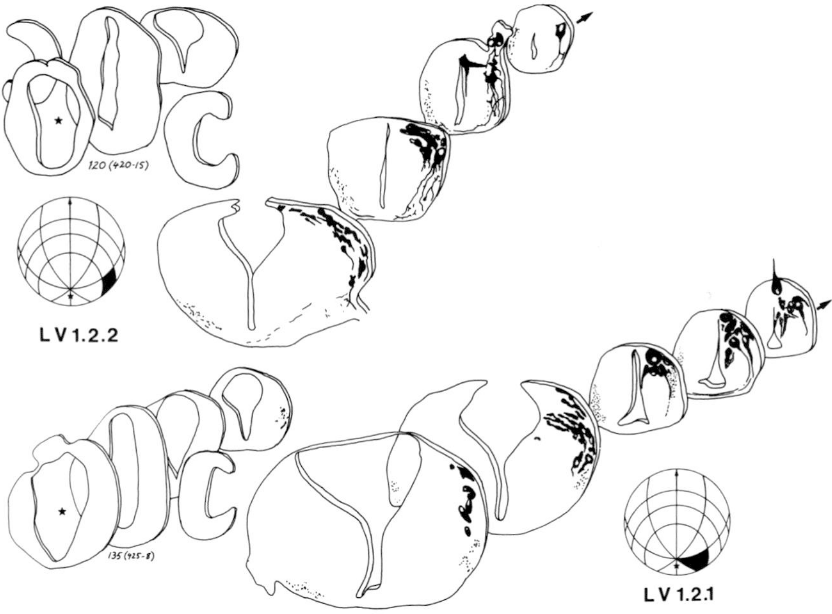

Figure 9. Serial section reconstructions of the CNS of larval *Xenopus* at stage 39 that had received an injection into blastomere LV1.2.2 (upper specimen) and LV1.2.1 (lower specimen) at the 32-cell stage. Sections of telencephalon, diencephalon, retina, and mesencephalon are drawn to half the scale of sections of rhombencephalon and spinal cord. Labeled cells are shown black, unlabeled regions white. Note labeled Rohon–Beard neurons and commissural neurons, the latter projecting labeled axons across the ventral commissure of the spinal cord. (From Jacobson and Hirose, 1981.[44])

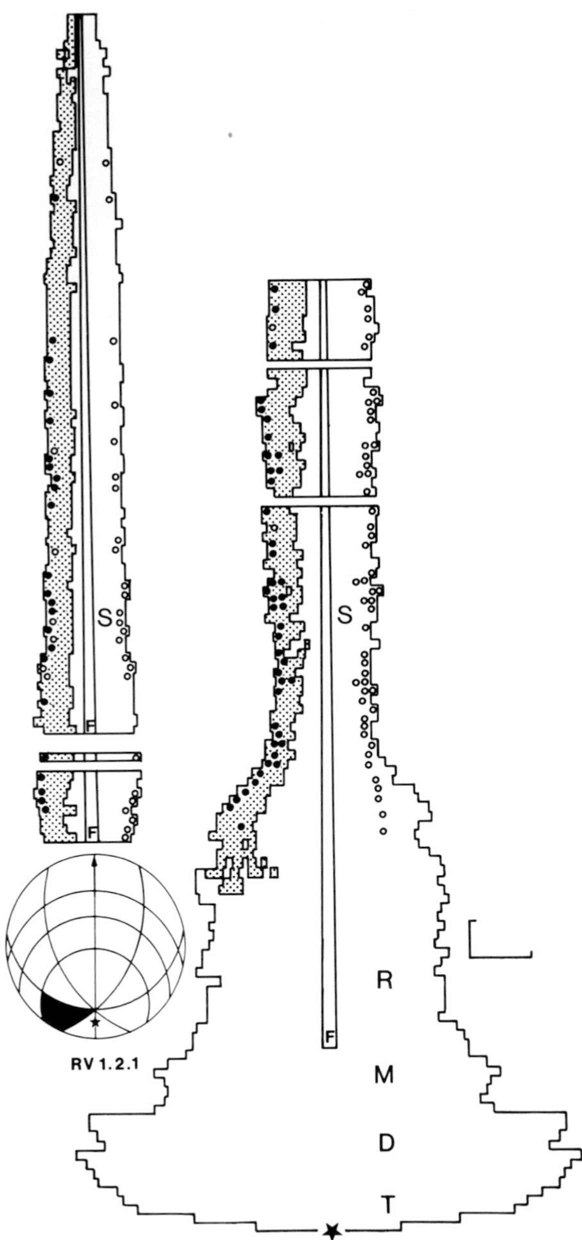

Figure 10. Topological map of the CNS of a *Xenopus* larva at stage 39 that had received an injection of HRP into blastomere RV1.2.1 at the 32-cell stage. The CNS is shown as if opened along the dorsal midline and folded out with the ventral midline forming the axis

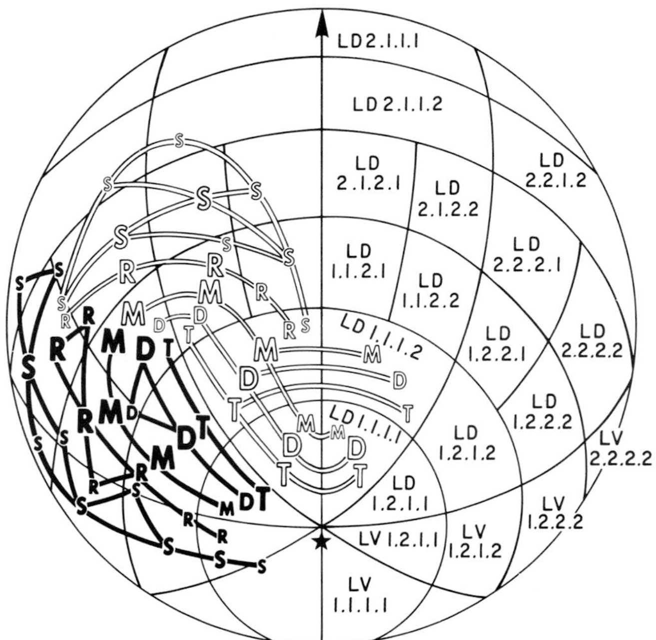

Figure 11. Fate map showing the regions of CNS populated by descendants of blastomeres of the 64-cell embryo. The embryo is viewed from the animal pole (star) and dorsal side. The tip of the arrow is at the vegetal pole. Blastomere designations are given on one side, while on the other side are shown the regions of CNS to which each blastomere contributed descendants. *Black letters* indicate dorsal regions of the CNS; *white letters* indicate ventral regions. The *sizes* of the letters (small, medium, or large) over each blastomere show the number of labeled cells found in each region after labeling that blastomere. See Fig. 10 for key. (From Jacobson and Hirose, 1981.[44])

stages. The primordial arrangement of founder cell groups in the blastula has been deduced from these results on the assumption that cell mingling starts only after the time of foundation of the compartments in the blastula.

The method of deducing the time of onset of compartmentation, that is, the foundation time, is based on two premises. The first is that coherent clonal growth occurs up to the foundation time[49,50]; the second

of symmetry. Labeled regions are stippled; unlabeled regions are white. Each black dot shows the position of a labeled Rohon–Beard neuron. Each white dot shows the position of an unlabeled Rohon–Beard neuron. The continuity of the map is broken by the absence of six sections. To fit the entire CNS on the diagram, the caudal end of the spinal cord is shown separately on the left. D, diencephalon; F, floor plate; M, mesencephalon; R, rhomencephalon; T, telencephalon; S, spinal chord. (From Jacobson and Hirose, 1981.[44])

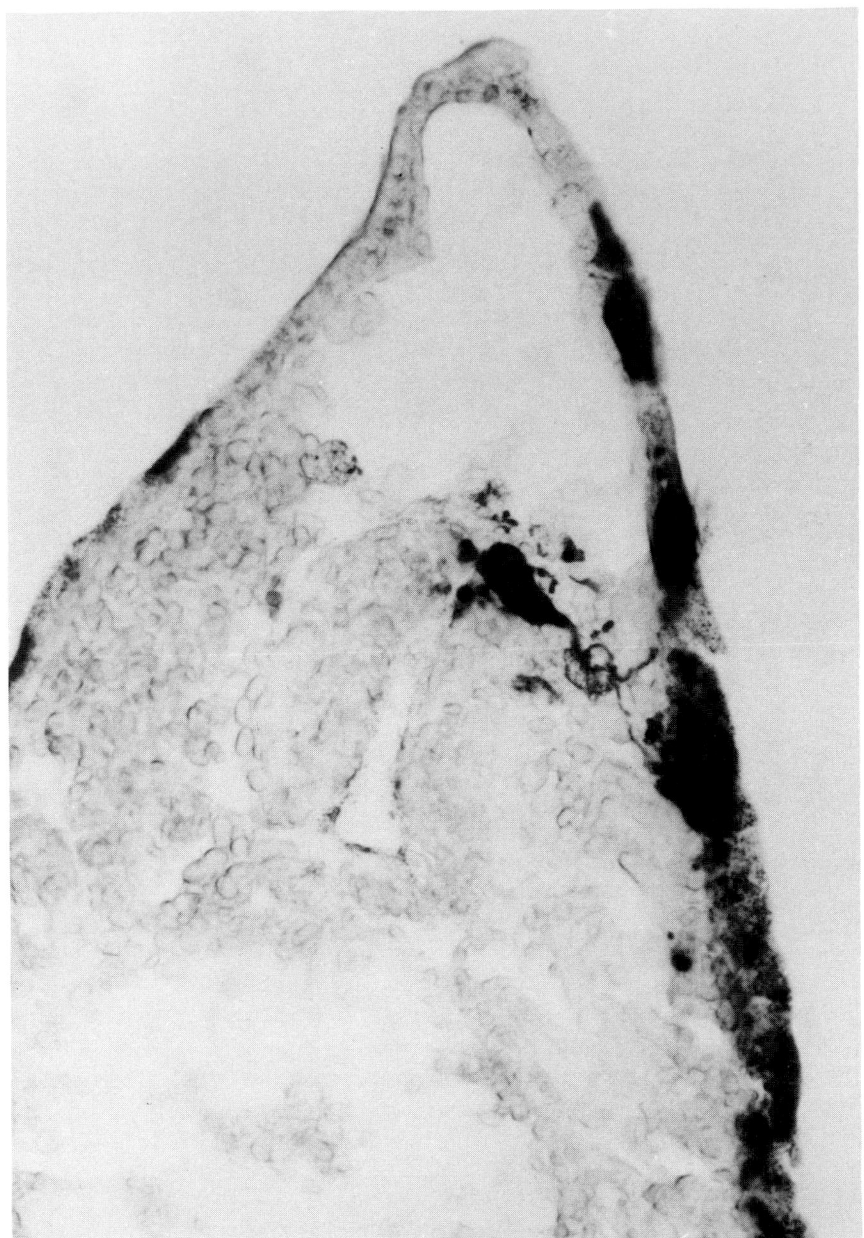

Figure 12. Coronal section at the level of thoracic spinal cord in a stage 34 *Xenopus* larva that had received an injection of HRP into blastomere RV1.2.1 at the 32-cell stage. Both the soma and neurites of a Rohon–Beard neuron are filled with the label. Several cells in the epidermis are also labeled.

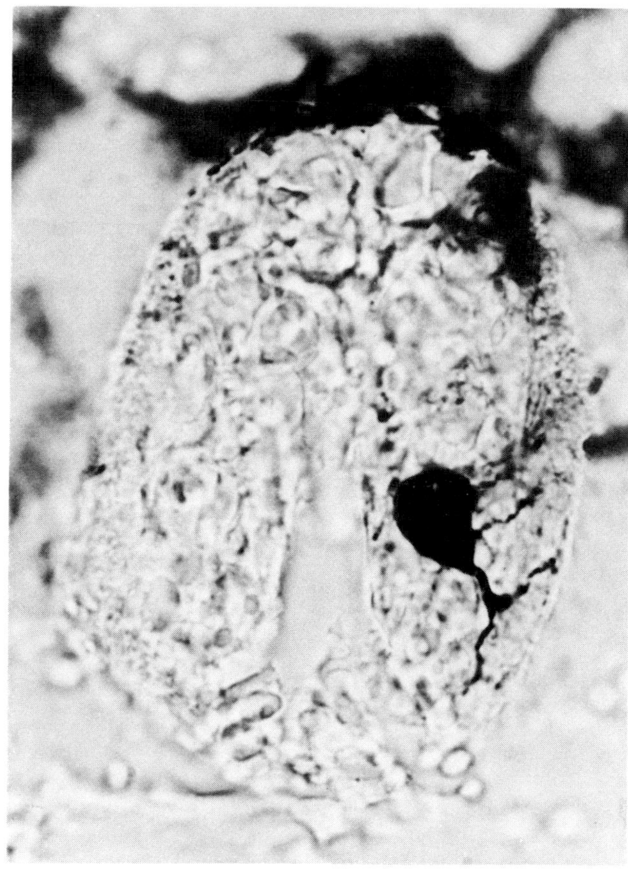

Figure 13. Coronal section through the spinal cord in a stage 34 *Xenopus* that had received an injection of HRP into blastomere LD2.2.1.2 at the 64-cell stage. A labeled neuron with labeled neurites is seen in the ventrolateral motor column of the spinal cord.

is that cells rapidly disperse after foundation time, as shown in Figs. 14 and 15, so that any cell labeled after foundation time will disperse its labeled descendants into a large part of the compartment, reaching but not crossing the compartment boundaries. Because coherent clonal growth occurs in *Xenopus* during cleavage stages until the 1024-cell stage, it was possible to observe compartment boundaries in some cases after labeling single cells at any stage. If the initially labeled cell contributed all its descendants to a single founder cell group, its descendants would remain entirely inside a single compartment; this was observed in all cases after labeling single cells at the 512-cell stage, but only in some cases after labeling cells at earlier stages. Alternatively, if the initially labeled cell contributed its descendants to more than one founder cell group, later generations of its descendants would disperse into more than one compartment. This was never observed after starting labeling at the 512-cell stage but occurred frequently after injection of single cells at 2- to 256-cell stages. However, the positions of those initially labeled cells that distributed descendants to more than one founder cell group could indicate the positions of the boundaries which their descendants straddled at foundation time, as shown in Fig. 19. This figure also shows the outer boundary of the presumptive neural region, that is, the total population of founder cells that contributed descendants to the central nervous system, and indicates that at the 512-cell stage there are between 20 and 30 founder cells for each compartment.

It follows that a fate map cannot be at a greater level of resolution than is permitted by the amount of cell dispersal and mingling. The fate map can give the probability of a particular cell giving rise to any one

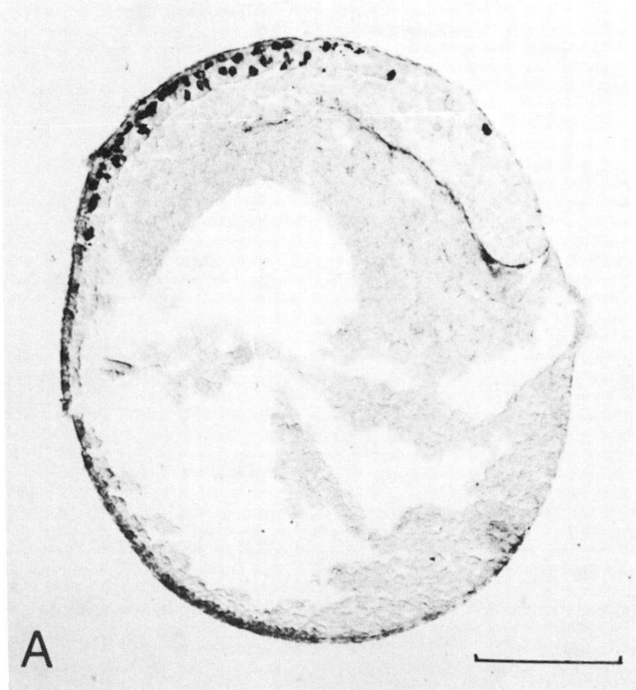

Figure 14. Sagittal section through a gastrula of *Xenopus* at stage 12 that had received an injection of HRP into blastomere LD1.1.1 at the 32-cell stage. The labeled cells containing the dark reaction product are dispersed and mingled with unlabeled cells in the ectodermal layer. B is a higher-power picture of the labeled region of A. Scale, 400 μm.

of the many types of cells that differentiate in the compartment. The fate map is a composite of the results of labeling single cells in a large number of individual embryos. Thus, it does not show the individual variability of the results. The significant variable in these results is the compartment as a whole, not the distribution of labeled descendants of any ancestral cell. According to the theory, any initially labeled cell, at any stage, can disperse its descendants at random within compartment boundaries. Therefore, any statistical evaluation of the theory would have to be restricted to an evaluation of the variability in the positions of compartment boundaries and not to a statistical treatment of the distribution of labeled cells within compartments.

3.2. Origins of Compartment-Specific Properties

The theory states that compartment-specific properties appear or become effective at the 512-cell stage and that those properties are responsible for restriction of mingling between descendants of different

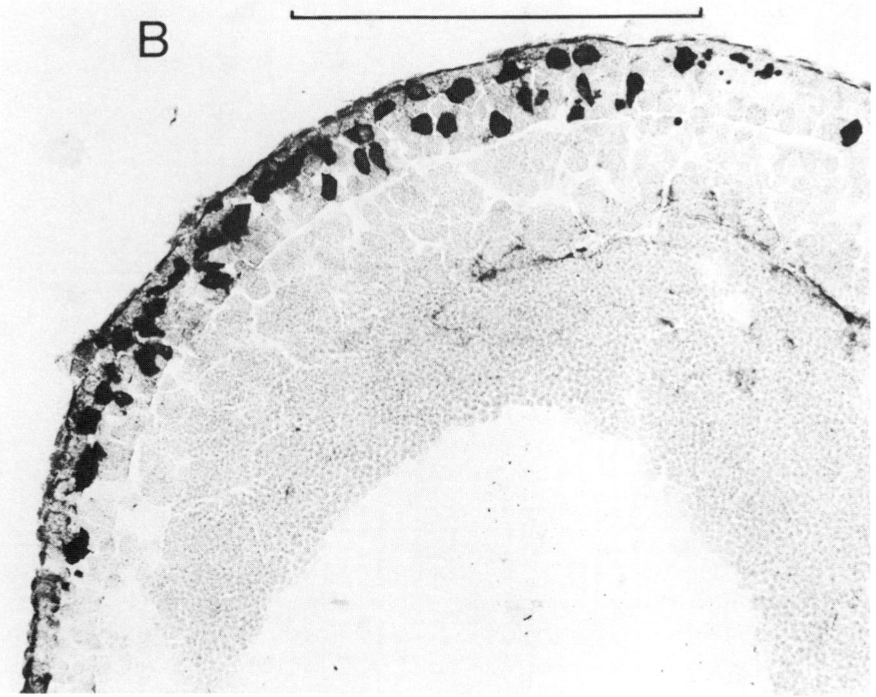

Figure 14 (*continued*).

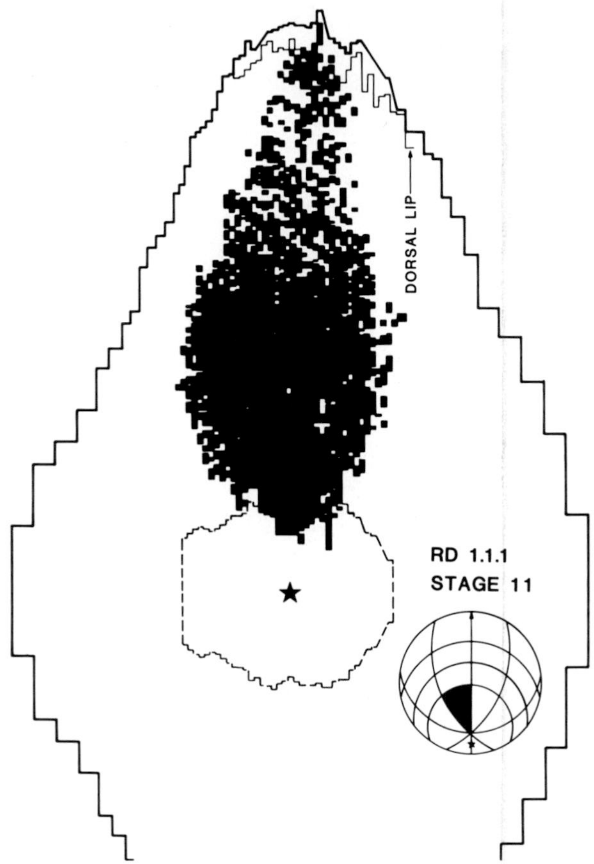

Figure 15. Topological map constructed from sagittal serial sections through a *Xenopus* gastrula (stage 11) that had received an injection of HRP into blastomere RD1.1.1 at the 32-cell stage. The embryo has been displayed by opening up each section at its posterior (vegetal) pole and flattening it out with the horizontal meridian of the animal half acting as the axis of symmetry. Labeled cells are projected onto the outer surface so that their superimposition gives the effect of greater coherence than was actually present. The star shows the animal pole; the dashed lines show tht blastocoele margin; the dorsal lip is indicated by a fine line. Labeled cells are black; unlabeled regions, white.

founder cell groups. The prediction from this is that there are biochemical properties shared by all cells belonging to the same compartment but different from one compartment to another. Development of these biochemical differences should be correlated with the time of foundation of compartments. However, one must bear in mind that determinants of compartments may be detectable as they become segregated into different lineages even before the time of foundation of compartments.

Table II. Compartments and Their Boundaries in the CNS and the Corresponding Compartments in the Blastula, Gastrula, and Neurula

Central nervous system	Blastula, gastrula, and neurula
(A) Boundaries	(A) Boundaries
(1) Dorsal midline (roof plate) between left dorsal and right dorsal compartments	(1) Lateral margins of prospective neural region
(2) Ventral midline (floor plate) between left and right sides of rhombencephalon and spinal cord	(2) Dorsal midline between left and right posterior-medial compartments
(3) Dorsal–ventral boundary between dorsal and ventral compartments along entire length of CNS on each side. Corresponds with sulcus limitans in rhombencephalon and spinal cord	(3) Medial–lateral boundary between lateral and medial compartments
(4) Anterior–posterior boundary between mesencephalon and rhombencephalon	(4) Anterior–posterior boundary between anterior and posterior compartments
(B) Compartments	(B) Compartments[a]
(1) Anterior–ventral compartment. Extends over ventral midline of telencephalon, diencephalon, and mesencephalon. Ventral parts of both retinae	(1) Anterior–medial compartment extends over midsagittal plane in anterior half of prospective neural region
(2) Anterior dorsal compartment on each side (L&R) includes dorsal telencephalon, diencephalon, mesencephalon, and retina	(2) Anterior-lateral compartment on each side (L&R)
(3) Posterior–ventral compartments on each side (L&R) includes ventral parts of rhombencephalon and spinal cord	(3) Posterior–medial compartment on each side (L&R)
(4) Posterior–dorsal compartment on each side (L&R) includes dorsal parts of rhombencephalon and spinal cord	(4) Posterior–lateral compartment on each side (L&R)

[a] Founder cell groups at the 512-cell stage, compartments at later stages.

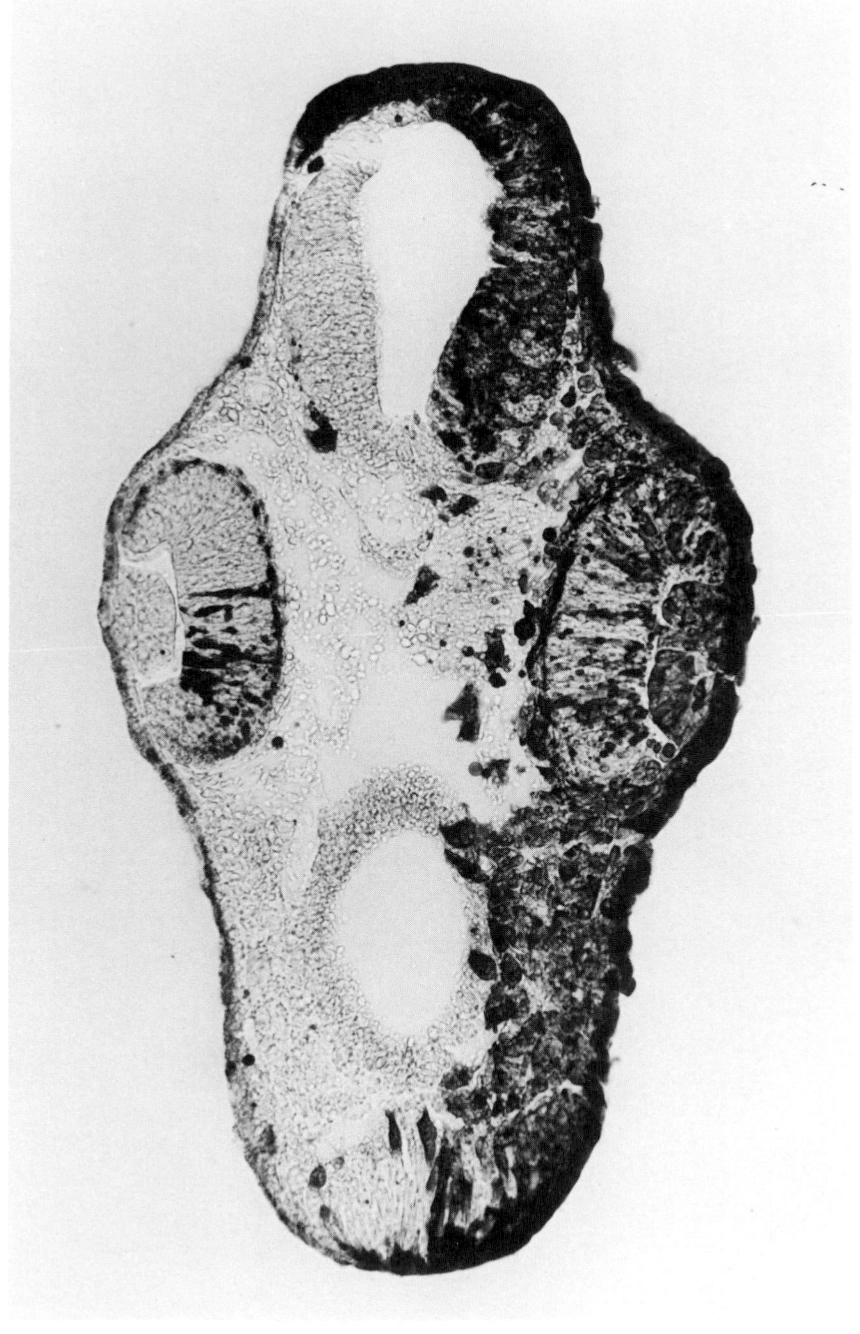

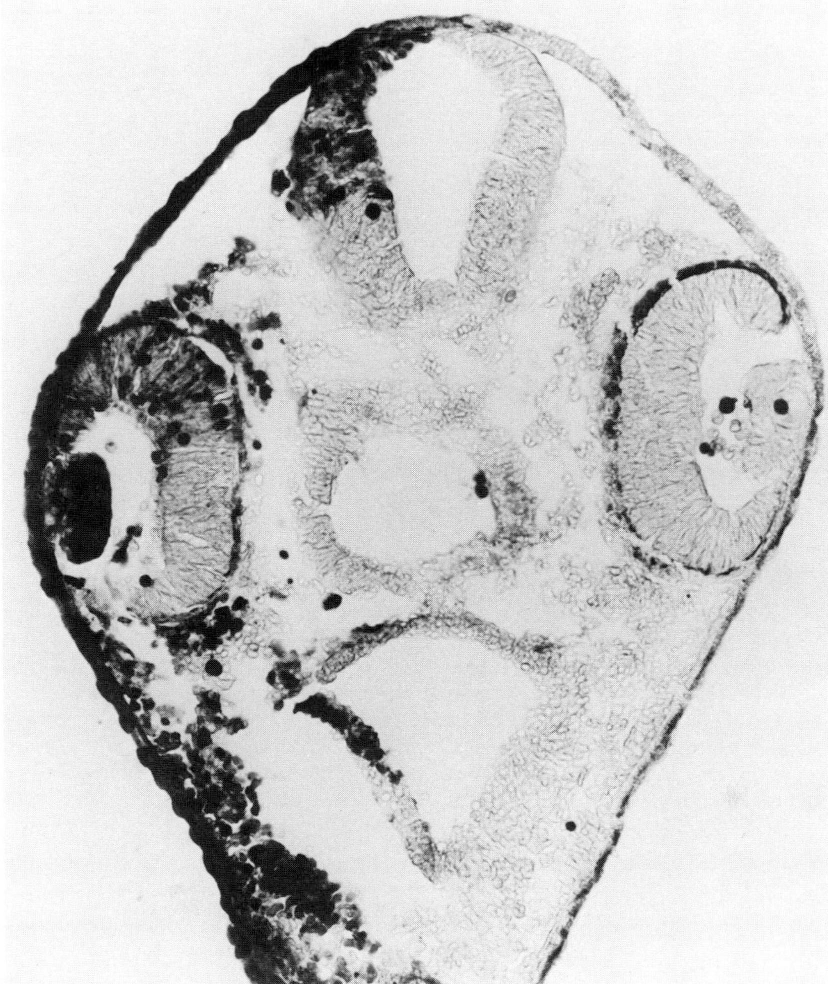

Figure 17. Coronal section at the level of the eyes and midbrain of a *Xenopus* larva at stage 34 that had received an injection of HRP into blastomere RD1.2 at the 16-cell stage. The labeled cells filled with dark reaction product are confined to the right anterior-dorsal compartment of the CNS and are seen in this section in the dorsal retina and dorsal mesencephalon on the injected side. Some neural crest cells are labeled and have migrated to both sides (not seen in this section). The distribution of labeled cells outside the CNS should be noted.

←

Figure 16. Coronal section at the level of the eyes of a *Xenopus* embryo at stage 34 that had received an injection of HRP into blastomere L at the two-cell stage. The entire retina on the injected side is labeled, but labeled and unlabeled cells are mingled in the ventral halves of both retinae. Some labeled cells have also crossed to the opposite side in the neural crest and in the ventral parts of the telencephalon, diencephalon, and mesencephalon (not seen in this section).

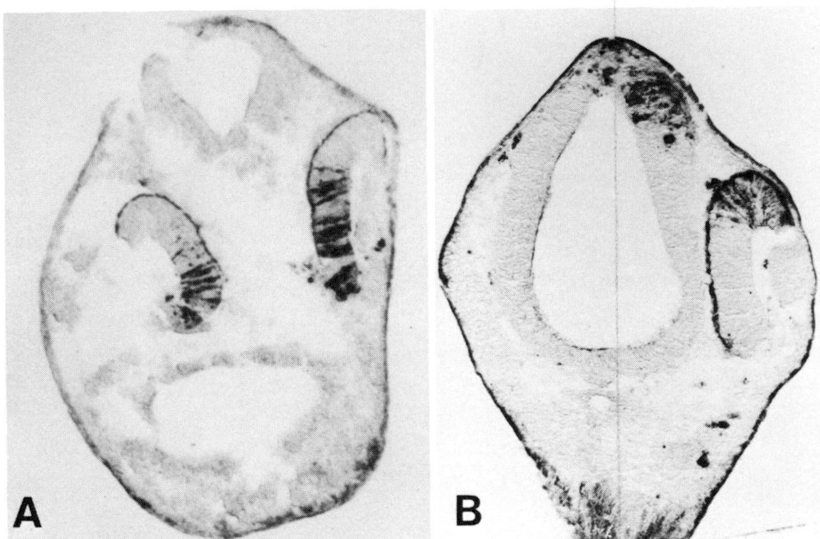

Figure 18. (A) Coronal section at the level of the eyes and isthmus through a *Xenopus* larva at stage 36 that had received an injection of HRP into a cell in the anterior-medial founder cell group at the 512-cell stage. Labeled cells in the CNS filled with dark reaction product are in the ventral parts of both retinae. These cells reach the ventral side of the boundary between anterior-dorsal and anterior-ventral compartments. (B) Coronal section at the level of eyes and midbrain of *Xenopus* larva at stage 36 that had received an injection of HRP into a cell in the anterior-lateral founder cell group at the 512-cell stage, showing the darkly labeled cells in the dorsal telencephalon and dorsal part of the retina on the side of the injection. These cells reach the dorsal side of the boundary between the anterior-dorsal and anterior-ventral compartments.

Moreover, the theory does not specify the magnitude of the differences between compartments, which may be very small, nor does it state whether the differences are qualitative or merely quantitative. Nevertheless, using the technique of Curie-point pyrolysis mass spectrometry,[51] we have detected qualitative differences between cells of the stage 13 neurula belonging to anterior-medial and anterior-lateral compartments (Fig. 20A). The chemical basis for such differences may eventually be determined by the incorporation of radio-labeled precursors into components of the cell surface and extracellular matrix, measured in different compartments rather than in the embryo as a whole.[25–27]

The theory states that compartmentation develops because of selective affinities between all descendants of the same founder cell group and disaffinities between descendants of different founder cell groups. One strategy for studying selective cell affinities in the intact embryo is to remove labeled cells from a particular compartment at late blastula stages and implant them into the blastocele or into other regions of an unlabeled host of the same stage, in order to determine at later stages how the implanted cells have formed associations with host cells. Experiments of this kind have shown a selective affinity between donor and host cells of homologous germ layers,[52–54] but those experiments were not designed to test the theory of compartmentation. This also applies to the large number of experiments that have shown selective reaggregation of disaggregated embryonic cells,[55,56] starting with the brilliant studies of Holtfreter on reaggregation of amphibian embryonic

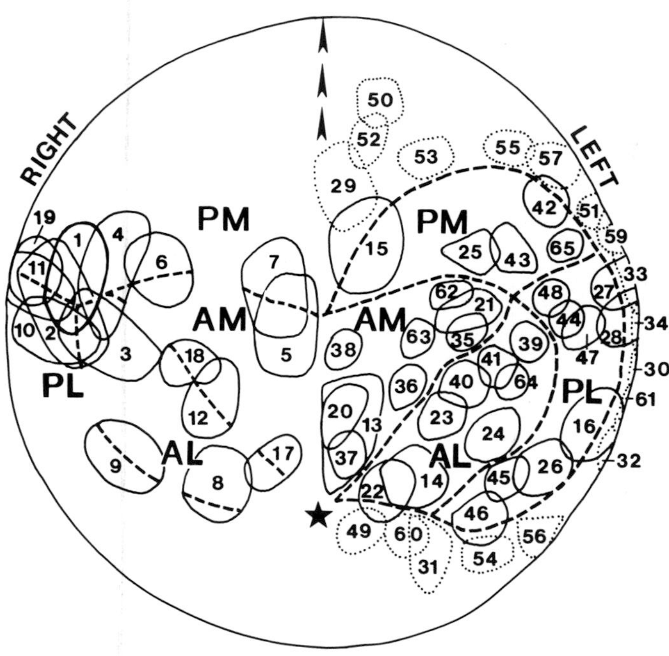

Figure 19. Composite diagram of the results of 65 experiments showing the positions of blastomeres at the 128-, 256-, and 512-cell stages of *Xenopus* that contributed descendants to the CNS (solid lines) or did not contribute to the CNS (dotted lines), although some contributed to the neural crest. Blastomeres that distributed their descendants into a single compartment of the CNS are shown on the left side of the embryo, and they form four founder cell groups, each populating a single compartment. Boundaries between the founder cell groups have been drawn with dashed lines. Blastomeres that distributed their descendants into more than one compartment of the CNS are shown on the right side of the embryo. Dashed lines over these blastomeres show the boundaries across which they distributed their descendants in the CNS. The blastomeres form four cell groups on each side: AL, anterior-lateral; AM, anterior-medial; PL, posterior-lateral; PM, posterior-medial. The star is at the animal pole, and the arrow points to the vegetal pole. The diameter of the embryo is about 1.3 mm.

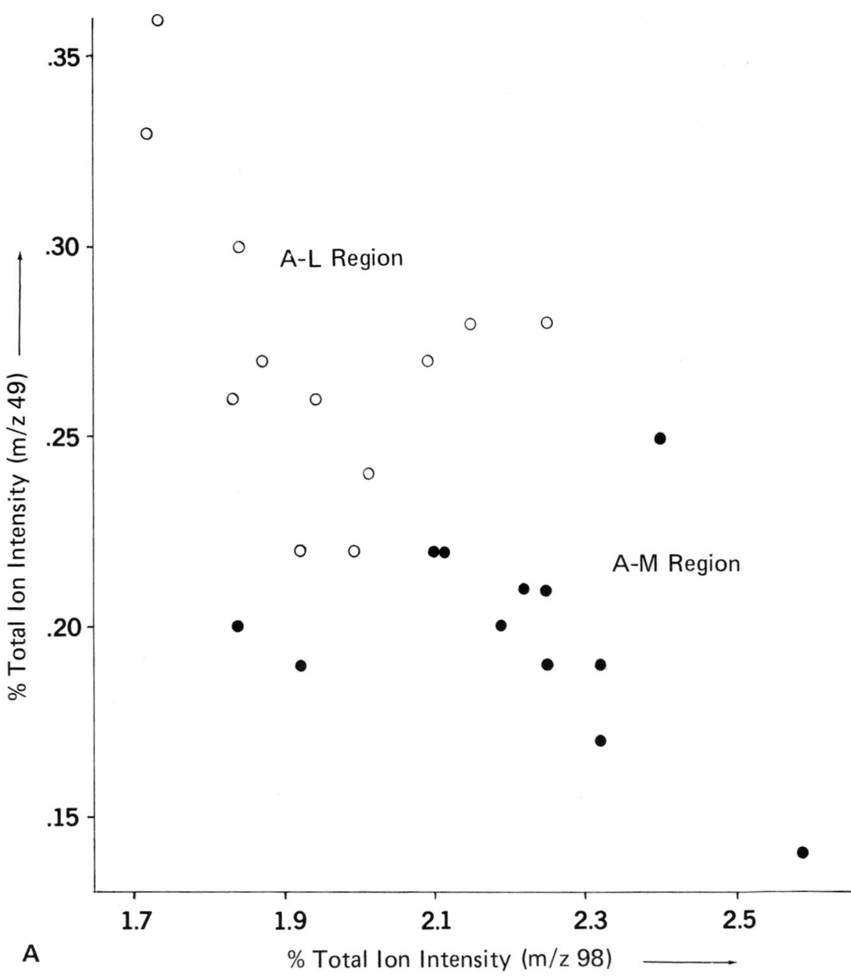

Figure 20. (A) Intensity distributions of two characteristic mass peaks in the Curie-point pyrolysis mass spectra of primordial brain tissue obtained at the neural plate stage from *Xenopus Laevis* embryos. Points represent single analyses of small (approximately 0.05 mm^3) pieces of tissue obtained from the antero-medial (●) and antero-lateral (○) compartments of 10 different embryos. The peaks at m/z 49 and 98 are believed to represent amino acid (methionine) and neutral saccharide or lipid fragments, respectively. Experimental conditions: Curie-point temperature 510°C, total heating time 0.8 sec, electron impact energy 12 eV. (B) Similar scatter plot as in A but now showing the intensities of the peaks at m/z 126 and 85 believed to be characteristic for neutral (poly)saccharides. Note the intermediate position of the four hindbrain (●) samples between the forebrain (○) and spinal cord (△) samples. See above (A) for experimental conditions (Meuzelaar and Jacobson, unpublished).

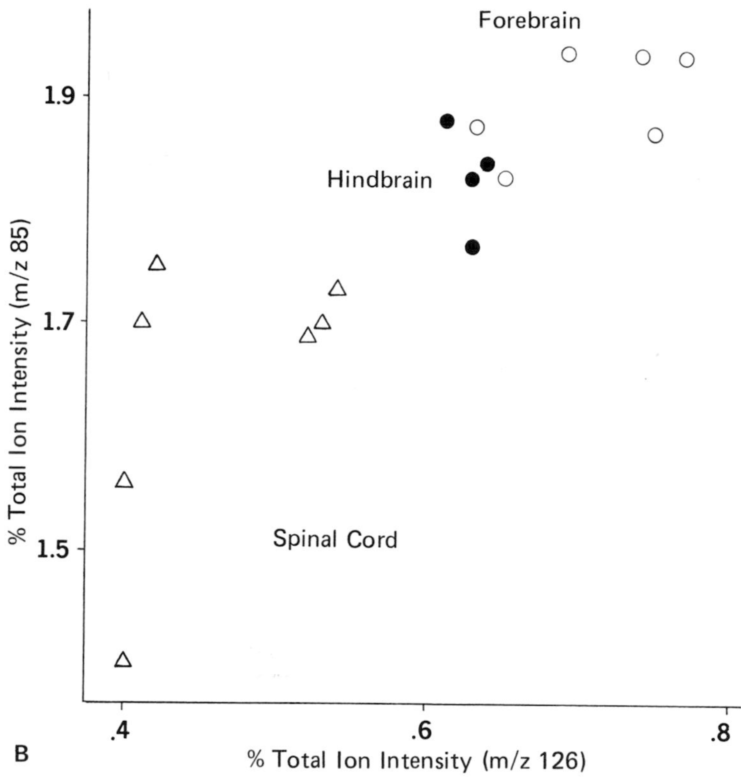

Figure 20 (*continued*).

cells that first showed how cell affinities could be the means of morphogenesis.[57,58] Experiments such as those are in progress to determine whether compartment-specific reaggregation occurs, as the theory predicts.

3.3. *Relation of Compartment Founder Cell Groups to Differentiated Cell Types*

According to the theory all the cells of the same founder cell group are equivalent in their probabilities of giving rise to all the types of cells that finally differentiate in their compartment. The descendants of a founder cell group mingle freely in a compartment so that commitment to differentiation of specific types of cells can occur only after mingling has ceased, or if the commitment occurs before cessation of mingling it must include mechanisms that enable the committed cells to migrate to their correct positions in the final pattern of differentiated cells. From the theory one can predict that complete regulation will occur after removal of parts of one or more compartments from the time of foundation until the time of irreversible commitment to specific programs of cell differentiation. After that time the theory predicts that removal of part of the compartment will result in absence of the cell types that have become committed, but only if those cell types are restricted to the part of the compartment that was removed. By contrast, the theory predicts that removal of an entire compartment at any time after the 512-cell stage will result in total and permanent absence of that compartment.

These predictions regarding removal of part or whole of a compartment have been verified experimentally. In a large series of cases I have removed precise numbers of ancestral cells at the 16- to 512-cell stages, and have in all cases found complete recovery of the normal pattern of differentiation in the CNS and also in all other systems.[59]

I have also obtained evidence that compartments as a whole, but not subpopulations within compartments, become irreversibly specified after the 512-cell blastula stage. The evidence comes from experiments in which pieces of 1024-cell blastula, ranging in size from fractions of one or more compartments to one complete compartment plus fractions of others, were removed or reimplanted in the same position but with the axes reversed. Complete regulation occurred after removal or axial reversal of fractions of compartments, but removal of an entire compartment always resulted in the corresponding deficit in the brain. Axial reversal of an entire compartment resulted in absence or severe abnormalities of the corresponding region of the brain. These results were found even when the sizes of the pieces were the same, but the compartment content of the pieces varied: permanent deficits always occurred if the ablated or rotated piece contained an entire compartment, while pieces of the same size which contained parts of two or more compartments could be removed or rotated without any permanent change in the final pattern of differentiation.

At first sight my results may seem to conflict with others showing regulation after removal or reversal of the axes of parts of the presumptive CNS as late as the neural plate stage. However, a goodly part of the earlier work may be reconciled with the theory of compartmentation. Thus, it has long been known that the amount of recovery was inversely proportional to the size of grafts: small grafts of rotated neurectoderm showed regulation, while larger grafts failed to do so.[60–62] Reversal of the axes of the neurectoderm in amphibians always resulted in corresponding reversal of the pattern of differentiation when the reversed piece was large enough to include an entire compartment, and when the operation was done at preneurula or neural plate stages, with or without the underlying mesoderm.[62–64] Smaller grafts, not large enough to include an entire compartment, done at the same stages, resulted in development of a normal brain.[65] None of the earlier workers planned their operations in relation to the positions of compartments; however, from the present vantage point it seems clear that most cases of failure of regulation involved operations large enough to include entire compartments, while most reports of complete regulation involved operations too small to include an entire compartment. However, there are reports of removal of large parts of the neural plate and neural tube that were followed by complete recovery[66–68] (see Chapter 11). Even in those cases in which the operation extended into several compartments it is likely that no compartment was entirely removed, so that complete recovery could be attributed to regeneration from the residual parts of several compartments rather than to regulation of the pattern within the residual cells.

With respect to the differentiative capacities of isolated pieces of neurectoderm, the theory predicts that pieces of compartments or entire compartments excised after the 512-cell stage, grafted to different positions outside the presumptive neural region of the embryo or grown under optimal conditions *in vitro*, should be capable of self-differentiation. Consistent with this prediction are many reports of the capacities of isolated pieces of blastula and neurula stages to differentiate into parts of the central nervous system when transplanted to the eye chamber or coelom of older hosts [69–72] or to other parts of the embryo.[68,73–79]

The times at which cells become committed to different pathways of terminal differentiation are not known. In theory, that may occur in two ways in relation to cell mingling. Either the commitment occurs before mingling has ceased, in which case there must be means for the committed cells to arrive at their correct final positions, or the commitment is delayed until the cells have arrived at their final resting places. In the case of neural crest cells, many of which continue to migrate until relatively late stages after closure of the neural tube, it has been shown that the final decision to adopt norepinephrine or acetylcholine as their transmitters depends on conditions of culture *in vitro*[80]; *in vivo* the decision appears to be made only after the neurons arrive at their final resting places.[81]

The times of irreversible commitment to development of specific types of nerve cells can, in principle, be investigated by removing a subpopulation of neural cell precursors in a series of embryos, starting at early blastula stages and progressing to later stages, until a time is found at which the operation results in failure of development of specific types of cells. Because this research strategy seems most likely to succeed when the type of cell being investigated is easily identified and can be easily counted I have chosen to study the time of commitment of Rohon-Beard neurons of *Xenopus.*

It is instructive to compare the Rohon–Beard neurons with primordial germ cells with respect to their origin, migration and differentiation and to ask whether there are determinants of Rohon–Beard cells localized in the cytoplasm of the egg as there are for the primordial germ cells.[82,83] Both these types of cells are large, originate from a discrete region of the early embryo, and later migrate some distance from their site of origin to their final positions. Rohon–Beard cells originate from 2 or 3 ancestral cells of the 16-cell stage located near the anterior (animal) pole of the embryo, but these neurons finally move caudally to take up positions in the dorsal part of the spinal cord along its entire length.[44,45] Germinal cells and Rohon–Beard cells are among the first to become recognizable during development—the Rohon–Beard cells are the first cells to be produced and to differentiate in the central nervous system.[84]

With these similarities in mind I have started a series of experiments to determine whether removal of some or all the Rohon–Beard ancestral cells would prevent the development of Rohon–Beard cells or reduce their numbers. However, one must remember that the ancestral cells of the 16- to 64-cell stages that produce Rohon–Beard neurons also give rise to other types of neurons, and probably also to glial cells in the dorsal spinal cord as well as to neural crest derivatives such as extramedullary neurons and dorsal root ganglion cells.[46] In the first experiment, unilateral removal of blastomere V1.2, from which more than 70% of Rohon–Beard cells arise on that side, did not alter the number of Rohon–Beard neurons.[47] I have also shown that after removal of V1.2 the Rohon–Beard neurons can be produced by blastomere D1.2, which is a neighbor of V1.2 but does not normally give rise to any Rohon–Beard neurons.[47] Those results suggest that there are no prelocalized determinants of Rohon–Beard cell differentiation; if there are such determinants they must be capable of redistribution at the 16-cell stage, or they must be widely distributed at that stage and later become localized to the Rohon–Beard cell lineage. Therefore, it becomes necessary to investigate the effects of removal at progressively later stages of development, of all ancestral cells giving rise to Rohon–Beard neurons, and those experiments are still in progress.

To test the stability of the developmental program that results in Rohon-Beard neuron differentiation, I did the following experiment. HRP was injected into blastomere V1.2, and when those embryos reached the late blastula stage I transplanted labeled precursors of Rohon–Beard neurons under the ectoderm or into the blastocoele of unlabeled host embryos at gastrula stages 10½–11½. Those animals were processed histologically about 24 hr later at early larval stages 22–26, when Rohon–Beard neurons can easily be recognized. In all cases, labeled cells with the appearances of Rohon–Beard neurons and commissural neurons were present in the dorsal and dorsolateral regions of the host's spinal cord (Fig. 21) where those types of neurons normally differentiate. Labeled cells were not seen in abnormal locations in the

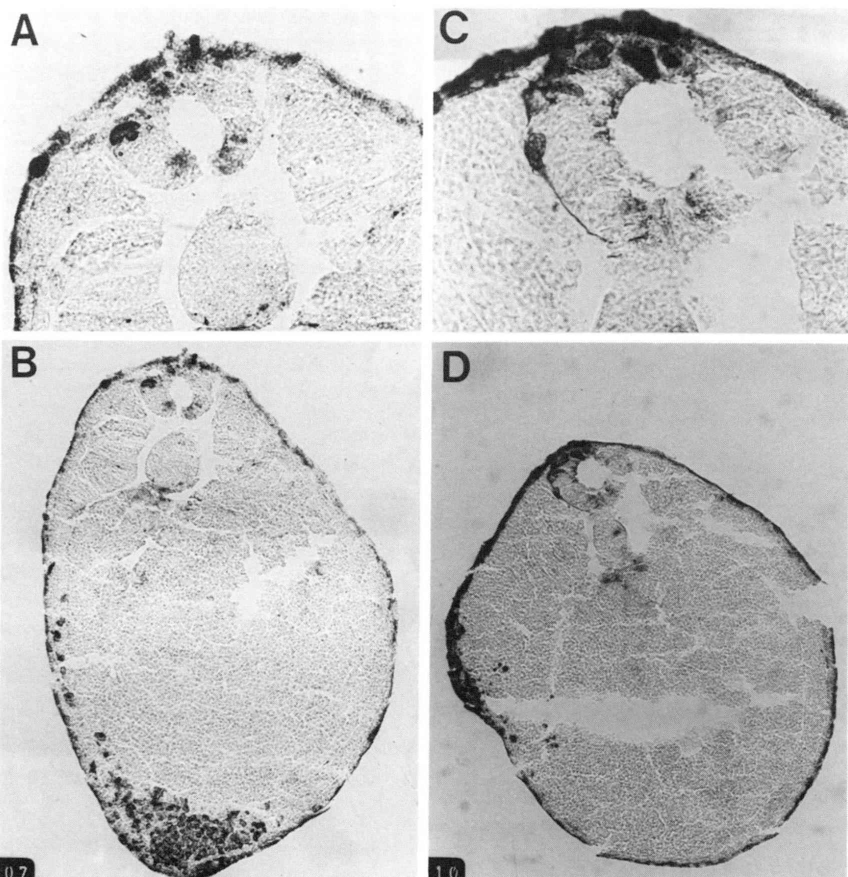

Figure 21. Migration of labeled neurons from a graft labeled with HRP into unlabeled host spinal cord. Two specimens are shown (left and right) in coronal section at the thoracic spinal cord level. The entire section (lower photographs) shows the position of the graft, while the upper photographs show the positions of labeled cells in the host's spinal cord. In both specimens the graft was taken from a late blastula (stage 9) that had received an injection of HRP into blastomere LV1.2 at the 16-cell stage, and the graft was placed inside the blastocoele of a host at gastrula stage 10½. The embryos were fixed at larval stage 26. See text for further details.

CNS, and there were no signs of death of labeled cells in the CNS. Therefore, the labeled neurons do not appear to have dispersed at random from the graft and to have survived in the host's CNS only in the correct positions. Rather, the Rohon–Beard and commissural neurons appear to have migrated selectively from the graft to their correct positions in the dorsolateral parts of the host's spinal cord. Control experiments in which labeled blastula cells from anterior-medial or posterior-medial compartments were grafted to unlabeled gastrula hosts have resulted in differentiation of various types of labeled cells, but none that resembled Rohon-Beard neurons. These experiments are still in progress, so that definite conclusions may be premature. Nevertheless, they suggest that Rohon–Beard neurons and commissural neurons of the dorsolateral spinal cord can complete their developmental program after they have been grafted from mid-blastula to later stages without having been in contact with the archenteron roof, and without having been involved in the processes of primary neural induction. Other results, to be discussed in the following section, also show that transplants of blastula prospective neural tissue can develop autonomously to form the appropriate parts of the central nervous system. Those observations are consistent with the theory of compartmentation but appear to be in conflict with the theory of the organizer.

4. CRITIQUE OF THE THEORY OF THE ORGANIZER

4.1. Preliminary Considerations

Since 1924 when Spemann and Mangold found that the region dorsal to the blastopore acts as an "organizer," it has been generally believed that the earliest events in development of the CNS occur during early gastrulation; the archenteron roof has been thought to "induce" a spatial pattern of developmental programs in the overlying ectoderm, which results in differentiation of a properly organized central nervous system. Evidence accumulated very rapidly in the next decade, apparently showing that the influence of the organizer on the prospective neural ectoderm was the first and absolute requirement for neural differentiation. It will be my purpose here to show that the primordial spatial pattern of the CNS originates during blastula stages, well before the beginning of gastrulation. I shall also show that Mangold and Spemann misinterpreted their original observations on the results of transplantation of the region dorsal to the blastopore. Their observation[85] was the first brick of an edifice that was rapidly built, an edifice in which the concepts of the "organization center" and of "primary embryonic induction" were enshrined.[48] To cap the elaborate construction with a gilded dome, all that remained to be discovered was the inductor itself, or at least, the mechanisms by which the organizer organized. The failure to discover the mechanism of action of the organizer has left the edifice without a roof. If the Mangold and Spemann experiment can be proved to be misconceived, and its conclusions shown to be false, the very foundation on which the entire edifice was built would crumble, and the entire structure would collapse. Accordingly I shall present the available evidence that the basic pattern of organization of the CNS exists in the blastula and probably originates in the newly fertilized egg.

The compartmentation theory[16] and the organizer theory[48] both attempt to account for the origins of the primordial pattern of differentiation in the embryo, but differ on the time at which the primordial pattern develops and on the mechanisms of its formation. According to the compartmentation theory the primordial pattern arises in the mid-blastula in the form of seven groups of 20 to 30 compartment founder cells, the descendants of each group remaining together to form a compartment at later stages. According to the organizer theory, the information necessary for development of the primordial spatial pattern of differentiation first develops in the mesoderm at the dorsal lip of the blastopore, the so-called organizer, and the information is transferred from mesodermal cells to the overlying ectodermal cells as the mesoderm moves into the roof of the archenteron during gastrulation. This process of "primary neural induction" has been the subject of much surmise and conjecture about the supposed cellular mechanisms and the presumed intercellular signals, a further review of which would be superfluous.[86–90] The problem of the origin of the spatial pattern of differentiation is not solved by the organizer theory, but the problem is merely transferred from ectoderm to mesoderm without dealing with the way in which the mesoderm originally develops regionally specific inductive powers. Attempts to explain the origin of the organizer as a product of a series of inductive interactions at earlier stages[88,89] have been unsuccessful and have only begged the question. More than 50 years of effort[91] have failed to reveal the putative inductor substances, nor has any progress been made in discovering the cellular mechanisms of release, transmission, reception, and interpretation of the developmental signals that are supposed to result in regional differentiation of the CNS. Proponents of the theory of the organizer are uncertain whether the effect of the organizer is instructive or merely permissive.[92] Nevertheless, it seems quite possible that the mesoderm has a necessary role in development of the neurectoderm (see Sections 4.2.2, 4.2.3, and 5.1) but that further investigations of its actual role are required.

My criticism of the organizer theory is based on the following three points. First, flaws in the design of the primary experiments on which the organizer theory is based reduce confidence in the validity of their results. These flaws include the use of inaccurate fate maps to interpret the result of experiments that are the main support of the organizer theory. Second, doubts about the predictive value of the theory arise because of the lack of progress in finding the putative "inductors" or in working out the cellular mechanisms of induction, despite intensive effort, using the most advanced techniques. Finally, other explanations of the experimental results are as good or better than those provided by the organizer theory.

In any critique of the theory of the organizer it is necessary to make a clear distinction between the organization of spatial patterns on a global scale and the differentiation of specific types of cells at particular locations as a result of a cell-to-cell interactions. In criticizing the validity of the theory of the organizer I am including primary embryonic induction, but I do not extend the criticism indiscriminately to all cases of cellular interactions during development.

4.2. *Early Experimental Tests*

The theory of the organizer is based on the crucial experiment reported by Spemann and Mangold in 1924.[85] They showed that a piece excised from the region above the dorsal lip of the blastopore of an early gastrula of the newt *Triturus*, transplanted into the blastocoele or into the ventral side of another early gastrula, resulted in the development of a secondary neural axis, more or less complete, in the host. There were considerable variations in the position and completeness of the secondary nervous system. Spemann and Mangold's observations were similar to those of Lewis,[93] who concluded that the secondary axis was derived from the graft. The crucial advance claimed by Spemann and Mangold was that the secondary neural axis was derived from host cells as well as graft cells, an observation made possible by the difference in pigmentation of host and graft cells. From this they deduced that the graft had "organized" a new axis, consisting of notochord, somites and neural tube, from host tissue which was completely reprogrammed from ventral mesoderm and epidermis. The observation that host and graft cells fitted together harmoniously into all parts of the new pattern assumed added significance when fate maps of the urodele early gastrula showed that the grafted tissue was fated to become chorda-mesoderm and not nervous system.[94,95] The graft cells had apparently changed their fates when integrated into the secondary neural tube.

The Spemann–Mangold experiment provided one of the central ideas of vertebrate embryology for the next half-century, namely, the idea of the "organization center" or "organizer," whose "inductive action" organizes the basic morphological pattern of the central nervous system. The hunt began, and has continued ever, since, for the substances that mediate the inductive effect.[87–92]

4.2.1. Two Criteria Not Met. When the Spemann–Mangold experiment is examined critically it is found to be seriously flawed and the experiment loses much of its force. The classical interpretation of this experiment depends on the following three conditions being satisfied. First, the cells of donor origin must be easily distinguished from those of the host. Second, it must be demonstrated that neither the host nor donor cells included in the neural tube of the secondary axis were originally fated to develop as neural tissue. Thus the secondary neural tissue must be shown not to have been derived from prospective neural cells, of either the host or the donor, that were originally located in the region of the graft or had migrated into the graft. And third, the structures identified as parts of the nervous system in the "induced" axis must be shown to be composed of nerve cells and belong to specific regions of the CNS. Only the first of these three conditions has been demonstrated.

It was not demonstrated that the ectodermal cells of the host which were included in the secondary neural axis were originally fated to be ventral epidermis. In the cases of apparent induction of neural tissue in pieces of ventral ectoderm cut out of early gastrulae and wrapped around putative inductors, it must be shown that the piece of ectoderm did not contain any neurectodermal cells from which the neural tissue could develop autonomously. This alternative is likely in view of the extension of the presumptive neural region into the ventral ectoderm, and the requirement for large pieces of ectoderm to wrap up the inductor. Furthermore, in the majority of cases reported by Spemann and Mangold the secondary axis was on the flank not far from the primary axis (although the best case of a secondary axis on the belly is most often illustrated). In many cases the primary and secondary axes were in direct contact at some point. The significance of this is that cells might have migrated from the primary to secondary axis if the secondary axis had been in direct contact with the primary at any stage of development. Spemann and Mangold did not consider that possibility, and therefore they did not do any controls to deal with cell migration from the primary neural axis to the region of the graft. Such migration of cells can occur from the graft into the primary CNS (see Sections 3.3 and 4.3.2) as well as from the latter into the graft. For example, the "induction" of neural tissue that has been observed after implantation of various mesodermal tissues (kidney, liver, bone marrow, living or dead)[87,91] might be due to migration of neural cells from other regions of the embryo into the region of the implanted "organizer." Or they might be due to selective survival of cells from an originally heterogeneous population.[96]

These possibilities were never considered by Spemann and Mangold or by any later reviewers of the subject. After Vogt[94,95] showed that the cells grafted from the dorsal lip were fated to become chordamesoderm, Spemann insisted on the accuracy and finality of Vogt's fate map. Spemann and his followers took it for granted that the grafts of the "organizer" did not contain any prospective neural cells. This has proved not to be so in *Xenopus* (see Section 4.3.1). In such cases, where induction is not the only means by which neural tissue could have differentiated, the burden of proof should be on those who claim to have demonstrated induction.

4.2.2. Accuracy of Fate Maps. An accurate fate map is an absolute prerequisite for the correct interpretation of the effects of transplanting, isolating or ablating pieces of the embryo. The interpretation of the Spemann–Mangold experiment depended on knowledge of the prospective significance of the piece of the dorsal lip that was transplanted. When the vital staining method of fate mapping showed that the dorsal lip region of the early to mid-gastrula consisted entirely of presumptive chorda-mesoderm in urodele as well as anuran embryos, Spemann was able to conclude that the secondary neural axis did not arise from presumptive neural ectoderm of the graft. The conclusion that the secondary neural axis developed mainly from the host tissue, under inductive influences from the implanted dorsal lip, was based on the conviction that the secondary neural axis originated from cells originally destined to form epidermis. This, in turn, was based on the belief that Vogt's fate maps were final and definitive. For that reason Spemann found it necessary to emphasize the accuracy of Vogt's fat map. Spemann[48] (p. 98) states that "I shall follow the important work of W. Vogt (1926–29) which may be considered fundamental and final." Referring to the fate map, Spemann (p. 11) writes: "Vogt has carried this down to the minutest particulars, with great exactitude, at first for the gastrula of the urodele and recently also for that of the anuran." Spemann insisted on the final and definitive status of Vogt's fate maps because he knew that all the experiments on neural induction would have to be reinterpreted if the fate maps were found to contain serious inaccuracies. As I shall show, Vogt's fate map was incorrect in several ways. It underestimated the region giving rise to the CNS, and especially failed to show the extent of presumptive neural region in the ventral half and in the vegetal half of the blastula and gastrula.[43,44] Vogt, as well as others who have relied on vital staining as a means of fate mapping in *Xenopus* embryos,[94,95,97–99] underestimated the amount of cell mingling in the presumptive neural region (see Section 4.3.1) and failed to observe the movement of cells across the midline which results in the ventral parts of the retina, telencephalon, diencephalon, and mesencephalon receiving cells from both sides (left and right) of the blastula and gastrula. Vogt also failed to consider the possibility that the presumptive neural region of the late blastula and early gastrula may be a mosaic of cells fated to become mesoderm as well as neural tissue.[45]

The theory of the origin of compartmentation in the blastula will eventually include both mesoderm and ectoderm because I have observed that the blastomeres of the 512-cell embryo that give rise to neurectoderm also give rise to mesoderm.[45] The questions, now under investigation, are whether there are clonal relationships between ectodermal and mesodermal elements, whether the neurectodermal compartments also include mesoderm, or whether any other form of compartmentation is in the mesoderm. Another question that has been raised in the past[100,101] and that can now be dealt with experimentally is what the spatial relationships are between mesoderm and ectoderm of the same ancestry during and after gastrulation. For example, is the mesoderm of the archenteron roof clonally related to the overlying neurectoderm? And, most important of all, what is the primary source of the developmental information eventually expressed as a program of regionally specific cell differentiations?

4.2.3. Identity of Induced Tissues. Finally, Spemann and Mangold[85] failed to prove that the cells of either host or graft origin in the "induced" neural tube eventually differentiated as nerve cells. Their figures show the structures of the secondary neural axis at stages before neurons can be recognized, and their histological techniques were inadequate to show the presence of neurons or of nerve fibers. In fact, it is usually difficult and often impossible to identify parts of the CNS in the secondary axis. This applies to tissues that develop *in vitro* as well as to the structures that develop after transplantation of dorsal lip into the blastocoele or other parts of the host embryo. Interpretation of such results depends on recognizing some histological organization that is typically neuronal or of identifying structures such as nasal placodes and optic or otic vesicles that are typically associated with particular subdivisions of the brain. Although most authors make such identification appear easy, their published photographs often fail to demonstrate that the induced tissues belong to any particular region of the CNS, and in some cases the photographs leave doubt whether the structures belong to the nervous system. Of course, the original histological preparations may be easier to interpret than the photographs. Nevertheless, no study has ever used a double blind method of evaluating the histological preparations so that the tendency to bias the interpretation in favor of the expected result has been controlled. Only a small minority of investigators[102–104] have expressed their skepticism about the identification of specific regions of the brain induced *in vivo* or *in vitro*. For example, Waddington[102] writes that "it usually requires a good deal of imagination to assign such masses to any particular part of the normal neural axis" and Eyal-Giladi[103] admits that "the identification of the different brain parts proper, has been . . . difficult . . . and, in many cases . . . it was impossible to make out their real identity." In contrast, Lehmann[105] went so far as to postulate three different inductors—"archencephalic," "deuterencephalic," and "spinocaudal"—on the basis of his ability to identify regions of CNS found in the induced tissues. Others have also identified different brain parts confidently, although from the evidence of their photographs it is difficult to concur with their identification of parts of the brain or even of associated structures such as nasal placodes, eye vesicles, or otic vesicles.

It is fair to state that all embryologists who have worked on the problem of neural induction have used extremely vague criteria for identification of regions of the CNS and even for identification of neural tissue. The identifications were based on general histological features of light-microscopic preparations that were not stained specially for neurons or glial cells. The results would have been far more compelling if histological methods for selectively staining or impregnating nerve cells had been used, but that has rarely been reported (see Chapter 11). It has now become possible to identify neural tissue by means of antibodies that react against specific types of neurons or glial cells[106–108] (see Chapter 3). Ideally, one should use monoclonal antibodies raised against neurons as markers to identify those neurons, first in normal embryos and then in the induced tissues. Identification of a region in an induced CNS is most often based solely on the thickness of the wall of the neural tubelike structure and not on its neuronal cytoarchitectonics. But there is considerable evidence that the thickness of the wall of the neural tube can be markedly altered by the amount of associated mesoderm: The more mesoderm the thicker the neural tube[109–111] (see Section 5.1). This has led many embryologists to call any thick-walled tube a spinal cord or rhombencephalon and any thin-walled tube a prosencephalon when there was no other evidence on which to base the regional identification. In an effort to find some objective method of identifying parts of the CNS before the time of histotypic differentiation, we have used Curie-point pyrolysis mass spectrometry and have shown that small pieces of presumptive forebrain, hindbrain, and spinal cord excised from the neural plate of *Xenopus* can be distinguished from each other (Fig. 20B).

4.3. *Recent Experimental Tests with HRP Label*

4.3.1. Fate Map Revision. By labeling single blastomeres of *Xenopus* at 64- to 512-cell stages, I have shown that the presumptive neural region is far more extensive than was revealed by the vital staining methods. I have found that blastomeres of the 64- to 512-cell stages that give rise to nerve cells also give rise to a variety of types of mesodermal cells. For example, somitic mesoderm and spinal cord neurons both arise from the same blastomeres of the 512-cell embryo.[45] I have also shown that widespread dispersal and mingling of cells, not revealed by the vital staining methods, occur during late blastula and gastrula stages.[49] These new findings necessitate a revision of the earlier fate maps of *Xenopus*,[97–99,101] and they throw a shadow of doubt on the accuracy of fate maps of other anuran and urodele amphibians.[94,95]

For any understanding of the development of patterns of cell differentiation for the purpose of constructing a fate map, it is essential to know how much cell dispersal and mingling occurs in the early embryo. The resolution of any fate map is limited by the amount of cell dispersal that occurs after application of the cellular marker. Thus, the fate maps obtained by the vital staining methods were limited by the fact that cell dispersal and mingling of labeled and unlabeled cells occurred after the stage of application of the vital stain. All investigators using the vital staining method have deduced their fate maps on the assumption that labeled cells remained together as a coherent patch, the entire patch merely undergoing changes in shape during morphogenesis. But this apparently coherent clonal growth was an artefact produced by the vital staining method, which only detects coherent patches of cells and cannot detect single labeled cells mingled with unlabeled ones. Such fate maps[94,95,97–99] not only underestimated the area of the embryo that gives rise to the nervous system but also underestimated the full range of prospective significance within an area from which cells migrate. If two groups of cells with different prospective significance originate from the same area but one group migrates out and disperses, the latter will not

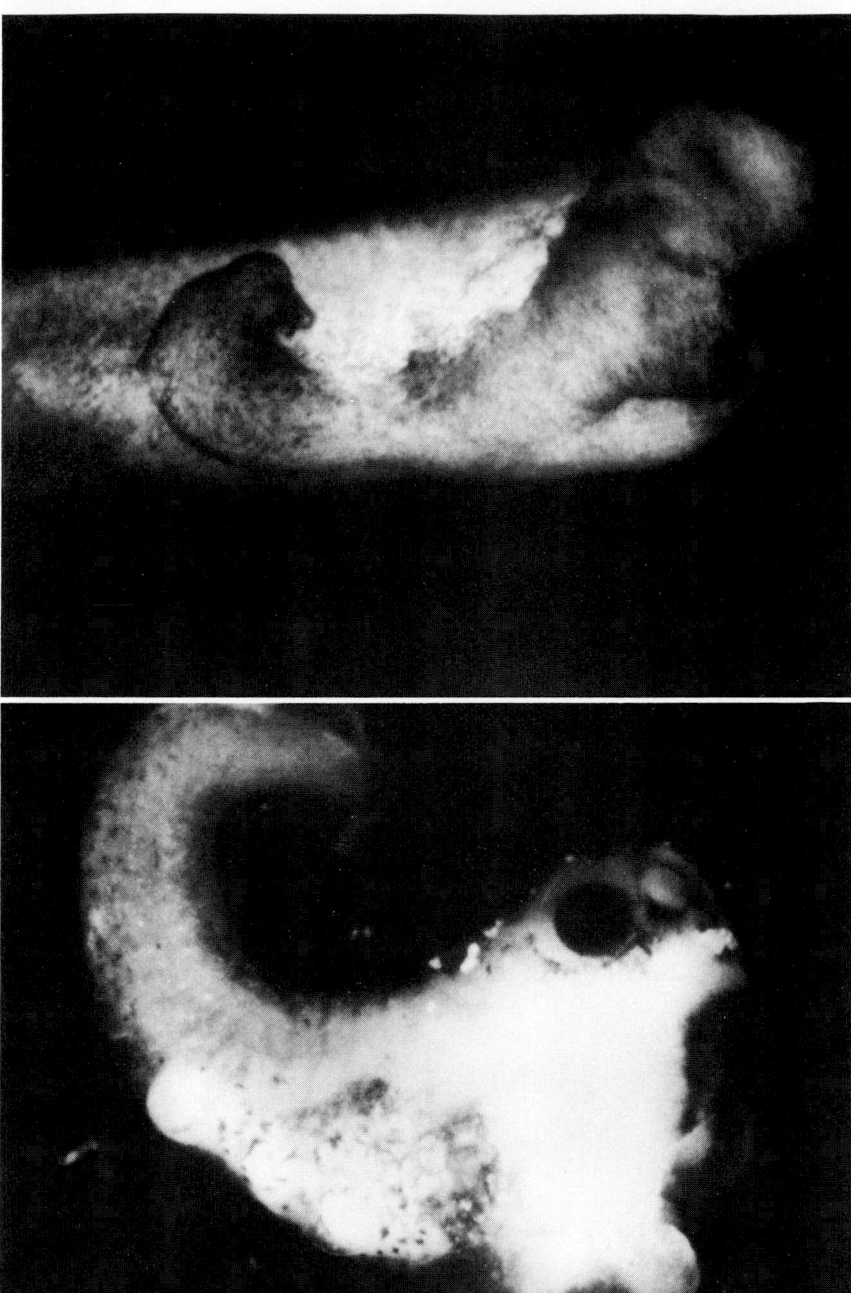

be detected by vital staining. The prospective significance given to such a vitally stained area will be limited to that of the cells that undergo coherent clonal growth.

It remains to be seen whether application of the HRP method to urodele embryos will result in a similar revision of their fate maps. If it does, the entire literature on primary neural induction that has relied on the accuracy of Vogt's fate maps will have to be reinterpreted. Such a revision would resolve many of the inconsistencies and difficulties in the literature on neural induction. For example, there is the inconsistency between Vogt's fate map obtained by vital staining of the urodele embryo and Holtfreter's fate map of the same embryos deduced from observations on the types of differentiation that occurred in explants taken from different regions of the early gastrula.[112] In Holtfreter's map the region giving rise to neural tissue is shown extending from the dorsal lip to the mid-dorsal region and also into the ventral region. If due allowances are made for the limitations of Holtfreter's methods (limitations due to primitive tissue culture methods and difficulties of identifying tissues, especially neurons, in such explants), it can be seen that Holtfreter's fate map of the presumptive neural region is much closer to the presumptive neural region that I have defined in *Xenopus* by the HRP method than it is to the presumptive neural region shown on any of the fate maps of urodele or anuran embryos obained by vital staining. Holtfreter's interpretation, which has been generally accepted, is that differentiation of neural tissue occurred in such explants of the organizer region as a result of the inductive action of the organizer on competent ectoderm. My interpretation is that the ectoderm was already programmed before the time of explantation, to become specific compartments of the nervous system, and that the presence of mesoderm in the explants permitted the ectoderm to complete its own program of development in a tissue culture medium that would not permit ectoderm alone to differentiate fully.

4.3.2. Second Neuraxis Derived from Graft. My experiments in which HRP was injected into single blastomeres of *Xenopus* at the 32- to 512-cell stages and the embryos were fixed at blastula and gastrula and larval stages, showed that clones known to contribute to the central nervous system had reached the region of the dorsal lip of the blastopore

←

Figure 22. Photographs of two *Xenopus* larvae that developed when a piece of the dorsal lip of the blastopore from a donor embryo had been grafted into the blastocoele. Both host and graft were at the onset of gastrulation (stage 10) at the time of grafting. The donor cells were totally labeled with HRP injected into both blastomeres at the two-cell stage. In both specimens the secondary neural axis was totally labeled with HRP.

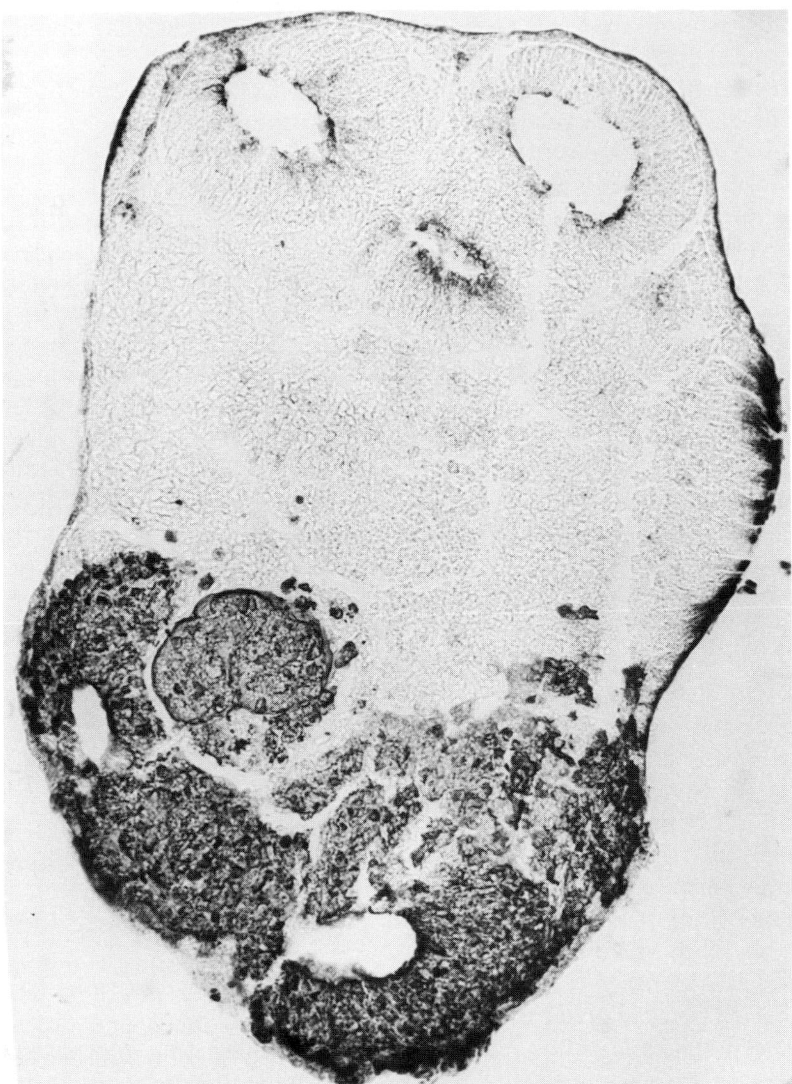

Figure 23. Coronal section through the level of the telencephalon of the embryo shown in the lower photograph of Fig. 22. A piece of dorsal lip of blastopore from an embryo at stage 10, totally labeled with HRP, was grafted into the blastocoele of the unlabeled host at stage 10. The specimen was fixed at stage 36 and processed to show the presence of HRP as a dark reaction product. All the cells of the secondary neural axis are labeled, showing that they originated from the graft. Note some dispersion of labeled graft cells into the host.

by early gastrula stages (Fig. 15). When I grafted those labeled cells from the dorsal lip of early gastrulae into the blastocoele or under the ventral ectoderm of unlabeled host gastrulae, well-formed secondary embryos developed (Figs. 22 and 23). These were identical in appearance to those which various authors claim to have "induced" by means of implants of dorsal lip.[85,87,88] However, in most of my cases all the cells of the secondary embryo were labeled if the graft had been taken from a completely labeled donor embryo. Thus, the graft contained cells that either were fated to become nerve cells or could alter their fates to become nerve cells, as Lewis originally concluded.[93] In a minority of cases I observed some unlabeled cells mingled with labeled cells in the CNS and other organs of the secondary embryo. However, in many of those cases labeled cells derived from the graft were also mingled in the host CNS and other organs. These results are not surprising in view of the extensive cell dispersal and mingling which occurs during normal development. Apparently, an exchange of host and graft cells had occurred at earlier stages of development. Experiments are in progress, using labeled hosts as well as labeled donors to determine the origins of the host cells as well as those of the donor in the secondary embryo.

5. COMPARTMENT vs. ORGANIZER THEORIES

5.1. *The Case for the Compartment Theory*

Support for the compartment theory comes primarily from the experiments discussed in Section 3 (see also Chapter 11). The case for the compartment theory is also strengthened by the extent to which it is consistent with older evidence, hitherto used to support the organizer theory. One of the results that can be explained by the compartment theory at least as well as by the organizer theory is Spemann's demonstration of the spatiotemporal specificity in the "inductive" activity of the dorsal lip.[113,114] He observed that dorsal lip of early gastrulae induced head structures while dorsal lip of late gastrulae induced trunk and tail structures. These results can be equally well ascribed to the presence in the grafts of neurectodermal cells already committed to regional neural differentiation, namely, compartments, taking into account the changes with time in the positions of the compartments relative to one another and to the dorsal lip of the blastopore.[16] I have observed that at the beginning of gastrulation the anterior medial and posterior medial compartments are nearest the dorsal lip of the blastopore but that as gastrulation advances, the anterior compartments move rostrally and the posterior lateral compartment moves from a lateral and ventral position toward the dorsal midline, so that at the end of gastrulation the posterior medial and posterior lateral compartments lie closest to the blastopore. In addition to the type of neurectoderm in the graft, the type and amount of mesoderm in the graft can greatly influence the form of the developing neural tube.[109–111] The presence of more mesodermal cells in the dorsal lip at the end than at the beginning of gastrulation (and more mesoderm in caudal than in rostral parts of the archenteron roof) would explain why a thin-walled neural tube develops in association with dorsal lip from early gastrulae or the rostral part of the archenteron roof ("head organizer"), while a thick-walled neural tube develops in association with dorsal lip from late gastrulae or in association with caudal parts of the archenteron roof ("tail organizer"). However, in the experiments that demonstrated the regional specificities of head and tail organizer,[115,116] no histological evidence was given to show that the histological structure of thin-walled and thick-walled neural tubes really corresponded with the types of nerve cells and nerve circuits characteristic of forebrain and spinal cord. Those experiments will have to be repeated, using grafts prelabeled with HRP and allowing the specimens to develop to stages at which neuronal differentiation has clearly occurred.

In my opinion, based on a review of several hundred papers that provide enough information to permit a reconsideration of their conclusions, alternative explanations can explain the results at least as well as the organizer theory. It is attractive to reinterpret this literature in terms of the compartmentation theory, according to which the neurectodermal cells have started their program of regional neural development before the beginning of gastrulation. However, it is quite likely that stabilization of those programs occurs as a result of interactions between neurectodermal and mesodermal cells, probably starting during gastrulation and continuing into the neural plate stages and later. The neurectodermal cells have reached the dorsal lip region at the beginning of gastrulation, and because grafts of that region inevitably include both neurectodermal and mesodermal cells, the neurectodermal cells can complete their development. Since considerable rearrangements of neurectodermal cells occur during gastrulation, the kinds of neural tissues that develop will depend on the types of cells in the graft at the time of grafting, on the numbers and types of neurectodermal cells that survive in the graft, and on the cells that migrate in or out of it. The different kinds of tissues reported to have been "induced" under various conditions can be attributed to variability in the conditions mentioned above. Indeed, variables in the methods and in the evaluation of the results, unsuspected by the authors, must have been responsible for the many contradictory and conflicting results reported in the literature.

5.2. *Difficulties with the Organizer Theory*

Attention has already been directed at some weaknesses in the evidence used to support the organizer theory such as the inaccuracies in the fate maps obtained by vital staining methods, the failure to take into account the extensive cell mingling and cell migration that occur during normal morphogenesis and that can occur in to or out of grafts, and the inadequate methods used to identify nerve cells and to characterize specific regions of nervous system in the "induced" tissues. Finally, a few examples should suffice to show how the prevailing mode of thought has become so deeply permeated by the concept of the organizer that alternative explanations of the evidence are not given full consideration.

Nakamura *et al.*[117,118] isolated groups of animal pole blastomeres of the 16- and 32-cell stages of *Xenopus*, in saline solution, and found that neural tissues differentiated in about 10% of explants from the 16-cell blastula and in about 25% of explants from the 32-cell blastula. When clusters of eight blastomeres were explanted from the 32-cell blastula, neural structures differentiated in 50–75% of cases from the dorsal blastomeres which normally give rise to the central nervous system, but in no cases from blastomeres that do not normally contribute to CNS. From these results they concluded that the organizer must have developed in the excised fragments that gave rise to CNS structures.[90,117,118] To save the hypothesis, it has been found necessary to postulate the existence of the organizer whenever neural differentiation occurs and to rule out in advance any possibility of self-differentiation of neural structures occurring without an organizer.

Similarly Spemann[48] argued that the capacity of isolated pieces of late blastula ectoderm to develop autonomously as neural and other structures when grown in the eye cavity or coelome of living embryos, but not when grown in salt solutions *in vitro*, must be due to the presence of inductors in the eye cavity or coelome. He did not discuss the possibility that the living embryo provided supportive and permissive conditions absent from the culture medium. Spemann was not aware that many nerve cells require conditioned medium[119–122] and nerve growth factor[123] for their normal development. Likewise Niu and Twitty[124] showed that pieces of ectoderm from early gastrula would develop into neural tissue when cultured in salt solution previously conditioned by axial mesoderm, while the same pieces of ectoderm merely formed epidermis in unconditioned salt solution. Holtfreter and Hamburger[125] regarded this result as a demonstration "that the inductive factors of living tissues are indeed diffusible."

Holtfreter's demonstration that pieces of ectoderm from any region of gastrula or early neurula stages of newt embryos always differentiated as indifferent epithelium when grown for days to weeks in salt solution[126] was taken to mean that the ectoderm is regionally unspecified before gastrulation. This, and Holtfreter's demonstration that no neural differentiation occurred in the prospective neural region in embryos that had undergone exogastrulation,[127] was the main evidence that made it necessary to regard primary neural induction as an instructive event. This apparently neat resolution of the problem was disturbed when Barth discovered that isolated pieces of ectoderm from early blastula stages of *Amblystoma punctatum* differentiated into neural tissues when cultured in saline.[128] Holtfreter, however, demonstrated that neural differentiation occurred only when some of the cells of the explant underwent cytolysis.[129] Those results should have led to further experiments to determine whether the dead cells enriched the saline medium sufficiently to allow the surviving cells to complete their development or whether disinhibition of differentiation had occurred as a result of neutralization of inhibitory factors(s). However, Holtfreter's interpretation of the results, designed to save the organizer theory, was that an inductive effect was caused by "stimuli emerging from the decaying free cells," and he then complained that "we are faced with the regrettable situation that the search for the chemical principle of neural induction has been blocked everywhere by the actual or suspected interference of cytolysis".[130] The theory of the organizer had to be saved at all costs, even if that required the invocation of a principle of uncertainty or indeterminacy that insulated the theory against experimental falsification.

Summing up the results of over 50 years of research on primary embryonic induction, three of the principal workers in the field were forced to "confess that progress in understanding embryonic induction has been slow."[131] Saxén, *et al.* ask whether "the poineering work of one great scientist has led his successors astray or along a pathway that will come to a dead end, despite the superb methods and wealth of information available today." They conclude "that future projects should still be based on the fundamental ideas of Spemann and his school,"[131] but it has been one of my purposes here to give reasons to doubt the validity of that conclusion. My other and main purpose has been to propose an alternative theory that has great predictive power, and so to point the way to new experiments on the origins of the spatial pattern of differentiation in the embryo.

6. REFERENCES

1. His, W., 1874, *Unserer Körperform und das Physiologische Problem ihrer Entstehung*, Engelmann, Leipzig.
2. His, W., 1901, Das Prinzip der Organbildende Keimbezirke und die Verwandtschaften der Gewebe, *Arch. Anat. Physiol. Leipzig Anat. Abt.* 724.
3. Bonnet, C., 1762, *Considerations sur les Corps Organisés*, Marc-Michel Rey, Amsterdam.
4. Wilson, E. B., 1886, *The Cell in Development and Inheritance*, Macmillan, New York.
5. Davidson, E. H., 1976, *Gene Activity in Early Development*, 2nd ed., Academic Press, New York.
6. Nieuwkoop, P. D., 1956, Are there direct relationships between the cortical layer of the fertilized egg and the future axial system in *Xenopus laevis* embryos? *Pubbl. Stn. Zool. Napoli* **28:**24.
7. Harris, T. M., 1964, Pregastrular mechanisms in the morphogenesis of the salamander *Ambystoma maculatum, Dev. Biol* **10:**247.
8. Gerhart, J. C., 1980, Mechanisms regulating pattern formation in the amphibian egg and early embryo, in: *Biological Regulation and Development*, vol. 2 (R. E. Goldberger, ed.), pp. 133–316, Plenum Press, New York.
9. Schultze, O., 1894, Die Künstliche Erzeugung von Doppelbildungen bei Froschlarven mit Hilfe abnormer Gravitation, *Roux Arch. Entwicklungsmech. Org.* **1:**160.
10. Penners, A., and Schleip, W., 1928*a*, Die Entwicklung der Schultzeschen Doppelbildungen aus dem Ei von *Rana fusca*, Teil I–IV *Z. Wiss. Zool. Abt. A* **130:**305.
11. Penners, A., and Schleip, W., 1928*b*, Die Entwicklung der Schultzeschen Doppelbildungen aus dem Ei von *Rana fusca*, Teil V und VI, *Z. Wiss. Zool. Abt. A* **131:**1.
12. Curtis, A. S. G., 1960, Cortical grafting in *Xenopus laevis, J. Embryol. Exp. Morpho.* **8:**163.
13. Curtis, A. S. G., 1965, Cortical inheritance in the amphibian *Xenopus laevis*: Preliminary results, *Arch. Biol.* **76:**523.
14. Tompkins, R., and Rodman, W. P., 1971, The cortex of *Xenopus laevis* embryos: Regional differences in composition and biological activity, *Proc. Natl. Acad. Sci. U.S.A.* **68:**2921.
15. Kirschner, M. W., Gerhart, J. C., Hara, K., and Ubbels, G. A., 1980, Initiation of the cell cycle and establishment of bilateral symmetry in *Xenopus* eggs, *Symp. Soc. Dev. Biol.* **38:**187.
16. Jacobson, M., 1980, Clones and compartments in the vertebrate central nervous system, *Trends Neurosci.* **1:**3.
17. Gurdon, J. B., and Woodland, H. R., 1969, The influence of cytoplasm on the nucleus during cell differentiation, with special reference to RNA synthesis during amphibian cleavage, *Proc. R. Soc. London Ser. B* **198:**211.
18. Subtelny, S., 1974, Nucleocytoplasmic interactions in development of amphibian hybrids, *Int. Rev. Cytol.* **39:**35.
19. Dworkin, M. B., and Dawid, I. B., 1980, Use of a cloned library for the study of abundant poly(A)$^+$RNA during *Xenopus laevis* development, *Dev. Biol.* **76:**449.
20. Brock, H. W., and Reeves, R., 1978, An investigation of *de novo* protein synthesis in the South African clawed frog, *Xenopus laevis, Dev. Bio.* **66:**128.
21. Bravo, R., and Knowland, J., 1979, Classes of proteins synthesized in oocytes, eggs, embryos and differentiated tissues of *Xenopus laevis, Differentiation*113:101.
22. Johnson, K. E., 1969, Altered contact behavior of presumptive mesodermal cells from hybrid amphibian embryos arrested at gastrulation, *J. Exp. Zool.* **170:**325.
23. Johnson, K. E., 1970, The role of changes in cell contact behavior in amphibian gastrulation, *J. Exp. Zool.* **175:**391.

24. Johnson, K. E., 1977*a*, Extracellular matrix synthesis in blastula and gastrula stages of normal and hybrid frog embryos. I. Toluidine blue and lanthanum staining, *J. Cell Sci.* **25:**313.
25. Johnson, K. E., 1977*b*, Extracellular matrix synthesis in blastula and gastrula stages of normal and hybrid frog embryos. II. Autoradiographic observations on the sites of synthesis and mode of transport of galactose- and glucose-labeled materials, *J. Cell Sci.* **25:**323
26. Johnson, K. E., 1977*c*, Extracellular matrix synthesis in blastula and gastrula stages of normal and hybrid frog embryos. III. Characterization of galactose- and glucose-labeled materials, *J. Cell Sci.* **25:**335.
27. Johnson, K. E., 1978, Extracellular matrix synthesis in blastula and gastrula stages of normal and hybrid frog embryos. IV. Biochemical and autoradiographic observations on fucose-, glucose- and mannose-labeled materials, *J. Cell Sci.* **32:**109.
28. Johnson, K. E., and Smith, E. P., 1976, The binding of concanavalin A to dissociated embryonic amphibian cells, *Exp. Cell Res.* **101:**63.
29. Kosher, R. A., and Searles, R. L., 1973, Sulfated mucopolysaccharide synthesis during the development of *Rana pipiens, Dev. Biol.* **32:**50.
30. Fraser, B. R., and Zalik, S. E., 1977, Lectin-mediated agglutination of amphibian embryonic cells, *J. Cell Sci.* **27:**227.
31. Gaskell, W. H., 1889–90, On the origin of the central nervous system of vertebrates, *Brain* **12:**1.
32. His, W., 1892, Zur allgemeinen Morphologie des Gehirnrohres, *Arch. Anat. Physiol. (Leipzig) Anat. Abt.* 363.
33. His, W., 1893, Vorschläge zur Einteilung des Gehirns, *Arch. Anat. Physiol. (Leipzig) Anat. Abt.* 172.
34. Von Kupffer, C., 1906, Die Morphogenie des Centralnervensystems, in: *Handbuch der Vergleichende und experimentelle Entwicklungslehre der Wirbeltiere,* Bd. 2, Teil 3 (R. Hertwig, ed.), Fischer, Jena.
35. Johnston, J. B., 1902, An attempt to define the primitive functional divisions of the central nervous system, *J. Comp. Neurol.* **12:**87.
36. Herrick, C. J., 1908, The morphological subdivision of the brain, *J. Comp. Neurol.* **18:**393.
37. Kingsbury, B. G., 1920, The extent of the floor-plate of His and its significance, *J. Comp. Neurol.* **32:**113.
38. Kingsbury, B. G., 1922, The fundamental plan of the vertebrate brain, *J. Comp. Neurol.* **34:**461.
39. Kingsbury, B. G., 1930, The developmental significance of the floor-plate of the brain and spinal cord, *J. Comp. Neurol.* **50:**177.
40. Kuhlenbeck, H., 1973, *Overall Morphologic Pattern,* Vol. 3, Pt. II, *The Central Nervous System of Vertebrates*, Karger, Basel.
41. Morata, G., and Lawrence, P., 1977, Homoeotic genes, compartments and cell determination in *Drosophila, Nature* (*London*), **265:**211.
42. Jacobson, M., and Hirose, G., 1978, Origin of the retina from both sides of the embryonic brain: A contribution to the problem of crossing at the optic chiasma, *Science* **202:**637.
43. Hirose, G., and Jacobson, M., 1979, Clonal organization of the central nervous system of the frog. I. Clones stemming from individual blastomeres of the 16-cell and earlier stages, *Dev. Biol.* **71:**191.
44. Jacobson, M., and Hirose, G., 1981, Clonal organization of the central nervous

system of the frog. II. Clones stemming from individual blastomeres of the 32- and 64-cell stages, *J. Neurosci.* **1:**271.
45. Jacobson, M., 1982, Clonal organization of the central nervous system of the frog. III. Clones stemming from 128-, 256- and 512-cell stages, in preparation.
46. Jacobson, M., 1981*a*, Rohon–Beard neuron origin from blastomeres of the 16-cell frog embryo, *J. Neurosci.* **1:**918.
47. Jacobson, M., 1981*b*, Rohon–Beard neurons arise from a substitute ancestral cell after removal of the cell from which they normally arise in the 16-cell frog embryo, *J. Neurosci.* **1:**923.
48. Spemann, H., 1938, *Embryonic Development and Induction*, Yale University Press, New Haven, CT.
49. Jacobson, M., 1982, Dispersal and mingling of cells in late blastula and gastrula stages of *Xenopus* demonstrated by intracellular labeling with horseradish peroxidase, in preparation.
50. Hara, K., 1977, The cleavage pattern of the axolotl egg studied by cinematography and cell counting, *Wilhelm Roux Arch. Entwicklungsmech. Org.* **181:**73.
51. Meuzelaar, H. L. C., Haverkamp, J., Hileman, F. D., 1981, *Curie-Point Pyrolysis Mass Spectrometry of Biomaterials,* Elsevier, Amsterdam.
52. Boucaut, J.-C., 1973, Autoradiographic analysis of *Pleurodeles waltlii* embryos injected with labelled embryo donor cells, *Differentiation* **1:**413.
53. Boucaut, J.-C., and Gallien, L., 1973*a*, Chimères allophéniques intergénériques entre *Pleurodeles waltlii* Michah et *Ambystoma mexicanum* Shaw (Amphibiens urodeles). Mise en évidence du chimérisme integumentaire, *C. R. Acad. Sci. Ser. D,* **276:**1757.
54. Boucaut, J.-C., and Gallien, L., 1973*b*, Analyse autoradiographique des chimères allophénique intergénériques obtenues entre deux Amphibiens urodeles: *Ambystoma mexicanum* Shaw et *Pleurodeles waltlii* Michah, *C. R. Acad. Sci. Ser. D.*, **276:**1895.
55. Maslow, D. E., 1976, *In vitro* analysis of surface specificity in embryonic cells, in: *The Cell Surface in Animal Embryogenesis and Development* (G. Poste and G. L. Nicholson, eds.), pp. 697–745, North-Holland, Amsterdam.
56. Moscona, A. A., and Houseman, R. E., 1977, Biological and biochemical studies on embryonic cell recognition, in: *Cell and Tissue Interactions* (J. W. Lash and M. M. Burger, eds.), pp. 173–186, Raven Press, New York.
57. Holtfreter, J., 1939, Gewebeaffinität, ein Mittel der embryonalen Formbildung, *Arch. Exp. Zellforsch. Besonders Gewebezuecht.* **23:**169.
58. Townes, P. L., and Holtfreter, J., 1955, Directed movements and selective adhesions of embryonic amphibian cells, *J. Exp. Zool.* **128:**53.
59. Jacobson, M. in preparation.
60. Alderman, A. L., 1935, The determination of the eye in the anuran *Hyla regilla, J. Exp. Zool.* **70:**205.
61. Nicholas, J. S., 1957, Results of inversion of neural plate material, *Proc. Natl. Acad. Sci. U.S.A.* **43:**542.
62. Jacobson, C.-O., 1964, Motor nuclei, cranial nerve roots, and fibre pattern in the medulla oblongata after reversal experiments on the neural plate of Axolotl larvae. I. Bilateral operations, *Zool. Bidr. Uppsala* **38:**241.
63. Spemann, H., 1912, Über der Entwicklung umgedrehter Hirnteile bei Amphibienembryonen, *Zool. Jahrb. Suppl. 15* **3:**1.
64. Roach, F. C., 1945, Differentiation of the central nervous system after axial reversals of the medullary plate of *Amblystoma, J. Exp. Zool.* **99:**53.
65. Sládeček, F., 1955, Regulative tendencies of the central nervous system during embryogenesis of the Axolotl (*Amblystoma mexicanum* Cope). II. Regulation after

simultaneous inversion of anteroposterior and mediolateral axes of medullary plate, *Acta Soc. Zool. Bohemoslav.* **19:**138.
66. Lewis, W. H., 1910, Localization and regeneration in the neural plate of amphibian embryos, *Anat. Rec.* **4:**191.
67. Harrison, R. G., 1947, Wound healing and reconstitution of the central nervous system of the amphibian embryo after removal of parts of the neural plate, *J. Exp. Zoo.* **106:**27.
68. Corner, M. A., 1963, Development of the brain of *Xenopus laevis* after removal of parts of the neural plate, *J. Exp. Zool.* **153:**301.
69. Dürken, B., 1926, Das Verhalten embryonalen Zellen im Interplantat. Mit Berüksichtigung des Geschwulstproblems, *Wilhelm Roux Arch. Entwicklungsmech. Org.* **107:**728.
70. Kusche, W., 1929, Interplantation umschriebener Zellbezirke aus der Blastula und Gastrula der Amphibien. I. Versuche an Urodelen, Wilhelm Roux Arch. Entwicklungsmech. Org. **120:**192.
71. Bautzmann, H., 1929, Über bedeutungsfremde Selbsdifferenzierung aus Teilstücken des Amphibienkeimes, *Naturwissenschaften* **17:**818.
72. Bytinski-Salz, H., 1929, Untersuchungen über das Verhalten des praesumptiven Gastrulaektoderms der Amphibien bei heteroplastischer und Xenoplastischer Transplantation ins Gastrocoel, *Wilhelm Roux Arch. Entwicklungsmech Org.* **114:**594.
73. Mangold, O., 1931, Das Determinationsproblem. III. Das Wirbeltierauge in der Entwicklung und Regeneration, *Ergeb. Biol.* **7:**193.
74. Mangold, O., 1933, Isolationsversuche zur Analyse der Frage der Entwicklung bestimmter Kopforgane, *Naturwissenschaften* **21:**394.
75. Aufsess, A. von, 1941, Defeckt und Isolationsversuche an der Medullarplatte und ihrer Unterlagerung an Triton alpestris—und Amblystoma-Keimen, mit besonderer Berücksigtigung der Rumpf-und Schwantzregion, *Wilhelm Roux Arch. Entwicklungsmech. Org.* **141:**248.
76. Ter Horst, J., 1947, Differenzierungs und Induktionsleistunger verschiedener Abschnitte der Medullarplatte und des Urdarmdaches von Triton im Kombinat, *Wilhelm Roux Arch. Entwicklungsmech. Org.* **143:**275.
77. Von Woellwarth, C., 1952, Die Induktionsstufen des Gehirns, *Wilhelm Roux Arch. Entwicklungsmech. Org.* **145:**582.
78. Waechter, H., 1953, Die Induktionsfähigkeit der Gehirnplatte bei Urodelen und ihr medianlaterales Gafälle, *Wilhelm Roux Arch. Entwicklungsmech. Org.* **146:**201.
79. Källén, B., 1958, Studies on the differentiation capacity of neural epithelium cells in chick embryos, *Z. Zellforsch. Mikrosk. Anat.* **47:**479.
80. Landis, S. C., 1980, Developmental changes in the neurotransmitter properties of dissociated sympathetic neurons: A cytochemical study of the effects of medium, *Dev. Biol.* **77:**349.
81. LeDouarin, N. M., Teillet, M., and LeLievre, C., 1977, Influence of the tissue environment on the differentiation of neural crest cells, in: *Cell and Tissue Interactions* (J. W. Lash and M. Burger, eds.), pp. 11–27, Raven Press, New York.
82. Beams, H. W., and Kessel, R. G., 1974, The problem of germ cell determinants, *Int. Rev. Cytol.* **39:**413.
83. Eddy, E. M., 1975, Germ plasm and differentiation of the germ cell line, *Int. Rev. Cytol.* **43:**229.
84. Lamborghini, J. E., 1980, Rohon–Beard cells and other large neurons in *Xenopus* embryos originate during gastrulation, *J. Comp. Neurol.* **189:**323.

85. Spemann, H., and Mangold, H., 1924, Über Induktion von Embryonalanlagen durch Implantation artfremder Organisatoren, *Wilhelm Roux Arch. Entwicklungsmech. Org.* **100:**599.
86. Dalcq, A., and Pasteels, J., 1937, Une conception nouvelle des bases physiologiques de la morphogénesè, *Arch. Biol.* **48:**669.
87. Saxén, L., and Toivonen, S., 1962, *Primary Embryonic Induction,* Logos Press, London.
88. Nieuwkoop, P. D., 1973, The "organization center" of the amphibian embryo; its origin, spatial organization, and morphogenetic action, *Adv. Morphog.* **10:**1.
89. Nakamura, O., and Toivonen, S., eds., 1978, *Organizer. A Milestone of a Half-Century from Spemann,* Elsevier/North-Holland, Amsterdam.
90. Nakamura, O., 1978, *Epigenetic Formation of the Organizer,* pp. 179–220, in Nakamura and Toivonen.[89]
91. Nakamura, O., Hayashi, Y., and Asashima, M., 1978, A half-century from Spemann—Historical review on the organizer, pp. 1–48, in Nakamura and Toivonen.[89]
92. Saxén, L., 1977, Directive versus permissive induction: A working hypothesis, in: *Cell and Tissue Interactions* (J. W. Lash and M. M. Burger, eds.), Raven press, New York.
93. Lewis, W. H., 1907, Transplantation of the lips of the blastopore in *Rana palustris, Am. J. Anat.* **7:**137.
94. Vogt, W., 1925, Gestaltungsanalyse am Amphibienkeim mit örtlicher Vitalfärbung. I. Methodik und Wirkungsweise der örtlichen Vitalfarbung mit Agar als Farbträger. *Wilhelm Roux Arch. Entwicklungsmech. Org.* **106:**542.
95. Vogt, A., 1929, Gestaltungsanalyse an Amphibienkeim mit örtlicher Vitalfarbung. II. Gastrulation und Mesodermbildung bei Urodelen und Anuren, *Wilhelm Roux Arch. Entwicklungsmech. Org.* **120:**384.
96. Ave, K., Kawakami, I., and Shameshima, M., 1968, Studies on the heterogeneity of cell populations in amphibian presumptive epidermis, with reference to primary induction. *Dev. Biol.* **17:**617.
97. Nakamura, O., and Kishiyama, K., 1971, Prospective fates of blastomeres at the 32-cell stage of *Xenopus laevis* embryos, *Proc. Jpn. Acad.* **47:**407.
98. Nakamura, O., Takasaki, H., and Nagata, A., 1978, Further studies of the prospective fates of blastomeres at the 32-cell stage of *Xenopus laevis* embryos, *Med. Biol.* **56:**355.
99. Keller, R. E., 1975, Vital dye mapping of the gastrula and neurula of *Xenopus laevis.* I. Prospective areas and morphogenetic movements of the superficial layer, *Dev. Biol.* **42:**222.
100. Nieuwkoop, P. D., and Ubbels, G. A., 1972, The formation of mesoderm in urodele amphibians. IV. Quantitative evidence for the purely "ectodermal" origin of the entire mesoderm and of the pharyngeal endoderm, *Wilhelm Roux Arch. Entwicklungsmech. Org.* **169:**185.
101. Keller, R. E., 1975, Vital dye mapping of the gastrula and neurula of *Xenopus laevis.* II. Prospective areas and morphogenetic movements of the deep layer, *Dev. Biol.* **51:**118.
102. Waddington, C. H., 1952, On the existence of regionally specific evocators, *J. Exp. Biol.* **29:**140.
103. Eyal-Giladi, H., 1954, Dynamic aspects of neural induction in amphibia, *Arch. Biol.* **65:**179.
104. Løvtrup, S., 1975, Fate maps and gastrulation in amphibia—A critique of current views, *Can. J. Zool.* **53:**473.

105. Lehmann, F. E., 1945, *Einfuhrung in die Physiologische Embryologie*, Birkhauser, Basel.
106. Barnstable, C. J., 1980, Monoclonal antibodies which recognize different cell types in the rat retina, *Nature* (*London*) **286:**231.
107. Zipser, B., and McKay, R., 1981, Monoclonal antibodies distinguish identifiable neurons in the leech, *Nature* (*London*) **289:**549.
108. Lagenauer, C., Sommer, I., and Schachner, M., 1980, Subclass of astroglia in mouse cerebellum recognized by monoclonal antibody, *Dev. Biol.* **79:**367.
109. Tokaya, H., 1956, Two types of neural differentiation produced in connection with mesenchymal tissue, *Proc. Jpn. Acad.* **32:**282.
110. Tokaya, H., and Watanabe, T., 1961, Differential proliferation of the ependyma in the developing neural tube of amphibian embryo, *Embryologia*, **6:**169.
111. Toivonen, S., and Saxén, L., 1968, Morphogenetic interactions of presumptive neural and mesodermal cells mixed in different ratios, *Science* **159:**539.
112. Holtfreter, J., 1938, Differenzierungspotenzen isolierter Teile der Urodelengastrula (Anurengastrula), Wilhelm *Roux Arch. Entwicklungsmech. Org.* **138:**522.
113. Spemann, H., 1927, Neue Arbeiten über Organisatoren in der tierischen Entwicklung, *Naturwissenschaften* **15:**946.
114. Spemann, H., 1931, Über den abteil vom Implantat und Wirtskeime an der Orientierung und Beschaffenheit der induzierten Embryonalanlage, *Wilhelm Roux. Arch. Entwicklungsmech. Org.* **123:**389.
115. Mangold, O., 1933, Über die Induktionsfähigkeit der verschiedenen Bezirke der Neurula von Urodelen, *Naturwissenshaften* **21:**761.
116. Ter Horst, J., 1948, Differenzierungs—und Induktions-Leistungen verschiedener Abschnitte der Medullarplatte und des Urdarmdaches von Triton im Kombinat, *Wilhelm Roux Arch. Entwicklungsmech. Org.* **143:**275.
117. Nakamura, O., Aochi, M., and Shiomi, H., 1970, Association of blastomeres as a basic factor in differentiation of cell species in amphibian morulae, *Proc. Jpn. Acad.* **46:**965.
118. Nakamura, O., Takasaki, H., and Mizohata, T., 1970, Differentiation during cleavage in *Xenopus laevis*. I. Acquisition of self differentiation capacity of the dorsal marginal zone, *Proc. Jpn. Acad.* **46:**971.
119. Patterson, P. H., and Chun, L. L. Y., 1977, The induction of acetylcholine synthesis in primary cultures of dissociated rat sympathetic neurons. I. Effects of conditioned medium, *Dev. Biol.* **56:**263.
120. Collins, F., 1980, Neurite outgrowth induced by the substrate associated material from nonneuronal cells, *Dev. Biol.* **79:**247.
121. Collins, F., 1978, Induction of neurite outgrowth by a conditioned medium factor bound to culture substratum, *Proc. Natl. Acad. Sci. U.S.A.* **75:**5210.
122. Coughlin, M. D., Bloom, E. M., and Black, I. B., 1981, Characterization of a neuronal growth factor from mouse heart-cell-conditioned medium, *Dev. Biol.* **82:**56.
123. Thoenen, H., and Barde, Y.-A., 1980, Physiology of nerve growth factor, *Physiol. Rev.* **60:**1284.
124. Niu, M. C., and Twitty, V. C., 1953, The differentiation of gastrula ectoderm in medium conditioned by axial mesoderm, *Proc. Natl. Acad. Sci. U.S.A.* **39:**985.
125. Holtfreter, J., and Hamburger, V., 1955, Embryogenesis: Progressive differentiation, amphibians, in: *Analysis of Development* (B. H. Willier, P. A. Weiss, and V. Hamburger, eds.), pp. 230–296, Saunders, Philadelphia.
126. Holtfreter, J., 1929, Über die Aufsucht isolierter Teile des Amphibienkeimes. I. Methode einer Aufsucht *in vitro, Wilhelm Roux Arch. Entwicklungsmech. Org.* **117:**422.
127. Holtfreter, J., 1933, Die totale Exogastrulation, eine Selbstablosung des Ektoderms von Entomesoderm, *Wilhelm Roux Arch. Entwicklungsmech Org.* **129:**669.

128. Barth, L., 1941, Neural differentiation without organizer, *J. Exp. Zool.* **87:**371.
129. Holtfreter, J., 1944, Neural differentiation of ectoderm through exposure to saline solution, *J. Exp. Zool.* **95:**307.
130. Holtfreter, J., 1945, Neuralization and epidermization of gastrula ectoderm, *J. Exp. Zool.* **98:**161.
131. Saxén, L., Toivonen, S., and Nakamura, O., 1978, Concluding remarks—Primary embryonic induction: An unsolved problem, pp. 315–320, in Nakamura and Toivonen.[89]

3

Monoclonal Antibodies to Embryonic Neurons

Cell-Specific Markers for Chick Ciliary Ganglion

KATE F. BARALD

1. INTRODUCTION

1.1. *Formation of Complex Connections in the Nervous System*

Both genetic and epigenetic events are involved in the generation of precise connections in the nervous system. Vast numbers of individual interactions between single neurons and their microenvironments contribute to the formation of complex neuronal pathways. Environmental cues may come to a developing neuron from many different sources, but there are at least three for which there is good experimental evidence: (1) the insoluble intercellular matrix or substratum consisting of collagens, glycosaminoglycans, fibronectin, etc.[1]; (2) soluble diffusible factors (neurotrophic factors, growth factors, hormones)[2]; and (3) the cell surfaces of other neuronal and nonneuronal cells with which a developing neuron comes in contact.[3] The cell surface of the target tissue or material associated with it such as the basal lamina probably serves to trigger the formation of the synapse[4] and, at least in amphibians,[5] its specific regeneration.

KATE F. BARALD · Department of Anatomy and Cell Biology, University of Michigan Medical School, Neuroscience Program, Ann Arbor, MI 48109.

Clues to the molecular mechanisms that lead to the formation of precise connections are potentially available at the level of the cell surface. There is much evidence to implicate cell–cell recognition events in the development and regeneration of the nervous system (see the recent reviews by Gottlieb and Glaser,[6] Landmesser,[7] and Muller[8]).

The problem of identifying cell surface elements that may be important for neuronal differentiation and synapse formation has been greatly simplified by the recent development of antibodies and other neuron-specific reagents that bind to neuronal cells.[9–12] However, most of these cell surface markers recognize general features common to many or most neuronal cells.

The question of whether developing neurons have diverse and characteristic cell surface identities is still being investigated. However, recent applications of immunohistochemical techniques that employ unique cell surface markers in the form of monoclonal antibodies indicate that this is indeed the case for mature neurons. For example, Zipser and McKay[13] have used monoclonal antibodies to demonstrate the remarkable antigenic diversity of neuronal subpopulations in the relatively simple nervous system of the leech. Barnstable[14] has used monoclonal antibodies to reveal the differences in cell surface characteristics of subpopulations of retinal cells in the rat, and Trisler *et al.*[15] have used monoclonal antibodies to examine "gradients" of cell surface markers that are differentially expressed across the retina. The cell surfaces of neurons derived from the neural tube and the neural crest also differ, as demonstrated with two monoclonal antibodies, each specific for neural cells originating from the tube or the neural crest.[16,17] The differences in the surface components of central and peripheral neurons revealed by monoclonal antibodies confirm an earlier finding by Pfenninger and Maylié-Pfenninger[18] that neurites from these two sources have different carbohydrate "signatures" detectable with a variety of lectins.

1.2. *Antibodies as Cytochemical Markers of Neuronal Cells*

Antibodies to unique cell surface antigens have a great many potential applications. They can be used to isolate the surface antigens, permitting their molecular and functional characterization. Antigenic distributions on the cell surfaces of neurons and their neurites can be mapped. Developmental studies of cellular interactions in the nervous system may be feasible with these antibodies, since they are useful tools for functional perturbation (e.g., through complement-mediated cytotoxicity) as well as cell markers. Such antibodies can be used to examine morphological, biochemical, and functional properties of developing neuronal cell populations *in vitro* and *in vivo*.

Antibodies found in the sera of immunized animals are complex biological reagents. They contain mixtures of immunoglobulin molecules, since serum contains numerous species of antibodies, and many antibodies of each type recognize different chemical or configurational aspects of injected molecules or cells. Each animal injected contains a different mixture of antibodies made in the course of the immune response. For example, no two rabbits injected with the same purified protein make the same mixture of antibodies. For this reason, seral antibodies pose a variety of problems as cell markers, including the simple one of inability to duplicate the exact mixture after the death of the immunized animal.

The monoclonal antibody technique, first worked out by Kohler and Milstein,[19] simplifies the use of antibodies as biological tools by "immortalizing" cells that produce a desired antibody. This is accomplished by fusing the antibody-producing spleen cells with tumor cells, called myelomas, that are themselves tumors of antibody-producing cells. The resulting hybrid or "hybridoma cell" will secrete antibodies of the desired parental type in pure form, making possible the production of large quantities of chemically homogeneous labeling reagents. Descendents of this cell, the monoclone, are identical and produce the same antibody.

Since the technique allows identification of immunoglobulin-producing cells that make antibodies even to minor cell surface components, it provides probes for the subtle differences among neuronal cells that may be involved in recognition events in the formation of the nervous system. Monoclonal antibodies produced by this technique are presently being used to distinguish and characterize a wide variety of neuronal cell antigens associated with extracellular and intracellular elements in both invertebrate and vertebrate systems.[13–17,20,21]

1.3. *The Ciliary Ganglion, a Model of Neuronal Development in Vertebrates*

The ciliary ganglion (CG) of the embryonic chick is a parasympathetic ganglion of neural crest origin that contains two populations of neuronal cells, both cholinergic.[22,23] These two populations innervate unique targets: the ciliary neurons make synapses on the ciliary body and the striated muscle of the iris; choroid neurons make synapses on the smooth muscle of the vasculature of the choroid layer. Both neuronal populations survive well in tissue culture in conditioned medium[24,25] and have been shown by Nishi and Berg[25] to make synapses on skeletal myotubes from embryonic chick pectoral muscle in culture (see Chapter 9). Studies of the development of cell-specific functions in these neurons and the process of synapse formation with potential targets are likely to be facilitated by the availability of specific monoclonal antibodies. The discovery of specific cell surface markers would facilitate developmental studies of these two neuronal populations *in vivo*, as well as observations of the early cell–cell interactions that occur as synapses are formed *in vitro*. Antibodies generated against such unique surface antigens could be used to (1) identify these neuronal populations unequivocally even at very early times in development and in the presence of other neuronal cell types both *in ovo* and in tissue culture; (2) isolate and identify unique surface antigens that may play important roles in neuronal development or synapse formation, if these events are affected by the antibodies; and (3) eliminate the neuronal population with cytotoxic antibodies, enabling one to assess the effects of such elimination on pre- and postsynaptic cells.

Five hybrid clones have been produced[26] that secrete antibodies to cell surface components present on CG neurons. Two of these antibodies, CG–1 and CG–4, also bind to a subpopulation of cranial neural crest cells *in vitro* and are synergistically cytotoxic for these cells and for CG neurons in the presence of complement. In contrast, none of the cells from trunk neural crest tested *in vitro* binds detectable amounts of these antibodies; nor are they cytotoxic for these cells. The antibodies bind to chick ciliary ganglion neuronal cell bodies and neurites at all times tested in cell cultures isolated from embryos 1–18 days old. None of the other neuronal or nonneuronal cells tested expresses the antigen at any time. Although we have not ruled out the possibility that the antigens expressed by neural crest cells represent so called "jumping" antigenic determinants, i.e. those that occur on a number of functionally unrelated cell types, this evidence suggests that the neural crest contains a precursor population of cells that contributes to the formation of the CG. Such a population may be distinguished early in development by its cell surface components.

2. MATERIALS AND METHODS

2.1. *Dissociated Cell Cultures*

Cell cultures were prepared in essentially the same way whether used for immunizations, for screening of supernatants, or for mitogen-plus-antigen stimulation of spleen cells prior to hybridization. Cultures of CG neurons were prepared by dissection of ganglia from 8-day chick embryos (stage 34), from which cell suspensions were made.[20] Cells were plated on collagen-coated dishes as previously described[25,23] and were harvested for immunizations after 4–10 days in culture. After washing three times in Puck's phosphate buffered saline containing 1 g/liter glucose (PBSS),[23] a cold (4°C) solution of PBSS was added. The neuronal cells detached from the culture dish and floated. The nonneuronal cells remained attached to the substratum (provided only a small number of nonneuronal cells was present in the cultures). Cells were injected within 10 min of removal from the plates after centrifuging at 50*g*.

Neural crest cultures were prepared as described by Newgreen *et al.*[27] and others.[28,29] Cranial crest cultures were prepared from 31-hr embryonic chicks, and trunk crest from 3-day embryos. The neural tubes were removed after 8 hr in culture in nerve growth medium.[23]

2.2. *Immunological Procedures*

2.2.1. *Production of the Hybridomas.* Individual mice were given three injections of CG neurons prepared as described above.

BALB/c × C3H female mice 4 months of age were litter mates from the inbred mouse colony (Department of Biological Sciences, Stanford University). Each mouse received intraperitoneal (i.p.) injections on days 1, 22, and 36 consisting of 1.2×10^6 cells per injection in 200 μl of PBSS. Three days after the final injection, two mice were killed and a suspension of spleen cells prepared according to the method of Oi and Herzenberg.[30] The parental myeloma cell line used was the NS-1 variant of the P3 (MOPC 21) line.[30] A modification of the method of Robertson *et al.*[31] was used in which the isolated spleen cells were grown in the presence of the antigen-bearing cells and two mitogens: dextran sulfate (25 μg/ml) and lipopolysaccharide (10 μg/ml). Spleen cells in the presence of mitogens were incubated over a monolayer of CG cells (100 ganglion equivalents, 6.0×10^5 cells per 75-mm tissue culture flask). The bottoms of the flasks were collagen-coated prior to neuron addition.

Spleen cells were collected and washed after 4 days of mitogen–antigen stimulation and hybridized at 10^8 spleen cells per 10^7 myeloma cells. After fusion, 4×10^5 cells per well (of a 96-well microtiter plate) were maintained in modified HAT medium[32] until hybrid cells were detected in the wells (11 days). When supernatants had been tested for antibody production, cells were cloned by the limiting-dilution method of Oi and Herzenberg.[30]

2.2.2. *Screening Assays.* Other neuronal and nonneuronal cells were prepared for antibody screening. Spinal cord–neuronal cultures were prepared as described previously from 4- and 7-day embryos.[33] The cells were plated at 1000 cells per well in flexible microtiter plates (Cooke). Neuronal cells plated at similar densities included neuronal cells from trigeminal[34] and superior cervical ganglia[35]; dorsal root ganglion neurons (DRG's)[23]; brain[36]; Remak's ganglion[37]; and neurons of the sympathetic chain.[38] These cells were used only in fluorescence assays. Spinal cord neurons and cerebellum were dissociated by trituration without the use of trypsin[33] but all other preparations were trypsin-dissociated. Nerve growth factor (NGF) at 5 U/ml was included in DRG and sympathetic nerve cell cultures. Cultured nerve cells were tested in the plate-binding assays or fluorescence assays within 20 hr of plating, and then at various times up to 3 weeks in culture.

Eleven-day chick embryos were the source of skeletal muscle myotubes,[39] whole-body embryonic fibroblasts,[39] and heart fibroblasts,[24] for plate-binding and fluoresence experiments. Liver cells were prepared from 11-day chick and used only in fluorescence assays.

Hybridoma supernatants were tested for antibody production by a modification of the plate-binding assay of Tsu and Herzenberg.[40] Flexible 96-well microtiter plates were coated with a layer of rat-tail tendon collagen. CG cells from 8-day embryonic chick were prepared as described above and plated at 1000 cells per well. Initial results were obtained with live cells, but identical results were obtained with lightly fixed cells (0.125% glutaraldehyde)[41]; fixed cells were used in subsequent assays. After incubation of supernatants with either live or fixed cells, plates were washed three times in RIA buffer.[40] Plates were then incubated in ^{125}I-labeled protein A (from *Staphylococcus aureus*) or with ^{125}I-labeled goat-anti-mouse IgG prepared by the method of Mather.[42] In either case, 5×10^4 cpm per well were added in a volume of 50 μl at 21°C for 1–3 hr. After three washes in RIA buffer, wells were examined for cell loss, and random fields were counted in each well. The number of cells per well was recorded and bound radioactivity normalized for cell number. Assays were done in duplicate or triplicate. Wells were cut from the plates[40] and counted in a Beckman Gamma 4000 counter. Wells were scored as positive when they contained at least five times background.

Clones that produced antibody as detected in the plate-binding assays were tested in two-step immunofluorescence assays. Dilutions of the supernatants (1/2–1/500) were used as a first step with 24-hr cultures of live or fixed[41] cells from the CG of 8-day embryonic chick (8dCG) or other cell types plated on glass or quartz cover slips. Supernatant incubation at 21°C for 30 min was followed by three rinses in phosphate buffered saline (PBS), and a second step of 50 μg/ml rhodamine-conjugated goat-anti-mouse IgG.[42] Controls included use of the second-step fluorescent reagent alone and the application of the supernatants from the myeloma parent cell line followed by goat–anti-mouse IgG conjugated with rhodamine. Cells were observed with an Olympus fluorescence microscope.

IgG fractions were isolated from supernatants of hybrid cells that had been grown to stationary phase in 75-mm tissue culture flasks. The cells were removed by centrifugation and the pooled 500-ml lots of supernatants passed over a protein A sepharose column (bed volume, 25 ml) if the antibodies were protein A positive. IgG fractions were eluted in 0.2 M sodium acetate buffer. Hybrids yielded between 24 and 37 μg of pure IgG per milliliter of cell suspension. Purified IgG from supernatants was used at concentrations of 0.01 μg/ml in binding and fluorescence assays.

In some tests of the purified IgG fractions, the antibodies were coupled to biotin[44] and a rhodamine–avidin or fluorescein–avidin second step was used to characterize the binding to individual cells.[44] Optimal staining with most supernatants was achieved at 90–150 μg/ml with a rhodamine-conjugated avidin second step at 0.1 mg/ml. IgG fractions were considered positive if staining was observed with CG neurons but not with other neuronal or nonneuronal cells; the exception was the case of CG-5, the antibody that stains all neuronal but not nonneuronal cells. Controls included the use of anti-IgA antibody coupled with fluorescein in the cases where staining with biotin–IgG was observed.

2.2.3. Functional Tests: Cytotoxicity Assays. CG neurons and cranial and trunk neural crest cells were plated as previously described in 35-mm tissue culture dishes on glass cover slips. Cultures were incubated in the presence of antibodies (purified IgG's) and complement (rabbit or guinea pig) at either 22 or 37°C for various times, and then scored immediately for cell death as described by Oi and Herzenberg.[30] Alternatively, the numbers of surviving neurons were counted directly or assayed by staining with labeled antibody at later times. Controls included complement alone and antibody alone.

2.3. *Reagents*

RPMI 1640, trypsin, glutamine, nonessential amino acids, penicillin, streptomycin, fungizone, and fetal bovine serum (FBS) were obtained from MA Bioproducts. All lots of FBS from MA were screened for ability to support at least 90% clonal growth from both myeloma parents and 80% growth of hybridomas from single cells. Lipopolysaccharide and dextran sulfate were from GIBCO and DIFCO, respectively. Protein A and protein A sepharose were from Pharmacia. Biotin–succinimide ester was from Biosearch, San Raphael, CA. Rhodamine–avidin and fluorescein–avidin were from Vector, Burlingame, CA; or avidin was obtained from Sigma and conjugated with rhodamine or fluorescein isothiocyanate from Research Organics. Goat anti-mouse immunoglobulin and rabbit or guinea pig complement were from Miles-Yeda.

3. RESULTS

3.1. *Initial Selection and Cloning of Antibody-Producing Hybrids*

Of the 390 wells initially plated, 360 contained one or more hybrid colonies after 11 days in culture. We selected 38 antibody-producing wells for study from these cultures. These antibodies were selected on the basis of their binding to cell surface components of ciliary neurons, since live cells were used in the [^{125}I]protein A or ^{125}I–anti–IgG plate-binding assay. Cells were impermeable to trypan-blue after the binding of antibody and washing were completed.

Thirty-one of the initial 38 positives in this fusion were eliminated as nonspecific for ciliary neurons since they also bound to either skeletal muscle myotubes or DRG neurons in plate binding assays. Cells in the remaining 7 positive wells were transferred to 1-ml cultures and cloned.

One hundred sixty clones were derived from the seven hybrid wells, 42 of which were positive when tested with ciliary ganglion neurons and negative when tested with muscle or DRG's. Four high-activity clones (CG1–CG4, derived from four different wells) were selected for further study (Table I) and the rest frozen. This fusion produced the only CG–positive, other–neuron–negative clones. Previous screening of 10,000 isolates from ten other fusions were negative. Screening of the 4 clones with various cultured neuronal and nonneuronal cells was carried out as follows: (1) nonspecific clones were eliminated by plate binding assays with other neuronal cells, scored with [^{125}I]protein A or rabbit-anti-mouse IgG, and (2) those that passed this initial test were screened in the more sensitive fluorescence assays. Clone CG-5 was characterized along with the other 4 after it was shown to have very high activity in the initial ciliary and DRG screen but not in the muscle cell screen. Subsequent tests with other neuronal and nonneuronal populations showed that CG-5 labeled all neuronal cells tested but not nonneuronal cells of the embryonic chick.

Table I. Antibody Specificities

Cell type	CG-1	CG-2	CG-3	CG-4	CG-5
Neural crest derivatives					
Ciliary ganglion	+	+	+	+	+
Dorsal root ganglion	–	–	–	–	+
Remak's ganglion	–	–	–	–	+
Trigeminal ganglion	–	–	–	–	+
Superior cervical ganglion	–	–	–	–	+
Sympathetic chain	–	–	–	–	+
Spinal cord	–	12%	–	–	+
Brain	–	–	–	–	+
Muscle	–	–	small spots	–	–
Fibroblasts (whole embryo)	–	–	–	–	–
Heart	–	–	–	–	–
Liver	–	–	–	–	–
Mesencephalic neural crest	5%	–	–	5%	–
Trunk neural crest	–	–	–	–	–

3.2. *Monoclonal Antibodies Specific for CG Neurons*

Both antibodies CG-1 and CG-4 reacted with some antigenic determinants on the surface of embryonic CG neurons in culture. These neurons could be labeled with both antibodies at all stages tested from day 6 *in ovo* (stage 28) to day 14 (stages 40–41). None of the other cell types tested (Table I) reacted appreciably with CG-1 or CG-4.

The antibody distribution of either CG-1 or CG-4 on the surface of cell bodies of CG neurons in living or fixed cells was uniform although there was some punctate staining along the neurites (Fig. 1). At the level of light microscopy it was difficult to determine whether their distributions reflected surface features of neuronal processes such as varicosities or whether this distribution was the result of scattered patches of antigen. The punctate staining was similar to that observed with antiacetylcholinesterase (AChE), on the same neurons, visualized with antibody made in rabbits to purified AChE. However, CG-1 and CG-4 binding was not affected by antibodies to AChE (see Section 3.6 below).

3.3. *Staining of Cranial Neural Crest Cells in Vitro*

Antibodies made by clones CG-1 and CG-4 stain a small (5%) percentage of cultured mesencephalic neural crest cells from stage 9 em-

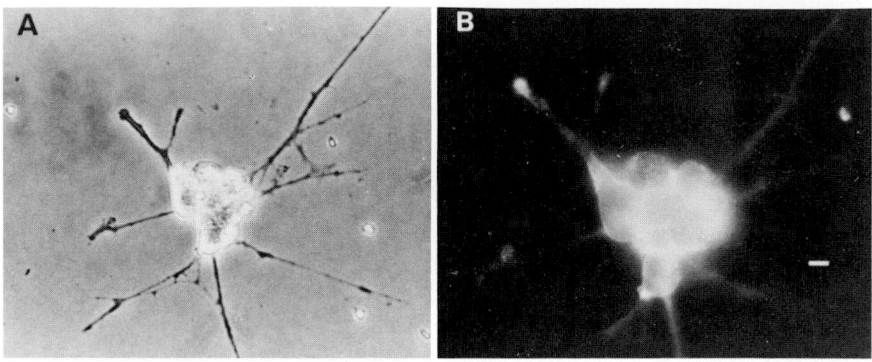

Figure 1. (A) Ciliary ganglion neurons from 8-day embryonic chick after 12 hours in culture. Well-developed growth cones and neurites are seen in this phase contrast micrograph. (B) The same view as in A, after treatment of the cultures with CG-1 monoclonal antibody (purified IgG isolated on a protein A affinity column) conjugated to biotin. After washing extensively, the cultures were then treated with fluorescein-linked avidin. Neurites and growth cones as well as the external cell surface are brightly labeled. Note that demarcations between neurons are more clearly seen in the fluorescence than in the phase contrast micrograph. The bar represents five microns.

bryos (31 hr *in ovo*). The mesencephalic crest is the region from which the CG neuron precursors are derived.[22] The neural tube was removed after 8 hr in these cultures, and testing was begun just after removal and up to 1 week in culture. A constant proportion of cells was labeled during this time. Explanted trunk neural crest cells from 3- or 4-day embryos were not stained. Antibody CG-1 conjugated to biotin and followed by rhodamine–avidin could be seen in a nonuniform distribution on the surface of the mesencephalic crest cells.

3.4. *Cytotoxicity of CG-1*

Antibody CG-1 was cytotoxic for ciliary ganglion cells in culture if small amounts of antibody CG–4 (in ratios of 8:1) and complement were present. Neither antibody alone was cytotoxic for either neural crest or CG neurons. Cells from 8–14 day (in ovo) embryos maintained in culture for 1–7 days were killed. In the absence of complement, however, or if the serum was heat inactivated, neuronal cells were able to extend long neurites even in high concentrations of the antibody. Cell death in the presence of antibody and complement was rapid. Nearly 95% of all the CG neurons in culture died within 30 min of addition of complement (Fig. 3A, B). Cell death was assessed by the ethidium bromide–acridine orange fluorescence assay.[30]

The antibodies were also synergistically cytotoxic for a small fraction of the cultured mesencephalic neural crest cells (<5%). If a culture were treated with complement in the presence of as little as 0.2 mg/ml of the purified IgG from CG-1 and 25 μg of CG-4, about 5% of the cells could be killed within 40 min of complement addition (Fig. 3C, D). No cells were stained with CG-1 antibodies or CG-4 antibodies in these cultures at later times, although sister cultures that were either untreated or

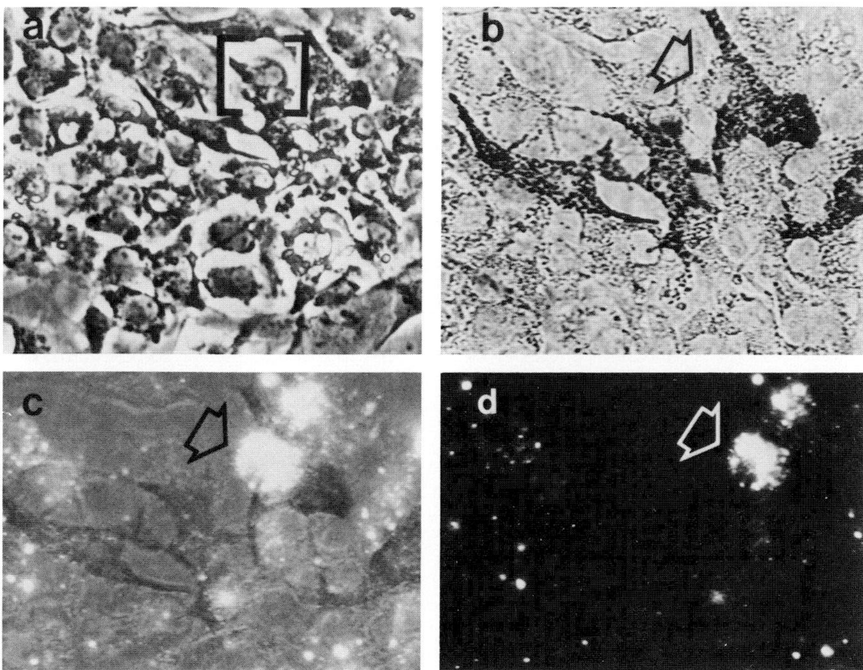

Figure 2. Neural crest cells from a 31-hour embryo (mesencephalic region) explanted into culture with the neural tube. The neural tube was removed after eight hours in culture and neural crest cells allowed to grow out on polyornithine-collagen coated cover slips. The cells had been in culture for three days when the phase contrast micrograph in A. was taken. B., the cell boxed in A., is indicated by an arrow in this brightfield micrograph of the migrating crest population. Note that the cell indicated is next to a cell containing pigment granules that are easy to see in the brightfield micrograph. In C. the same field as in B. is revealed after treatment with a monoclonal antibody CG-1 conjugated with biotin. The cell indicated by the box in A. and arrow in B. stains brightly with rhodamine-linked avidin after the biotin-antibody step. Both transmitted and fluorescent light were used simultaneously to demonstrate that the labeled cell and the pigment-containing cell are distinguishable from one another. In D. only fluorescent light is used to view the rhodamine-labeled cells in the field. This antibody stains about 5% of the mesencephalic neural crest cells in culture.

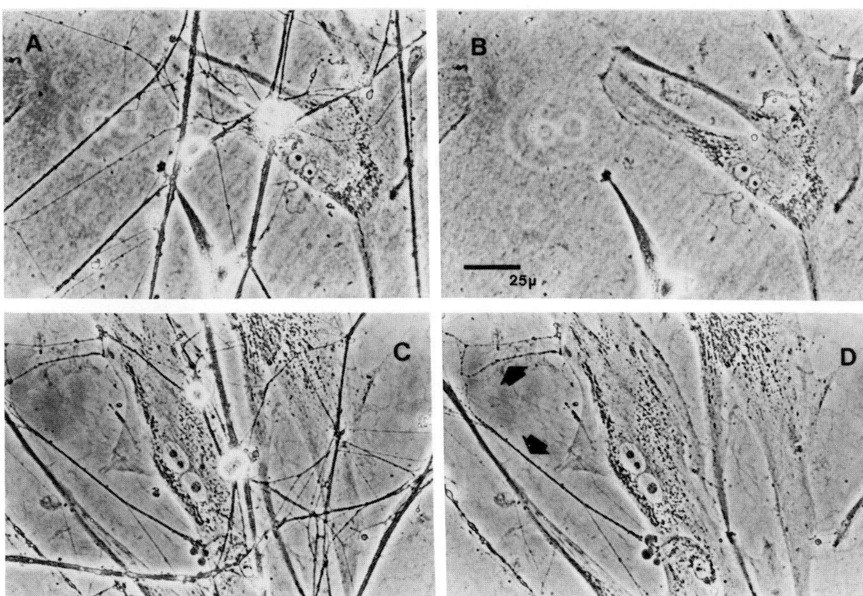

Figure 3. Cytotoxicity of antibodies CG-1 and CG-4 in the presence of complement. A. and C.: Ciliary ganglion-muscle cultures from embryonic chick after one week in culture. Pectoral muscle myotubes are prepared from 12-day embryos and allowed to fuse on a collagen-coated cover slip. The cells were treated with 10^{-5}M cytosine arabinoside for 48 hours and then the antimetabolite was removed and the cultures, relatively free of contaminating fibroblasts, allowed to grow for two more days prior to the addition of ciliary ganglion neurons from 8-day embryonic chick. In A., 0.2 mg/ml of purified IgG from CG-1 and 25 μg of antibody CG-4 (purified in the same manner) have been added. Even after one hour all of the cells are healthy and when ethidium bromide and acridine orange are added, all of the neuronal cells are seen to be alive. B. and D.: The same fields of view after addition of guinea pig complement 30 minutes later. Note that the neuronal cells and processes have been lysed but that the muscle cells are intact. No live neurons are revealed by fluorescence microscopy when acridine orange and ethidium bromide are applied to the cultures. In D., the arrows indicate neurites that have not lysed but have developed swellings prior to lysis.

treated with complement alone could be stained to reveal the presence of the antigens on a small percentage of the cells (<5%). Trunk crest and other neuronal and nonneuronal cells were unaffected by the CG-1 antibody or the CG-4 antibody, separately, or in combination, in the presence or absence of complement.

3.5. *Other Monoclonal Antibodies*

Clone CG-5 produced an antibody that labeled all embryonic chick neuronal populations tested (Table 1). None of the nonneuronal cells screened in either cell-binding or immunofluorescence assays was labeled, including the nonneuronal cells from the various ganglia. The cytotoxic properties of CG-5 have not been tested.

Clone CG-2 labeled CG neurons and a small population (12 ± 3%, SEM, n = 6) of neurons in dissociated spinal cord cultures from embryonic chick (day 4).

Antibody produced by CG-3 also bound to discrete small patches on living cultured skeletal muscle myotubes in addition to labeling CG neurons. The stained regions on the myotubes were not sites over nuclei over the synaptic regions, or regions containing acetylcholine receptors. The latter were visualized by fluorescent-labeled α-bungarotoxin or with an antibody to AChE. Neither bungarotoxin binding sites nor AChE sites coincided with the small patches of antibody binding.

3.6. *Blocking Studies*

In these experiments, the ability of a given monoclonal antibody to bind to CG neurons was tested after neuronal cells had been exposed to one of the following reagents: (1) one of the other four monoclonal antibodies, (2) 10^{-8}M α-bungarotoxin, (3) the anti-AChE antibody, (4) a monoclonal antibody to Thy-1 made in rats, or (5) phosphorylcholine-binding proteins (immunoglobulins) from a myeloma cell line that has been reported[12] to stain neuronal cells specifically. These PCB proteins are immunoglobulins of the IgA class and can be visualized with a goat-anti-mouse IgA antibody. The reverse competition experiments were also performed to see if any of the monoclonal antibodies interfered with the binding of these components.

None of the above reagents blocked the binding of any of the monoclonal antibodies to the CG neurons, even at a 100-fold excess concentration, and none of the monoclonal antibodies blocked the binding of these various reagents in similar tests. (CG-1 did not block the binding of the CG-4 antibody and vice versa.) However, each monoclonal antibody, in unlabeled form, blocked the binding of its own biotin-conjugated purified IgG. Furthermore, when one component was fluorescently labeled with rhodamine and the other with fluorescein, the distributions of the two components were not affected.

The labeling of the phosphorylcholine-binding immunoglobulins to chick cells was not as specific for chick neuronal cells as it was previously shown to be in the mouse.[12] Many nonneuronal cells were brightly stained by these phosphorylcholine-binding proteins. It is evident that both antibodies CG-1 and CG-4 seem to be more specific for CG neurons than the PCB proteins. CG-5 antibody also stains neuronal cells more selectively than the PCB immunoglobulins. None of the other monoclonal antibodies (including CG-5) could block the binding of CG-2 to the small population of spinal cord neurons.

4. DISCUSSION

4.1. *The Specificity of These Monoclonal Antibodies*

These monoclonal antibodies made to surface components of the CG neurons are among the first markers for a specific population of neuronal cells in vertebrates. Furthermore, the markers recognize components that are present throughout a fairly lengthy period in the development of these neurons, during the time when other neuronal phenotypes first appear. Barnstable[14] has shown that monoclonal antibodies that recognize different subpopulations of cells in the rat retina, recognize different cell surface antigenic distributions on the same cell. Whether these are quantitative or qualitative distributions remains to be shown. A recent report by Cuello *et al.*[45] describes the use of a monoclonal antibody to substance P for the identification of several populations of substance-P-containing neurons in the rat.[45,46] The monoclonal antibody technique has been used in invertebrate systems to demonstrate that small populations of neuronal cells have unique cell associated components. Zipser and McKay,[13] in benchmark experiments with the leech nervous system, have demonstrated that the diversity may be such that each subpopulation has a unique set of cell markers.

Among the markers reported to label neuronal cells preferentially are neuron-specific enolase,[9] tetanus toxin,[10] anti-Thy-1 antibodies,[11] and the recently reported phosphorylcholine-binding immunoglobulins from certain myeloma cells.[12] However, none of these is specific for a given type of neuronal cell, such as cholinergic neurons, or for neuronal cells with a specific function or location, such as the motoneurons of the spinal cord or DRG neurons.

It will be important to establish whether the antigenic components recognized by the antibodies described here are truly unique to CG neurons or only present on their cell surfaces in greater quantity or unique configuration. It will also be important to test additional neuronal cells from other species to see if the antigen is present and to test additional neuronal populations from the chick. The latter approach may be simplified by using frozen sections of early embryonic material rather than by culturing each neuronal type. Such approaches will be needed to determine whether there are subtle differences in the distribution of the antibody binding sites on the surface of the ciliary and choroid populations, since the location and therefore identity of these two cell types can be distinguished *in vivo* but not unambiguously *in vitro*.[22]

4.2. *Possible Identification of CG Neuron Precursors*

An interesting finding is that the monoclonal antibodies made by clones CG-1 and CG-4 label a small proportion of mesencephalic neural crest cells *in vitro* (<5%). These results suggest the intriguing hypothesis that these cells are precursors of the CG neurons *in vivo*. This population can be identified in cultures in which the mesencephalon is explanted at 31 hr of embryonic life, and at all times between 24 hr and 1 week in culture following removal of the mesencephalon after 24 hr *in vitro*. None of the neural crest cells from the trunk spinal cord explanted on days 3–4 labels with the antibody. It will be necessary to attempt to reproduce this finding *in vivo* since there may be selective survival of some crest cells in culture. It is also important to determine whether this antigen's presence on neural crest cells is entirely fortuitous, and without morphological or functional significance (a so-called "jumping determinant").

The cytotoxicity of the antibodies CG-1 and CG-4 for this small population of cranial crest cells *in vitro*, in the presence of complement, will permit tests of the precursor hypothesis. It is possible to kill cells in the early embryo and examine chicks at later stages for effects on the subsequent appearance of the CG. Chapters 1, 2, and 5 detail other approaches to the analysis of neuronal lineage. It should be noted that antibodies CG-1 and CG-4 do not react with any of the other neural crest derivatives that have been tested (Table I).

4.3. *Independence and Identity of the Antigenic Determinants*

The blocking studies demonstrate that neither CG-1 nor CG-4 can prevent the other antibody from binding. This indicates that although both antibodies selectively label CG neurons, but not seven other neuronal cell types, the antigenic determinants they recognize are different. The fact that both antibodies need to be present for complement–mediated cytotoxicity to occur, may indicate that either the two antibodies recognize different determinants on the same molecule or molecules that are closely associated on the cell surface.[47,48] The possibility that either antibody is to AChE is unlikely, since neither can be used to label spinal cord neurons or DRG's both of which can be stained for AChE histochemically.[23] It is also unlikely that CG-5 is directed to AChE, since it does not stain 11-day chick myotubes, which can be stained for AChE. The antigenic determinant recognized by CG-2, which is present on a small fraction of spinal cord cells as well as CG neurons, has not yet been characterized, and it has not been correlated with the electrophysiological properties of subpopulations of spinal cord neurons.

4.4. *Potential Heterogeneity of CG Neurons*

In cytoxicity studies, the CG-1 antibody in company with CG-4 has been shown to kill both ciliary and choroid cells in tissue culture in the presence of complement. This conclusion is based on the fact that under the culture conditions, all of the neuronal cells from the ganglion survive,[25] but that 95% of the cells in culture can be killed within 30 min of the addition of complement after the antibodies are added in proportions of 8:1. Since it is difficult to identify the two neuronal cell types unambiguously in culture, these results also need to be repeated *in vivo* using frozen sections to see if the small number of surviving cells may all be of one type.

The question of whether the neural crest population contains one or more heterogeneous subpopulations is currently a matter of controversy.[49–51] However, Smith *et al.*[52] have recently reported that as soon as the mesencephalic crest cells begin to migrate, they can synthesize acetylcholine (ACh). Although these authors did not test crest cells from other axial levels, specifically identify the cells that synthesize the ACh, or show whether all or only a small number of the cells do so, they postulate that their results may show early differentiation of the cells that will give rise to the CG neurons. Conceivably the cells that we have been able to label with the monoclonal antibodies CG-1 and CG-4 could be among the cells shown to synthesize ACh. We have preliminary evidence that some cells (12–15%) in the explanted cranial crest *in vitro* have a high-affinity choline uptake system, one of the characteristics of cholinergic neurons. It may be that the differentiation of these subpopulations of crest cells, like others that have been studied,[53] begins early in development, considerably in advance of the time when the cells aggregate to form the ciliary ganglion.

Acknowledgments

Part of this work was performed in the laboratory of Dr. Norman K. Wessells of Stanford University, to whom thanks are due for many helpful and enjoyable discussions.

I am grateful to Drs. Pat Jones and Vernon Oi for use of their facilities and for endless discussions. I thank Dr. Pat Jones for critical comments, and Bonita Johnson for expert typing of the manuscript. This work was supported by an NIH postdoctoral fellowship to KFB, by PHS Grant #HD04708 to NKW, and PHS Grant #NS17262 to KFB.

5. REFERENCES

1. Barondes, S. H., 1970, Brain glycomacromolecules and interneural recognition, in: *The Neurosciences Second Study Program,* (F. O. Schmitt, ed.), pp. 747–760, Rockefeller University Press, New York.
2. Greene, L. A., and Shooter, E. M., 1980, The nerve growth factor: Biochemistry, synthesis and mechanisms of action, *Ann. Rev. Neurosci.* **3**:353.
3. Rutishauser, U., Thiery, J.-P., Brackenbury, R., Sela, B.-A., and Edelman, G. M., 1976, Mechanism of adhesion among cells from neural retina of chick embryo, *Proc. Natl. Acad. Sci. U.S.A.* **73**:577.
4. Jacob, M., and Lentz, T.-L., 1979, Localization of acetylcholine receptors by means of horseradish peroxidase-α-bungarotoxin during formation and development of the neuromuscular junction in the chick embryo, *J. Cell Biol.* **82**:195.
5. Sanes, J. R., Marshall, L. M., and McMahan, U. J., 1978, Reinnervation of muscle fiber basal lamina after removal of muscle fibers, *J. Cell. Biol.* **78**:357.
6. Gottlieb, D. T., and Glaser, L., 1980, Cellular recognition during neural development, *Ann. Rev. Neurosci.* **3**:303.
7. Landmesser, L. T., 1980, The generation of neuromuscular specificity, *Ann. Rev. Neurosci.* **3**:279.
8. Muller, K. J., 1979, Synapses between neurones in the central nervous system of the leech, *Biol. Rev.* **54**:99.
9. Schmechel, D., Marangos, P. J., Athanosios, P. Z., Brightman, M., and Goodwin, F. D., 1978, Brain enolases as specific markers of neuronal and glial cues, *Science* **199**:312.
10. Mirsky, R., Wendon, L. B., Black, P., Stolkin, C., and Bray, D., 1978, Tetanus toxin: A cell surface marker for neurones in culture, *Brain Res.* **148**:251.
11. Fields, K. L., Brockes, J. P., Mirsky, R., and Wendon, L. B., 1978, Cell surface markers for distinguishing different types of rat dorsal root ganglion cells in culture, *Cell* **14**:43.
12. Hooghe-Peters, E. L., Fowlkes, B. J., and Hooghe, R. J., 1979, A new neuronal marker identified by phosphorylcholine-binding myeloma proteins, *Nature* (*London*) **281**:376.
13. Zipser, B., and McKay, R., 1981, Monoclonal antibodies distinguish identifiable neurones in the leech, *Nature* (*London*) **289**:549.
14. Barnstable, C. J., 1980, Monoclonal antibodies which recognize different cell types in rat retina, *Nature* (*London*) **286**:231.
15. Trisler, G. D., Schneider, M. S., and Nirenberg, M., 1981, A topographic gradient of molecules in retina can be used to identify neuron position. *Proc. Natl. Acad. Sci. USA* **78**:2145.
16. Cohen, J. and Selvendren, S. Y., 1981, A neuronal cell-surface antigen is found in the CNS but not in peripheral neurones. *Nature* **291**:421.

17. Vulliamy, T., Rattray, S., and Mirsky, R., 1981, Cell surface antigen distinguishes sensory and autonomic peripheral neurones from central neurones, *Nature* (*London*) **291**:418.
18. Pfenninger, K. H., and Maylié-Pfenninger, M.-F., 1979, Properties and dynamics of plasmalemmal glycoconjugates in growing neurites, *Progr. Brain Res.* **51**:83.
19. Kohler, G., and Milstein, C., 1975, Continuous cultures of fused cells secreting antibody of predefined specificity, *Nature* (*London*) **256**:495.
20. Eisenbarth, G. S., Walsh, F. S., and Nirenberg, M., 1979, Monoclonal antibody to a plasma membrane antigen of neurons, *Proc. Natl. Acad. Sci. U.S.A.* **76**:4913.
21. Cuello, A. C., Milstein, C., and Priestly, J. V., 1980, Use of monoclonal antibodies in immunocytochemistry with special reference to the central nervous system, *Brain Res. Bull.* **5**:575.
22. Marwitt, R., Pilar, G., and Weakly, J. N., 1971, Characterization of two ganglion cell populations in avian ciliary ganglia, *Brain Res.* **25**:317.
23. Barald, K. F., and Berg, D. K., 1979, Ciliary ganglion neurons in cell culture: High affinity choline uptake and autoradiographic choline labeling, *Dev. Biol.* **72**:15.
24. Helfand, S. L., Smith, G. A., and Wessells, N. K., 1976, Survival and development in culture of dissociated parasympathetic neurons from ciliary ganglia, *Dev. Biol.* **50**:541.
25. Nishi, R., and Berg, D. K., 1977, Dissociated ciliary ganglion neurons *in vitro*: Survival and synapse formation, *Proc. Natl. Acad. Sci. U.S.A.* **74**:5171.
26. Barald, K., 1981, Cell surface specific monoclonal antibodies to chick ciliary ganglion neurons, *Soc. Neurosci. Abstr.*, Vol. **7**:120.
27. Newgreen, D. F., Ritterman, M., and Peters, E. A., 1979, Morphology and behavior of neural crest cells of chick embryo *in vitro, Cell Tissue Res.* **203**:115.
28. Cohen, A. M., 1977, Independent expression of the adrenergic phenotype by neural crest cells *in vitro, Proc. Natl. Acad. Sci. U.S.A.* **74**:2899.
29. Norr, S. G., 1973, *In vitro* analysis of sympathetic neuron differentiation from chick neural crest cells, *Dev. Biol.* **34**:16.
30. Oi, V. T., and Herzenberg, L. A., 1980, Immunoglobulin producing hybrid cell lines, in: *Selected Methods in Cellular Immunology* (B. B. Mishell and S. M. Shiigi, eds.), pp. 351–372, W. H. Freeman, San Francisco.
31. Robertson, S. M., Mayfield, G., and Kettman, J. R., 1980, The use of polyclonal activators in the generation of monoclonal antibodies, *Microbiology* 1980. (D. Schlessinger, ed.), pp. 181–185. Washington.
32. Kohler, G. and Milstein, C., 1976, Derivation of specific antibody-producing tissue culture and tumor lines by cell fusion, *Eur. J. Immunol.* **6**:511.
33. Barald, K. F., and Berg, D. K., 1979, Autoradiographic labeling of spinal cord neurons with high affinity choline uptake in cell culture, *Dev. Biol.* **72**:1.
34. D'Amico-Martel, A., and Noden, D. M., 1980, An autoradiographic analysis of the development of the chick trigeminal ganglion, *J. Embryol. Exp. Morphol.* **55**:167.
35. Sorimachi, M., and Kataoka, K., 1974, Developmental change of choline acetyltransferase and acetylcholinesterase in the ciliary and the superior cervical ganglion of the chick, *Brain Res.* **70**:123.
36. Pettman, B., Louis, J. C., and Sensenbrenner, M., 1979, Morphological and biochemical maturation of neurons cultured in the absence of glial cells, *Nature* (*London*) **281**:378.
37. Le Douarin, N. M., Teillet, M. A., Ziller, C., and Smith, J., 1978, Adrenergic differentiation of the cholinergic ciliary and Remak ganglia in avian embryo after *in vivo* transplantation, *Proc. Natl. Acad. Sci. U.S.A.* **75**:2030.

38. McCarthy, K. D., and Partlow, L., 1976, Preparation of pure neuronal and non-neuronal cultures from embryonic chick sympathetic ganglia: A new method based on both differential cell adhesiveness and the formation of homotypic neuronal aggregates, *Brain Res.* **114**:391.
39. Barald, K. F., and Berg, D. K., 1978, High affinity choline uptake by spinal cord neurons in dissociated cell culture, *Dev. Biol.* **65**:90.
40. Tsu, T. T., and Herzenberg, L. A., 1980, Solid phase radioimmune assays, in: *Selected Methods in Cellular Immunology* (B. B. Mishell and S. M. Shiigi, eds.), pp. 373–397, W. H. Freeman, San Francisco.
41. Stocker, J. W., and Heusser, C. H., 1979, Methods for binding cells to plastic: Application to a solid-phase radioimmunoassay for cell-surface antigens, *J. Immunol. Methods* **26**:87.
42. Mather, E. L., 1980, Double antibody radioimmunoassay for the quantitation of cellular proteins, in: *Selected Methods in Cellular Immunology* (B. B. Mishell and S. M. Shiigi, eds.), pp. 307–324, W. H. Freeman, San Francisco.
43. Godding, J. W., 1978, Use of staphylococcal protein A as an immunological reagent, *J. Immunol. Methods* **20**:241.
44. Heggeness, M. H., and Ash, J. F., 1977, Use of the avidin-biotin complex for the localization of actin and myosin with fluorescence microscopy, *J. Cell. Biol.* **73**:783.
45. Cuello, A. C., Galfre, G., and Milstein, C., 1979, Detection of substance P in the central nervous system by a monoclonal antibody, *Proc. Natl. Acad. Sci. U.S.A.* **76**:3532.
46. Chan-Palay, V., 1979, Immunocytochemical detection of substance P-neurons, their processes and connections by *in vivo* microinjections of monoclonal antibodies, *Anat. Embryol.* **156**:225.
47. Howard, J. C., Butcher, G. W., Licence, D. R., Galfre, G., Wright, B. and Milstein, C., 1980, Isolation of six monoclonal antibodies against rat histocompatibility antigens: clonal competition, *Immunology* **41**:131.
48. Howard, J. C., Butcher, G. W., Galfre, G., Milstein, C., and Milstein, C. P., 1979, Monoclonal antibodies as tools to analyze the serological and genetic complexities of major transplantation antigens, *Immunol. Rev.* **47**:139.
49. Cohen, A. M., and Konigsberg, I. R., 1975, A clonal approach to the problem of neural crest determination, *Dev. Biol.* **46**:262.
50. Le Douarin, N. M., 1977, The differentiation of the ganglioblasts of the autonomic nervous system studied in chimaeric avian embryos, in: *Cell Interactions in Differentiation* (M. Karkinen-Jaaskelainen, L. Saxen, and L. Weiss, eds.), pp. 171–190, Academic Press, London.
51. Le Douarin, N. M., 1980, The ontogeny of the neural crest in avian embryo chimaeras. *Nature* (*London*) **286**:663.
52. Smith, J., Fauquet, M., Ziller, C., and Le Douarin, N. M., 1979, Acetylcholine synthesis by mesencephalic neural crest cells in the process of migration *in vivo, Nature* (*London*) **282**:853.
53. Rothman, T. P., Gershon, M. D., and Holtzer, H., 1978, The relationship of cell division to the acquisition of adrenergic characteristics by developing sympathetic ganglion cell precursors, *Dev. Biol.* **65**:322.

4

Genetic Manipulation of Sensory Pathways in *Drosophila*

JOHN PALKA

1. INTRODUCTION

1.1. *Levels of Analysis*

Like the other investigators contributing to this volume, I want to understand how nervous systems develop. Such a broad question can be approached on at least three levels of analysis: (1) the description of developmental events as they occur over time; (2) the formulation of rules—regularities of cellular behavior revealed by perturbation experiments; and (3) the identification of molecular mechanisms which underlie the rules.

These levels of analysis are all necessary. One obviously cannot describe mechanisms for events whose existence is not yet known; a detailed cellular description of developmental events is required. Rules reveal the range of functions or capabilities which mechanisms should explain. For example, suppose that cell A normally only synapses with cell B. If B is unavailable A may (1) form no synapses at all, (2) show a graded preference for C more than D more than E, or (3) synapse haphazardly. Different mechanisms would need to be invoked to explain these alternative behaviors, so knowing the rules aids in the search for mechanisms and helps us sort between plausible and unlikely ones.

JOHN PALKA · Department of Zoology, University of Washington, Seattle, WA 98195.

Knowing just the rules, however, without the mechanisms, is incomplete and unsatisfying. If we know the rule that a muscle fiber normally innervated only by a single axon from a particular source will accept a foreign axon when the original one is cut, how could we not wonder why this is, what mechanisms underlie such specific cellular behavior? (See Chapter 10.)

1.2. *Advantages of Different Organisms*

Different organisms offer special advantages for studies using particular techniques or aimed at different levels of analysis. For example, leeches have been used for elegant descriptions of very early events in embryogenesis, because their cells are large and can be injected with stable and noninjurious marker materials so that the structures to which they give rise can be identified (see Chapter 1). The neuroblasts and freshly formed neurons of grasshoppers have been studied intensively because they are accessible to both electrophysiological and dye injection techniques, and a rather detailed chronological account of their anatomical, physiological, and pharmacological development has been provided (see Chapter 5). Young mammals respond especially well to Golgi techniques, and a rich literature on mammalian neural development dates back to Ramón y Cajal.[1] Such a list of examples could be extended (see also Chapter 2), and is in the best tradition of developmental biology.

Among the techniques potentially available to an experimental biologist are genetic ones. As a practical matter, however, their use is especially narrowly restricted to particular species; in fact there are only three in which diverse genetic tools can currently be applied to the study of developmental neurobiology: the nematode worm *Caenorhabditis elegans*,[2] the fruit fly *Drosophila melanogaster*,[3] and the mouse *Mus musculus*.[4] In this group *Drosophila* is intermediate in size and complexity. The available repertoire of genetic variants and techniques is the widest. It has been studied intensively by developmental biologists, often using genetic methods and applying genetic thinking and models to developmental problems, and this background enriches studies on the nervous system. It is a large enough animal to permit the use of standard light-microscopic techniques and small enough to be convenient for work with the electron microscope in both transmission and scanning modes. Electrophysiology is easy in many of its muscle cells, and feasible though difficult in a variety of neurons. Methods for cell and tissue culture have been worked out, and a good deal is known of the endocrine influences on development. Thus, in spite of real limitations imposed by the small size of its nerve cells, it has proved to be a suitable species for studies in developmental neurobiology at all three levels of analysis, and it offers the special opportunity of genetic manipulation. During the past several years my laboratory has sought to exploit this special opportunity.

1.3. *What Understanding Can We Gain from Genetic Manipulation?*

There is a dispute among students of development, including developmental neurobiology, about basic goals. Everyone agrees that genetic variants and techniques provide useful *tools* for analyzing biological processes, including development. However, it has also been argued that a basic *goal* of developmental studies with genetic techniques is to understand how genes control development.[5] The extreme alternative view has recently been championed by Stent,[6,7] who believes that such a goal is misconceived because the relationship between the synthesis of a polypeptide directed by a gene and the acquisition of ordered form and function is very remote and indirect. To repeat his favorite example, we know that albinos lack melanin, usually because in these animals the tyrosinase gene does not function properly. But knowing in great detail the biochemistry of albinism does not explain why a lack of tyrosinase or of melanin results in the abnormal crossing of some ganglion cell axons at the optic chiasm, let alone explain the normal role of the tyrosinase gene in neural development. The important events to understand are the molecular and cellular interactions that follow the direct action of genes, which is merely to encode the primary structure of polypeptides.

This view highlights an old issue. Waddington, for example, articulated it in his classic textbook.[8] He described the manipulative approach of experimental embryology and the genetic approach as quite different but complementary, and advocated making the best use of both, a position which I wholeheartedly endorse:

> The science of genetics has clearly shown that when an animal differs from nearly related forms, the nature of these differences is nearly always controlled by genes carried on its chromosomes. It is clear then that genes must be amongst the most important causal entities which play a role in guiding development. We have so far discussed the question of why an organ, such as a limb, develops as it does in terms such as organisers, fields, competence, etc. Genetics, following a quite different mode of analysis, formulates its answer to the same question in a quite different way. It finds that the development of the organ is dependent on the activities of certain genes in the fertilized egg. The task [of this chapter] is to present the picture of the development of an organ or tissue as seen in terms of genes. This will provide

a view of the epigenetic system which we must take as being complementary to that derived from experimental embryology.

I suggest that an operational criterion can be applied to decide whether the genetic approach has contributed more than tools. It has often been said that a theory is useful if it generates experiments. Let us examine whether developmental theories formulated in genetic terms have led to *experiments which reveal previously unknown and unexpected attributes of developmental processes.* Further, let us ask whether new, testable hypotheses about development have been formulated because of studies with genetic techniques, specifically *hypotheses which could not have been derived from surgical and other nongenetic experiments.* I will argue that the answer to both questions is yes: new, revealing experiments have been done because questions about the action of genes have been asked; and genetic experiments have led to new, testable hypotheses which are different in kind from those based on simple observation, surgical intervention, and other nongenetic techniques.

2. THE EXPERIMENTAL MATERIAL

In order to take serious advantage of genetic materials and methods in developmental neurobiology, it is obviously first necessary to become familiar with them. This section presents just a glimpse of what is possible: a few mutants and a few techniques for producing genetic mosaics, together with an argument for why studies on mosaics are essential in the genetic analysis of developing nervous systems.

2.1. *Mutants*

We start with a consideration of the material available for study in *Drosophila*—a constantly increasing library of mutants in which form and/or function has been altered in ways potentially useful to the investigator.

2.1.1. The Richness of the Material. The number of genes in the genome of *Drosophila* has been estimated at 5000–10,000.[9] The catalogue of Lindsley and Grell[10] lists mutations at over 1000 loci, most of them recognizable by external inspection and hence having some effect on the form of the animal. This large number is reasurring in that it represents a significant fraction of the total, but is also bewildering. How can one make a rational approach to such diversity?

2.1.2. Some Classes of Mutations. Classifying at least some of the hundreds of mutants available from various laboratories and stock centers helps in choosing the right material for experiments—an ordered list is much easier to keep in mind than a random list.

A classification of mutants also prompts us to think about the role which the corresponding wild-type alleles might play in development, indirect though such an inference is. By analogy with bacterial systems, we would expect that not all genes have functions of equal logical value: structural genes encode the amino acid sequence of enzymes and other proteins with a direct role in cell metabolism or structure, but the task of regulatory genes is to control the operation of the structural genes. There are some aspects of a hierarchical or branching organization in the genome of *E. coli*. It is rapidly becoming clear that genetic control mechanisms in all eukaryotes including *Drosophila* are much more elaborate than in prokaryotes, and we do not yet understand them in any detail. But for our present purposes it is sufficient to state the presumption that different genes will prove to occupy different levels in the thus far unknown logical tree which relates the genome of the fly to its form.

Trying to deduce the wild-type roles of genes by studying mutants is somewhat similar to making guesses about evolution by studying modern organisms. For example, we cannot firmly establish the evolutionary relationships among the animal phyla by studying only living animals, but such a study does provide clues to past events. Similarly, studying the phenotype of an animal one of whose 10,000 genes is not working properly does not directly reveal how that phenotype came about during development. However, studying mutants according to the kind of effect seen in the phenotype gives clues to the control functions through which genes might determine biological form. The following highly abbreviated classification is adapted from García-Bellido.[11]

2.1.2.a. Mutations Affecting Mitotic Rate. Mutations at many loci on all the chromosomes of *Drosophila* produce a slowing of the rate of cell division. The adult flies look normal except that many of their bristles are more slender or perhaps shorter than usual, but the time required for development is much increased. These *Minute* mutations are very useful as an adjunct to the technique of clonal analysis, described below. In addition, mutations have been described which seem to influence the orientation of mitotic spindles or the relative probability of cell division occurring in different planes.

2.1.2.b. Mutations Affecting Cellular Differentiation. The visible external structures of flies are made of a chitinous cuticle secreted by epidermal cells. The pattern of secretion can be modified in various ways. For example, in the mutant *multiple wing hairs* (*mwh*) each epidermal cell that should produce a single hairlike process produces several (Fig. 1); in the mutant *forked* (*f*) the sensory bristles, whose shafts are likewise secreted by single cells, are branched rather than simple; in *yellow* (*y*) the pigmentation of the cuticle is altered.

How such effects are brought about is not known in most cases, but all these mutations share an important property—*cell autonomy*. Individual cells either do or do not express the mutant phenotype according to their own genotype, independently of the genotype of other cells in the animal. Thus, for example, a single cell which is homozygous mutant for *multiple wing hairs* (mwh^-/mwh^-) will produce mutant cuticle even if it is surrounded by a sea of cells which are heterozygous (mwh^-/mwh^+) and therefore produce normal cuticle. Cell autonomy enables us to use these mutations as markers in mosaic experiments (see Section 2.2 below), a technical feature of great importance.

2.1.2.c. Mutations Affecting Developmental Pathways. In contrast to the mutations just described, recognized by the abnormal appearance of a cuticular product of a specific epidermal cell, there are others in which the secretion products are well made but inappropriately located.

The best examples are the *homeotic mutations* in which entire complex structures assume a form appropriate to some other part of the body (for extensive reviews, see Postlethwait and Schneiderman[12]; Ouweneel[13]). For example, in *Antennapedia* a leg develops in the location normally occupied by an antenna (Fig. 2); in *Ophthalmoptera* part of what should be the compound eye develops as a wing; and in *bithoraxoid* the

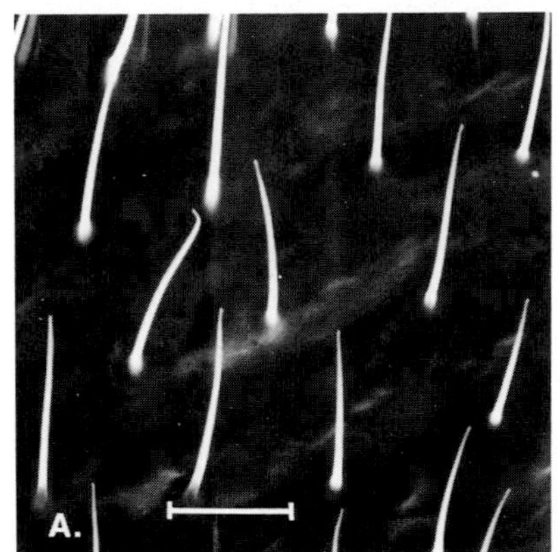

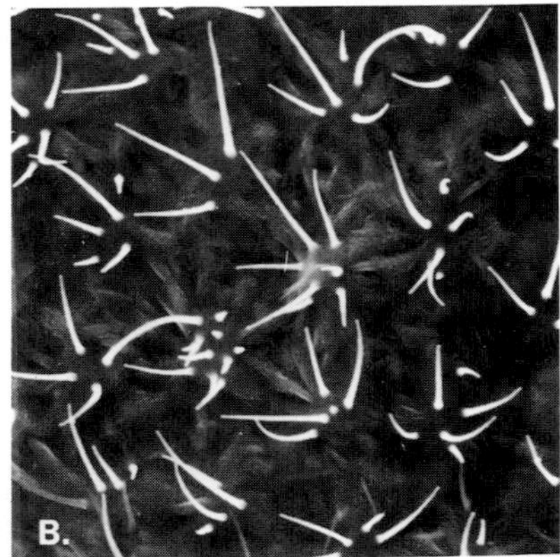

Figure 1. Scanning electron micrographs of cuticle in a mosaic wing. (A) Cells which are mwh^-/mwh^+ produce a single hairlike process or trichome whose morphology is indistinguishable from that in wild-type flies. (B) Cells which are mwh^-/mwh^- because of mitotic recombination produce starbursts of several trichomes per cell. Scale, 10μm.

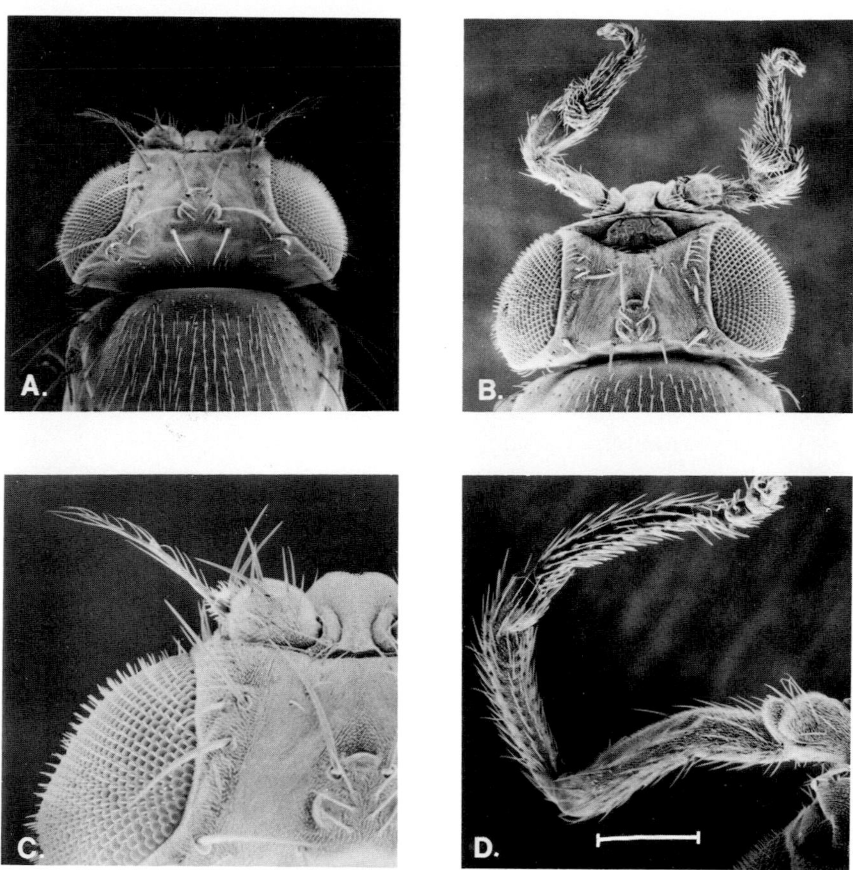

Figure 2. Head morphology. (A) Dorsal view of the head of a wild-type fly. (B) Dorsal view of the head of an *Antennapedia* fly ($Antp^-/Antp^-$). (C) A higher-magnification view of the eye and normal antenna. (D) A higher magnification view showing the details of the homeotic appendage, a well-formed mesothoracic leg. Scale, 150 μm (A, B); 300 μm (C, D).

first abdominal segment displays modified hind legs and halteres, indicating that it has assumed a thoracic quality but with mixed meta- and mesothoracic attributes. The novel structures are very well formed: there is no question of their morphological identification, and the cuticular pattern elements, such as various bristles, are well developed and appropriate to the overall structure. Intermediate or novel cuticular structures do occur, but only rarely. This either/or character of the homeotic phenotypes underlies much of the current speculation that these mutations affect "genetic switches," genes whose products regulate the activities of many other genes in a coordinated fashion. The activity of the entire regulated set ultimately results in the production of one out of a limited set of alternative forms.

2.2. *Mosaics*

A genetic mosaic is an organism constructed of cells of more than one genotype. Mosaics have been known and studied both for their own sake and as tools in other investigations since long before the present century. Stern[14] presents a masterful and engaging account of the biology of mosaics and the history of their study.

2.2.1. *The Importance of Mosaics in Developmental Neurobiology.* There is a simple reason why mosaic animals are essential in studies on neural development in which the manipulation of genotypes is an integral part of the experimental design. If an animal is mutant, all of its cells are mutant, and any of them may express one effect or another of the mutation. Until direct evidence is provided to the contrary, we must assume this as the probable case.

In many of my own studies, as well as those from other laboratories, the central questions revolve around the establishment of neural pathways and synaptic relationships. Mutants are employed to perturb the developing system, changing the normal relationship between axons, their growth substrates, and their targets. If one and the same mutation affects the growing cells, its targets, and the cells which it bypasses or upon whose surfaces it grows, the observed result cannot be interpreted in any detail. It is like trying to solve a single equation in four unknowns. Critical studies seeking to take advantage of genetic mutations must find ways to deal with this built-in ambiguity.

The phenotypic effects of some mutations do appear to be limited to discrete parts of the body. Unfortunately, appearances can be deceiving, especially since most mutants have been described on the basis of characteristics easily seen under a dissecting or, at best, a compound microscope. This does not include neural connections, and thus the information essential to a neurobiologist is generally not available.

A much safer procedure is to study genetic mosaics in which only one set of cells in the system of interest is mutant and the remainder are wild type. It may then be possible to link any change in neural development to the effect of the mutation, though, as we will see below, the details of the argument may still be complex.

2.2.2. *Types of Mosaics.* Mosaics having applications in studies of neural development can be produced in several ways. The following classification is taken from an earlier summary.[15]

2.2.2.a. Gynandromorphs. These are individuals containing both male and female tissues. They occur occasionally in natural populations and were historically the first kind of mosaic to be studied. They can arise in a variety of ways, and the prevalent mechanisms differ according to species (see Stern[14]). A detailed account of gynandromorphs and other types of genetic mosaics in *Drosophila* is given by Hall *et al.*[16]

In neurobiology the value of a gynandromorph may lie directly in the segregation of male and female territories, as in studies of neural and hormonal influences on reproductive behavior (e.g., Hall *et al.*[17]). It may also lie in the simultaneous segregation of cells carrying a particular genotype of interest. If a recessive allele is located on the X chromosome and the XX zygote is heterozygous, cells in the female territory will express the dominant allele; but cells in the male territory, being XO, may express the recessive allele. For example, the mutation *hairy* results in the overproduction of sensory bristles and sensilla campaniformia (s.c.) (sensory structures illustrated in Fig. 8). In a gynandromorph whose male–female line coincides with the midline, one side of the CNS would receive several times as many sensory axons as the other; other individuals might have extra axons in one segment but not another. Such animals could prove useful in studies of the consequences of hyperinnervation or of competition.

2.2.2.b. Grafts. Grafts in insects can be made between individuals of the same species, different species, and even more or less distantly related genera. They can be made at any stage of development including the adult, though the best integration of donor and host tissues occurs in young animals. Grafting in *Drosophila* is not easy but can be done following the method developed for much larger flies by Bhaskaran and Sivasubramanian[18]; appendages such as wings, halteres, and legs can be made to grow in various places on the abdomen (M. Schubiger, unpublished). The graft can come from an animal of genotype different from the host, so that a genetic mosaic is produced by surgical methods.

2.2.2.c. Mitotic Recombination Mosaics. Genetic recombination normally occurs during meiosis when homologous chromosomes pair intimately and physical exchange of pieces of sister chromatids can occur. In some animals, including *Drosophila*, recombination can also occur during ordinary mitotic divisions, perhaps because pairing of homologous chromosomes also occurs during mitosis. The spontaneous frequency of such recombination events is extremely low, but can be greatly increased by X-irradiation. In a suitable stock, mitotic recombination will give rise to a recognizable genetic mosaic. It is a considerable advantage that, within reasonably wide limits, the time at which the potential effects of a difference in genotype will start to take effect is set by the time of irradiation and is thus under experimental control.

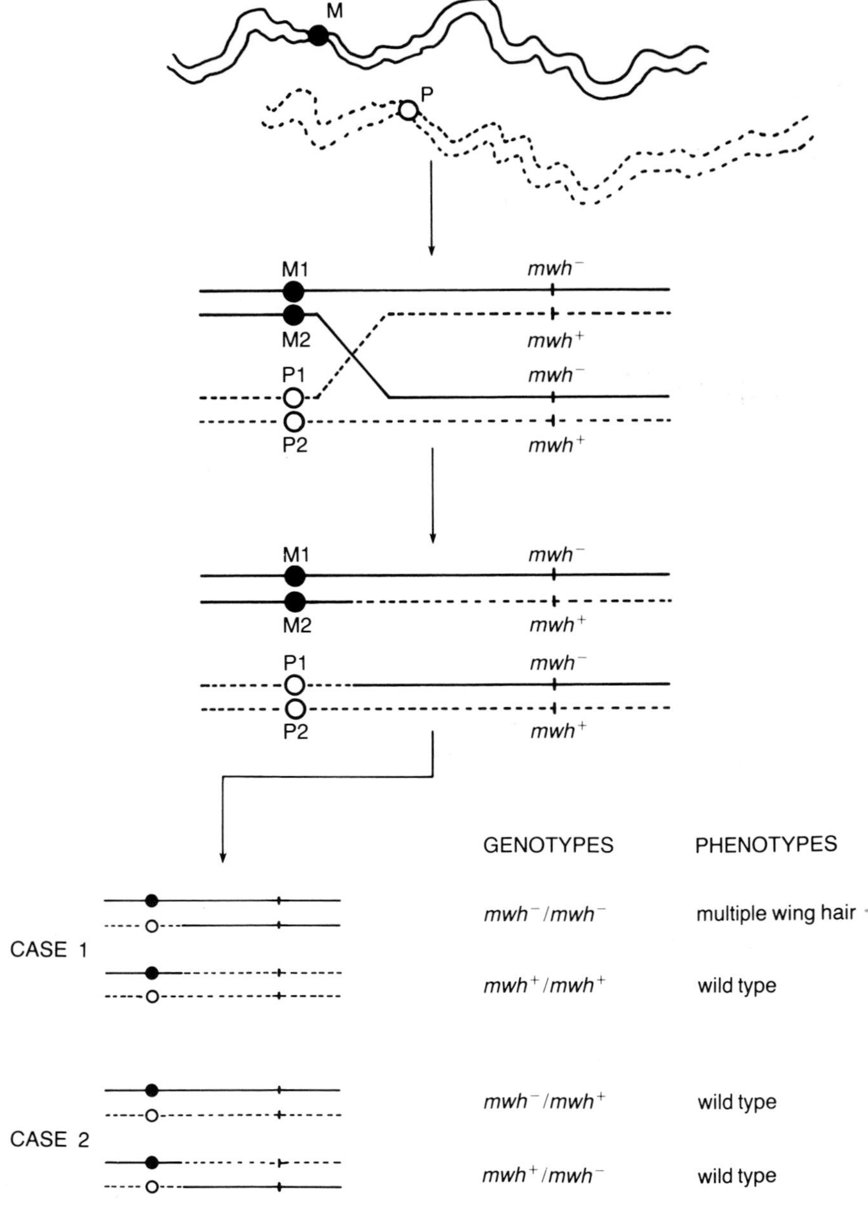

Figure 3. Mitotic recombination. During mitosis in *Drosophila*, homologous chromosomes pair and exchange pieces of their chromatids. This occurs with highest probability close to the centromere. When the chromatids segregate, two pairings are possible: an intact and a recombined chromosome in each daughter cell (m_1p_1 and m_2p_2, Case 1 in the figure);

This has been an extremely important technique in developmental studies, so I have illustrated it in considerable detail in the example of Fig. 3. We start with a fly heterozygous for a recessive mutation such as *multiple wing hairs* (mwh^-/mwh^+); the phenotype, of course, is wild type. It is believed, by analogy with meiosis, that once DNA replication has occurred in a cell preparing to divide, the new chromatids can intertwine, form chiasmata, and exchange pieces at one or several points. This occurs preferentially close to the centromere. If exchange does take place, the possibility for recombination of the alleles of interest is established. In the scheme of Fig. 3, if the chromatids assort so that centromeres m_1 and p_1 (derived from the maternal and paternal homologues respectively) go to one daughter nucleus and m_2 and p_2 go to the other, the resulting genotypes will be mwh^-/mwh^- (recognizable by the multiple wing hair phenotype) and mwh^+/mwh^+ (wild-type phenotype and hence not distinguishable from the original heterozygous condition). If the other possible combination occurs, m_1 and p_2 to one daughter, m_2 and p_1 to the other, the occurrence of recombination will not be recognized.

Suppose that detectable recombination does in fact occur. Then the progeny of the homozygous recessive daughter cell will constitute a clone of a genotype different from that of the rest of the fly, so a genetic mosaic will have been produced at a known time and made visible for study. With suitable markers the other, simultaneously produced clone can also be made visible, yielding a so-called twin spot. See Becker[19] for a detailed review of this technique.

In many cases it is important to have very large clones. These can be produced with the aid of *Minute* mutations[20] (Section 2.1.2.a). The principle of the method is to start with a fly which is not only heterozygous for the recessive mutation of which a homozygous clone is desired, but is also heterozygous for a *Minute*. Inasmuch as the *Minutes* are dominant, all the cells of the fly will divide at a slow rate. If the selected *Minute* is located close to the recessive allele being studied, then the same recombination event which produces a homozygous recessive cell will simultaneously produce a cell lacking the *Minute*, and hence dividing at a normal rather than a reduced rate. This gives the

---

or two originals and two recombinants (m_1p_2 and m_2p_1, Case 2 in the figure). In case 1 a cell homozygous for the recessive mutation is generated, and it and its progeny are made visible; case 2 would pass undetected. In this scheme, if mwh^- is on a maternal chromosome which also carries a wild-type allele of a *Minute* (M^+), and the paternal chromosome carries mwh^+ and a dominant *Minute* allele (M^-), the m_1p_1 daughter cell will be not only mwh^-/mwh^- but also M^+/M^+, and hence will have a growth advantage over the M^-/M^+ or M^-/M^- cells.

clone a growth advantage which can be very strong. In the wing, as we shall see, nearly half of the whole appendage can be a clone derived from a single cell.

2.2.2.d. Temporal Mosaics. A number of mutations have the property that they are expressed at some temperatures but not at others. Temperature-sensitive (TS) alleles of many apparently unrelated genes are known. If a fly carries such a mutation, it can be raised for part of its life so that the mutation is not expressed, then shifted to a new temperature which permits the expression of the mutation. Thus, the animal can be thought of as a mosaic in time rather than space. A detailed account of TS mutations is given by Suzuki *et al.*[21]

3. A THEORETICAL FRAMEWORK

3.1. *Binary Decisions*

Several phenomena in the development of *Drosophila* exhibit an either-or character, in that the cells in a given place form either one structure or another, but not something in between or totally novel. Kauffman[22] suggested that the determination of a cell is the result of the combined binary states (0 or 1, on or off) of a small set of biochemical switches, and reversing one of those switches causes the cell to assume an alternate but equally specific determination. The primary data for this model came from studies of the phenomenon of transdetermination, which we will not discuss here (see the review of Hadorn[23]), but the general idea appears also in the analysis of homeotic transformations and the theory of compartmentalization. In fact, all of the current models seeking to explain homeosis and compartmentalization employ the basic notion of binary decision making (see Kauffman *et al.*[24]).

Homeosis and compartmentalization are phenomena that have played a major role in the neurobiological studies, in my laboratory as well as in several others, that form the substance of this chapter. The following sections provide a framework of data and theory from general developmental biology for the neurobiological results and interpretations of Sections 4, 5, and 6.

3.2. *The Bithorax Complex*

Most of the genes whose mutations result in homeotic effects on thoracic and abdominal segments are clustered close together in a small region of the right arm of the third chromosome. This cluster is known as the bithorax complex (BX-C); it has been studied by Lewis in a classic series of papers[5,25–33] and more recently by a number of other investigators.

3.2.1. *Its Characteristics.* The phenotypes of animals with mutations in this region, a number of which are schematized in Fig. 4, include the following:

anterobithorax (*abx*):	anterior metathorax → anterior mesothorax, hence anterior haltere → anterior wing
bithorax (*bx*):	similar to *anterobithorax*
postbithorax (*pbx*):	posterior metathorax → posterior mesothorax, hence posterior haltere → posterior wing
Contrabithorax (*Cbx*):	mesothorax partially → metathorax, hence wing → haltere
bithoraxoid (*bxd*):	first abdominal segment → metathorax/mesothorax, and metathorax partially → mesothorax
Hyperabdominal (*Hab*):	metathorax and first abdominal → second abdominal
Ultrabdominal (*Uab*):	first and second abdominal partially → third abdominal

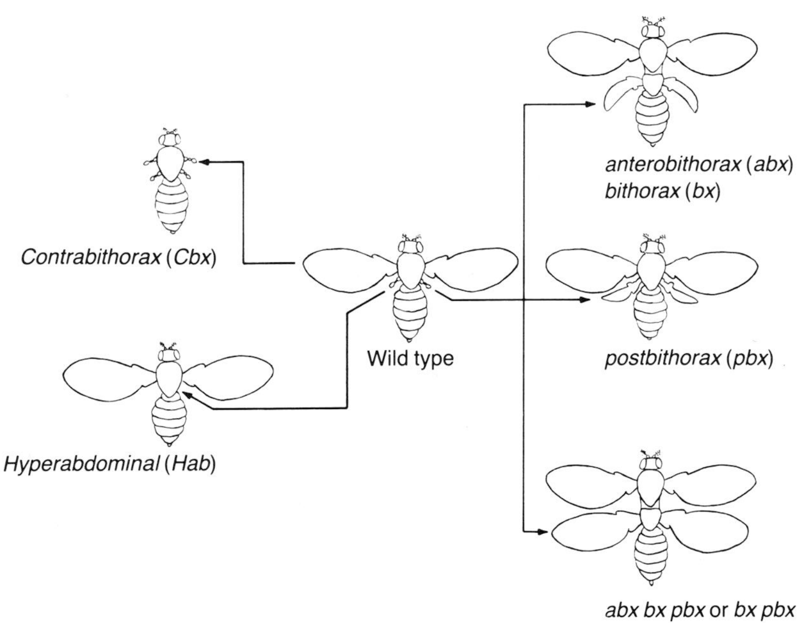

Figure 4. Mutants of the bithorax complex.

The genes occur very close together, the known map distances between them all being 0.01 map units or less. Since they are so closely linked and have related functions, they fit the definition of a complex locus or a pseudoallelic series. Their effects appear to be more or less additive, and multiple mutants can be spectacular (Fig. 5).

3.2.2. Its Possible Evolution. What might be the significance of such a tight cluster of genes whose mutations all effect alterations in segment morphology? Lewis[25] proposed the following evolutionary/developmental viewpoint. Suppose that the ancestral insect had a series of segments that were all alike (as are the segments of modern annelids or millipedes), and that each segment had both legs and dorsal, winglike appendages. In order to make any given segment different from this mesothoracic-like archetype, one or several genes were required whose products, through an unknown series of steps, suppressed the wings and/or legs in a segment-limited fashion. These are what we know as the genes of the BX-C. When they fail to function because of a mutation, the segment(s) which they influence tend to revert toward the archetypal mesothoracic state. Where did these genes come from? They arose by repeated duplication of an ancestral gene, and subsequent mutation giving the duplicates new functions; this is why they are so close together.

This argument predicts that if the whole BX-C were lacking, all the segments of the fly would look like mesothorax. The prediction can be tested, because long after the theory was formulated a physical deletion

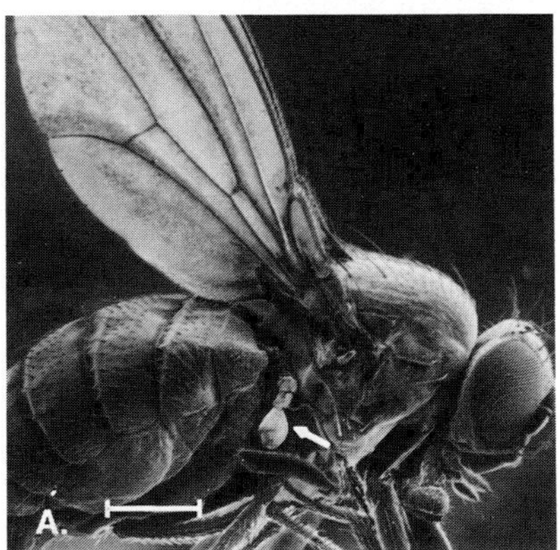

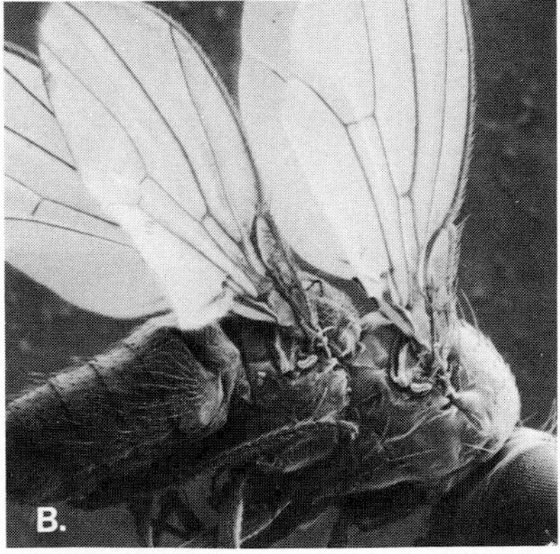

Figure 5. Scanning electron micrographs showing side view of (A) a wild type and (B) a four-winged fly of the genotype *abx* bx^3 *pbx*/*abx* bx^3 *pbx*. The haltere indicated by the arrow in (A) is absent in (B), and a virtually perfect wing has grown in its place. Scale, 500 μm.

of the entire BX-C region was obtained. Flies homozygous for the deletion die as late embryos or early first instar larvae. However, it is possible to distinguish one segment from another in the larvae, and the evidence is that all the segments except at the head and at the tip of the abdomen are indeed mesothoracic.[32]

3.2.3. How Does It Function in Development? How are these dramatic manipulations of segment quality brought about? Lewis has supposed that each gene codes for some substance, and that these substances act indirectly but in additive fashion to influence morphology. In any given segment some of the genes are repressed and others derepressed; the corresponding substances are absent or present, and the combination establishes the quality of the segment. A detailed model predicting precisely which genes should be on and which off in each segment is given by Lewis.[32,33]

What mechanism determines which genes shall be on and which off in a given segment? That is unknown, and unspecified in the theory. However, it is often supposed that molecules differentially distributed in the cortex of the egg, and hence influenced by the mother's ovarian tissue and genotype, are involved.[33–36]

3.2.4. Its Relevance to Neurobiology. For a neurobiologist, the central message is that a small number of genes in a well-defined cluster have profound and systematic influences on the differentiation of thoracic and abdominal segments from each other. The mutations of these genes cause selective alterations in the external morphology of particular segments, and concomitant changes in the arrays of receptors found on those segments. In effect, specific receptors are caused to differentiate in places where they normally would not, and their axons are found to enter the CNS at abnormal points.

At first glance this looks simply like a convenient, nontraumatic equivalent of transplantation—for example, of wings into the location of halteres. I will argue later, however, that this is only a partial picture and that other phenomena, which do not have direct surgical parallels, also occur.

3.3. The Antennapedia Complex

Evidence has recently been presented[37] that another cluster of genes on the third chromosome influences head and thoracic segments, somewhat as the BX-C influences thoracic and abdominal segments. This cluster has been named the Antennapedia complex (ANT-C), by analogy with the BX-C.

3.3.1. Its Characteristics. The following phenotypes exemplify the effects of mutations in this region:

proboscipedia (*pb*):	proboscis → distal prothoracic leg (raised at 28°) or → arista of antenna (17°)
Antennapedia (*Antp*):	antenna → mesothoracic leg (Fig. 2)
Multiple Sex Combs (*Msc*):	prothoracic leg → mesothoracic leg and meso- and metathoracic legs → prothoracic legs

Detailed genetic and developmental studies suggest a number of similarities between the ANT-C and BX-C, beyond a close clustering of homeotic genes.[38] How the two complexes interact with each other is not apparent at this time.

3.3.2. Common Features of the BX-C and ANT-C. There is no doubt that as additional work is done on both complexes, many surprises will be revealed. For the moment I want to emphasize the following points: (1) Nearly every segment of the fly can be changed quite specifically to some other segment by an already known homeotic mutation. (2) The homeotic genes are collected into clusters. (3) The clustering may reflect the evolutionary origin of the genes. (4) It affects the regulatory relationships among them, a point I have not discussed here but which helps to explain why some of the mutations are dominant and some recessive, and why not all of them produce transformations toward mesothorax.

3.4. Compartments

We have thus far considered genetic influences on segmental phenotypes. It has been argued that subsegmental regions called compartments are also under the control of small numbers of genes.[39–42]

3.4.1. The Operational Definition of Compartments. A compartment is a region whose boundaries, unlike those of a segment, cannot be seen by simple inspection. Compartment boundaries often occur in regions where no particular cuticular structures lead one to suspect a boundary of any sort. If its boundaries cannot be seen, how is the presence of a compartment established? By observing the boundaries of mitotic recombination clones. It is found empirically that clones initiated by a recombination event at a given time in development, and given a growth advantage by the *Minute* technique, may have any location and shape except that they do not cross certain lines. Some of these are segment boundaries, but others are not.

The location of the intrasegmental lines depends upon the time of induction of the clone. Clones can be induced by X-ray treatment as early as the blastoderm stage, when the embryo consists of just a single layer of cells at the surface of what used to be the egg. Even when induced at this early time, with most of the cell divisions producing adult structures still to take place, clones are observed not to cross a line which separates each thoracic segment into two regions, anterior and posterior (Fig. 6), even though they can include a large dorsoventral territory extending from the wing, say, through the thorax and onto the mesothoracic leg. Clones induced later are found to be confined to the wing and dorsal thorax, or leg and ventral thorax, as well as to the anterior or posterior hemisegment. In the wing, though not in the leg, still later clones are confined to still smaller areas.

3.4.2. The Developmental Role of Compartments. This behavior of clones defines compartments and compartment boundaries. It is natural to ask why intrasegmental compartments should exist. What is their function? An important suggestion has been that they are the territories of action of homeotic genes. For example, the *bithorax* mutation trans-

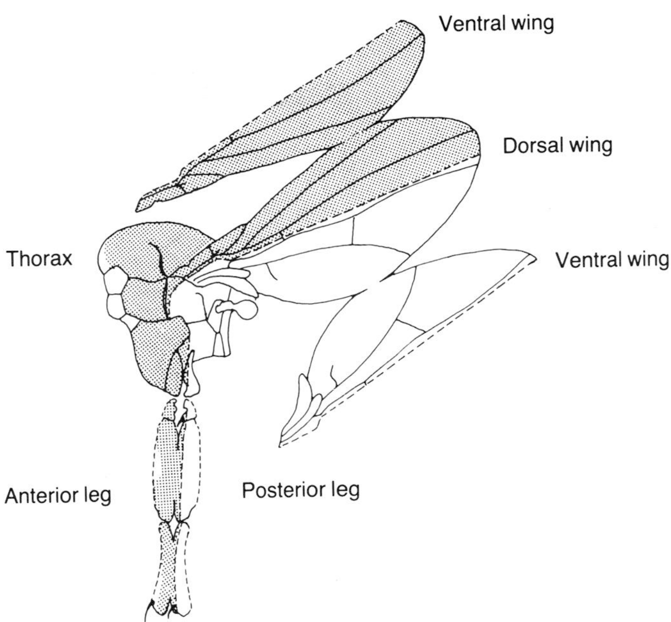

Figure 6. Very large clone (shaded) induced by X-irradiation during the blastoderm stage of the embryo and enhanced by the *Minute* technique. The clone includes virtually the entire anterior compartment—on both surfaces of the wing, on the thorax, and on the mesothoracic leg. The metathoracic segment bearing the haltere is not affected. From Steiner.[43]

forms not an arbitrary anterior region of the haltere into anterior wing, but precisely the anterior compartment as defined by clone marking experiments. Likewise, the *postbithorax* mutation transforms precisely the posterior compartment of the haltere into a posterior wing compartment.

There are also mutations which cause the substitution of structures within single segments. These have been interpreted as causing the homeotic transformation of one compartment of a given segment into a mirror image duplicate of its sibling compartment. Thus, the mutation *engrailed* introduces anterior wing structures into the posterior regions of the wing, and has been interpreted as being a homeotic mutation which transforms the posterior compartment into a second anterior one.[44,45] The *wingless* mutation eliminates the wing (or haltere) and replaces it with a duplication of part of the thorax; it has been interpreted as transforming a wing (or haltere) compartment into a second thoracic compartment.[46]

According to the compartment theory, a group of cells which are all alike at some point in development becomes subdivided into two populations which differ only in that a particular gene is switched on in one of them and switched off in the other. This gene is called a selector gene because its function is to select which of many other genes will be active in that compartment and which will be inactive. If the selector gene mutates and becomes ineffective, this makes no difference in the compartment in which it is switched off anyway. In the compartment in which it is switched on, however, it fails to function, so the difference between the compartments is destroyed and they assume a similar morphology.

The previously discussed homeotic genes have the properties expected of selector genes. In this model, *engrailed* is thought to be the selector gene which must be active in the posterior compartment to make it different from the anterior compartment; *wingless* is the selector gene whose activity is required to make the wing different from the thorax; and *bithorax* and *postbithorax* are selector genes required to make metathoracic segments different from mesothoracic segments. A given compartment has an identity specified by the combination of selector genes which are on or off in its cells.

3.4.3. *Why Do Compartments Have Sharp Boundaries?* Why should selector genes have such sharply defined geographical territories of action? Because if cells with different specifications (combinations of active and inactive selector genes) intermingled with each other, orderly structures could not develop.[41] Imagine what would happen if cells tightly specified to be wing intermingled with cells specified to be thorax. The components of the wing hinge, which is at the boundary, would hardly be expected to form properly if each little sclerite could have an arbitrary mixture of wing and thoracic cells. If cells are indeed assigned their morphogenetic roles in part by genetic switches, then these cells should be kept segregated.

How are the cells of different compartments prevented from intermingling? Possibly by adhesiveness differences which cause the cells at the compartment boundary to exert physical forces upon each other. It is found that in *engrailed* mutants clones will cross the antero-posterior (A–P) boundary which is rigidly respected in wild-type flies. This would be expected if adhesiveness differences were part of compartment quality; when compartments are rendered identical by a failure of the gene which produces the differences between them, adhesiveness differences also disappear and no barrier to the growth of clones remains.

3.5. *Evaluation*

Not all workers agree with the above ideas as I have presented them. Sharma and Chopra[47] and Deak[48] have argued that *wingless* is not a homeotic mutation, but rather brings about cell death and subsequent regeneration. Hayes *et al.*[49] have argued for a different way of looking at the interaction of *engrailed* with genes of the BX-C. Karlsson[50] challenges the idea that any of the known homeotic genes act as selector genes with compartment-limited territories of action. G. S. Stent (personal communication) regards all these interrelated hypotheses as so simplistic as to be misleading. Nevertheless, the ideas I have presented have been the most popular ones during the past decade and, right or wrong or soon to be modified, they embody a widespread concensus that some small group of genes exercises an especially profound effect on morphogenesis. How this is brought about at a biochemical level is not specified, but realistic hypotheses can be expected once the homeotic genes, especially the bithorax and antennapedia complexes, are sequenced and the wild-type gene products found. In brief summary, most workers now believe that while the relationship between genes and forms is undoubtedly complex and involves many epigenetic interactions, it is also true that the study of certain genes brings us especially close to the heart of the problem.

3.6. *Working Hypotheses and Questions for Neurobiologists*

Having reviewed a number of phenomena and ideas of interest in general developmental biology, let us summarize them as a small set of working hypotheses and then formulate a series of questions which extend this mode of thinking explicitly into studies of the nervous system.

3.6.1. Working Hypotheses. (1) Homeotic genes have a regulatory role in development. (2) Compartments, defined operationally, reflect the importance of establishing and maintaining discrete regions during development. (3) Homeotic mutations may (e.g., *bithorax* and *postbithorax*) but need not (e.g., *Antennapedia*) produce phenotypes limited to subsegmental compartments. Homeosis and compartmentalization are in principle independent phenomena, and whether they are causally or mechanistically linked in particular cases is an empirical question.

3.6.2. Questions. (1) Do compartment boundaries limit the growth of sensory axons in the periphery, as they limit the intermingling of ordinary epidermal cells? (2) Are peripheral sensory neurons affected by homeotic mutations, as are the neighboring epidermal cells which secrete the cuticle? (3) Are the paths taken by sensory axons within the CNS, and the destinations they reach, affected by the compartments in which the cell bodies are lodged? (4) Are there compartments in the CNS? If yes, what role do they have in the building of the CNS? (5) Is the CNS directly affected by the homeotic mutations that alter the external morphology of the fly?

4. COMPARTMENT BOUNDARIES AND PERIPHERAL NERVES

4.1. *General Neuroanatomy of Drosophila*

In *Drosophila*, as in other arthropods and indeed invertebrates generally, the cell bodies of motor neurons and interneurons are located within the CNS, but those of the vast majority of sensory neurons are peripheral (Fig. 7). There they may be closely associated with the epidermal cells, they may be suspended between two cuticular attachment points, or they may be associated with muscles. However, no matter what the precise geometry may be, with rare exceptions the cell bodies are peripheral and differentiate from peripheral precursor cells.

The CNS of *Drosophila* is highly condensed. In the head are found the usual structures: optic lobes, brain, and subesophageal ganglion. The three thoracic ganglia are fused, though their neuropilar regions are still distinguishable and are called neuromeres. The abdominal ganglia are also fused, and in addition are fused with the thoracic, forming a single thoracico-abdominal nerve mass. In all regions of the CNS the cell bodies are around the outside, primarily along the lateral and ventral

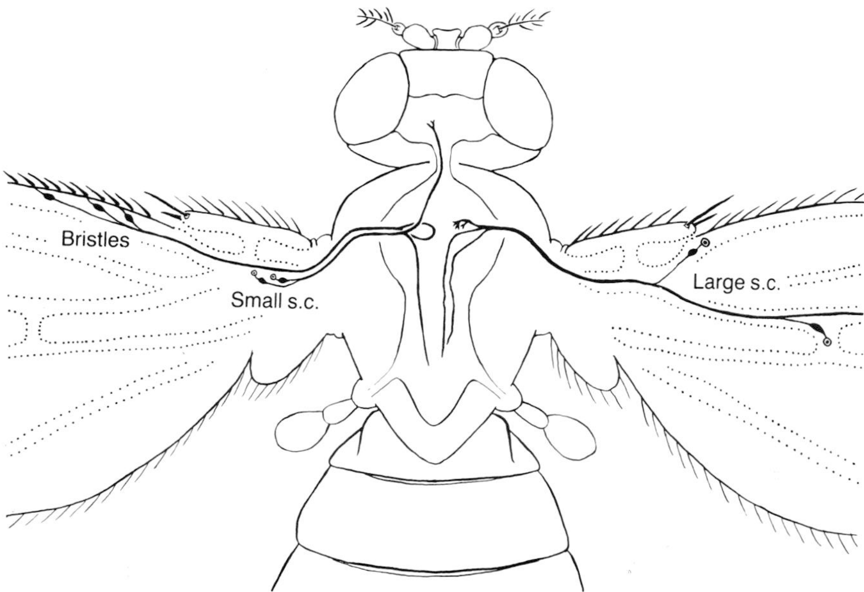

Figure 7. Sensory cells in *Drosophila* have peripheral cell bodies. Cells on the wing project into the thoracico-abdominal nerve mass. Axons from different classes of cells project to different tracts and termination areas.

surfaces; the neurites ramify in a central neuropil where all synaptic relationships are established and through which all fiber tracts run.

The nervous system of the adult, both central and peripheral, was described on the basis of reduced silver preparations by Power.[51–53] The most systematic modern account can be found in the review of Kankel *et al.*[54] The larval stages have not been explored in detail in recent years, and the most extensive study is still that of Hertweck[55]; an analysis of cell proliferation within the CNS, and the formation of adult optic lobe and brain centers from larval precursors, is given by White and Kankel.[56]

4.2. *Neuroanatomy of the Wing*

The wings of insects are thin cuticular blades reinforced by hollow struts, the veins, which carry blood and also the nerves composed of sensory axons travelling toward the CNS. There are no muscles, the movement of the wings being accomplished either by muscles attached to the wing base or indirectly by contraction-generated changes in the shape of the entire thoracic box, which are translated into wing move-

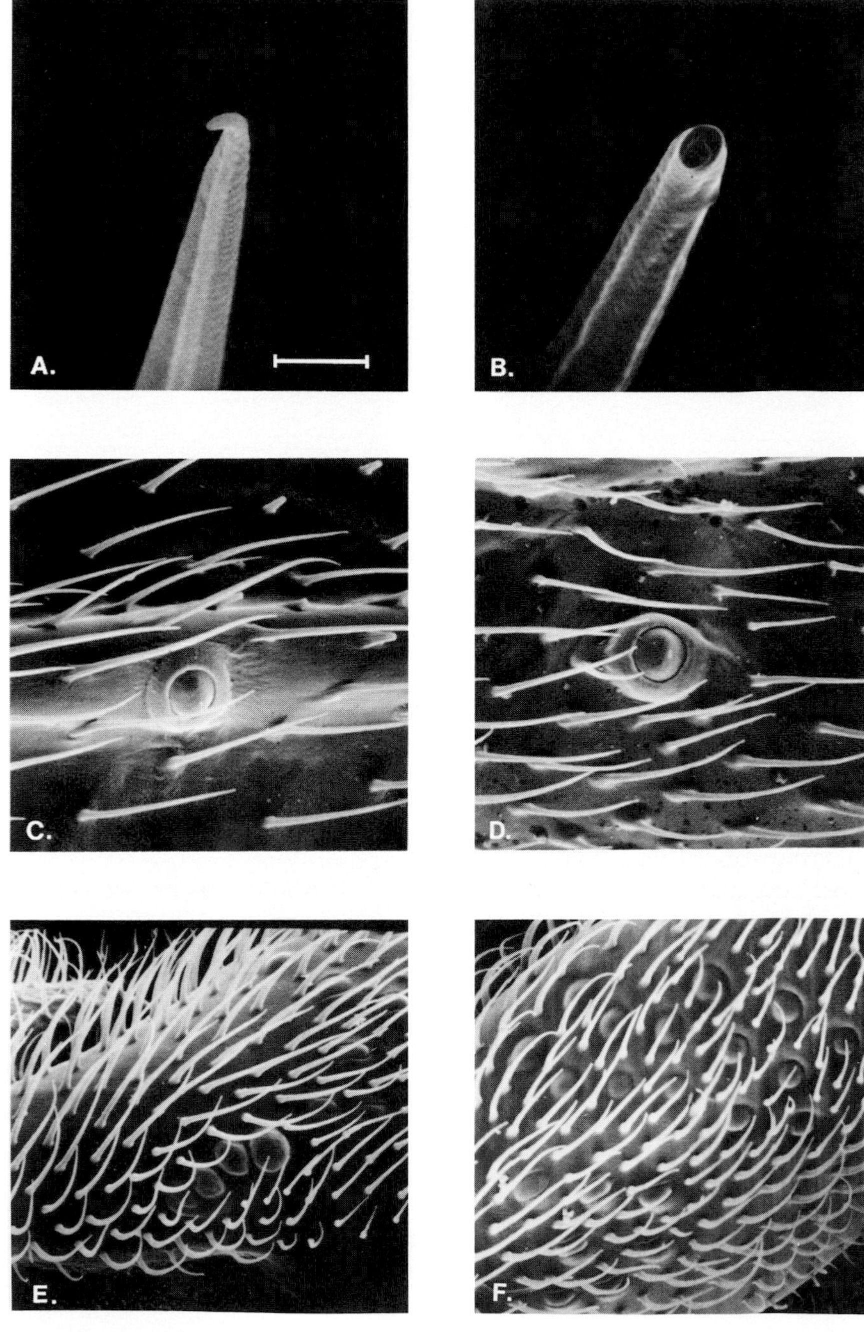
A.
B.
C.
D.
E.
F.

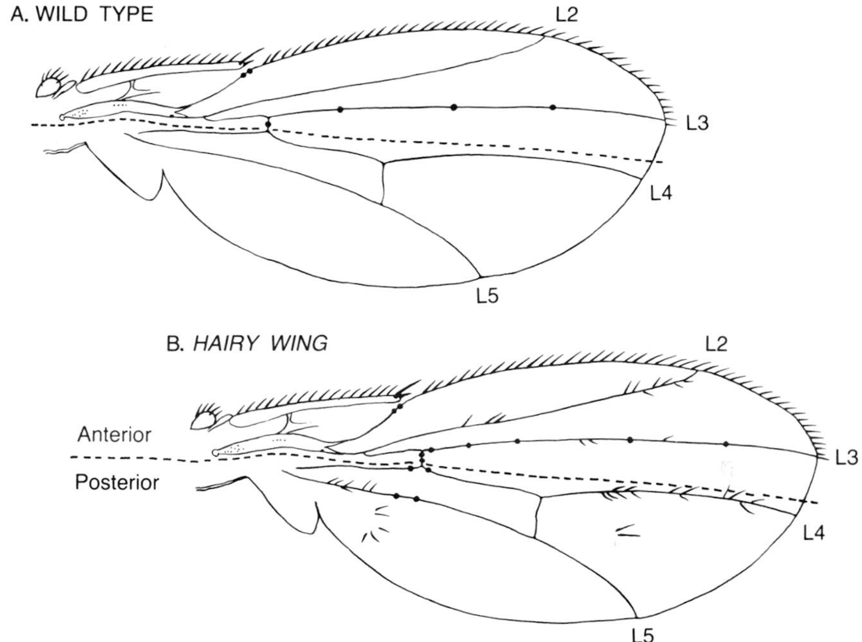

Figure 9. Distribution of sensory structures on the wing. (A) In wild-type *Drosophila* all receptors are in the anterior compartment. (B) In *Hairy wing* flies (in this case *Hw/Hw*), supernumerary receptors, including both bristles and s.c., develop in both compartments.

ments through the complex articulation between the wing and the thorax.

There are three morphological classes of receptors in the wings of *Drosophila*, all associated with the veins through which their axons travel: bristles, sensilla campaniformia (s.c.), and chordotonal organs. The bristles are conspicuous structures along the leading edge of the wing, which is formed by the marginal vein (Fig. 8A, B); the s.c. are disc-shaped receptors clustered in specific locations on a few veins (Fig. 8C–F); and the chordotonal organs are suspended across the lumen of the major proximal vein, the radius. All the receptors in the wing are in the anterior compartment (Fig. 9A).

The cell bodies and axons of the bristle and s.c. sensory neurons

←

Figure 8. Types of receptors found on the wing. (A) Thin mechanosensory and (B) chemomechanosensory bristles. (C) Large s.c. found distally on vein L3. (D) Large s.c. found on the anterior cross vein. (E and F) Different types of small s.c. found in discrete clusters on the radius. Scale, 1 μm (A, B); 5 μm (C–F).

can be stained with methylene blue injected into the body cavity. The wing is quite transparent and the stained cells can be seen beautifully, simply by mounting the wing in a drop of mineral oil under a coverslip.

4.3. *The Behavior of Axons at the A–P Compartment Border*

The first question we want to examine is, is the growth of axons through peripheral tissues restricted by compartment borders? Such a restriction has been claimed for another insect, the milkweed bug *Oncopeltus*,[57] and could reasonably be expected in view of the powerful restriction on the mixing of epidermal cells that occurs at these borders, possibly due to adhesiveness differences (Section 3.4.3). Therefore, we have examined the behavior of axons at the A–P boundary in the wing.[58]

The analysis cannot be done in wild-type flies, inasmuch as all of their wing receptors are in the anterior compartment. To obtain a suitable geometrical configuration we have used the mutant *Hairy wing* (*Hw*), which forms supernumerary receptors in both compartments (Fig. 9B).

In mature wings the only spaces normally used for axon growth are the veins, so we need to look for a vein crossing between the two compartments which a posterior axon would be able to use as a route into the anterior compartment, or vice versa. The anterior cross vein (ACV) between the longitudinal veins L3 (anterior compartment) and L4 (posterior compartment) is suitable for this purpose.

The outcome of this study is illustrated in Fig. 10. Axons originating from large s.c. situated distally on L3 grow toward the CNS through L3; on their way they pass the ACV but ignore it. The single sensillum located on the ACV is in the anterior compartment, and its axon always grows through L3. This description applies equally to wild type flies and to *Hairy wing* mutants.

Consider now the additional sensilla which form on the posterior vein L4 of *Hw* flies. If they form distal to the ACV, their axons travel through L4, but only until they reach the ACV. At the junction they make a right-angle turn and grow through the ACV, across the compartment border, and on to join the axons traveling through L3. The axons of sensilla just proximal to the ACV even travel distally for a short distance to cross through the ACV into the anterior compartment. The axons of more proximal sensilla, however, travel toward the CNS through L4.

If there were no special guiding factors influencing the growing sensory axons, we would expect that some reasonable proportion of cases in which axons starting in L4 would remain in L4 rather than

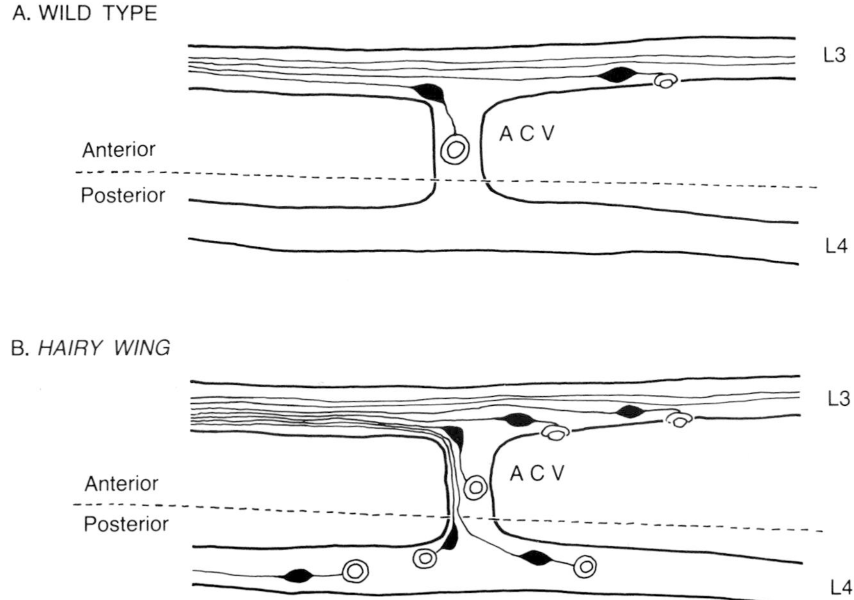

Figure 10. Axon paths in (A) wild-type and (B) *Hairy wing* wings. In the vicinity of the anterior cross vein (ACV), axons from sensilla in the posterior compartment (vein L4) always cross into the anterior compartment and join the nerve in vein L3. More proximally they travel in L4 toward the base of the wing.

turning out of it. We have not seen a single such case, however, and therefore suppose that some factor makes L3 particularly attractive to growing axons. This supposition is strengthened by the presence of axons taking shortcuts to L3 both from L4 in the posterior compartment and from L2 within the anterior compartment. This surprising behavior requires crossing the intervein regions in which axons normally never grow.

4.4. *Evidence That the Compartment Border Is Intact*

Hairy wing enabled us to make the analysis just described. But as emphasized earlier, one of the difficulties in using mutants as experimental material is that there is no way of knowing *a priori* all of the effects which a given mutation might have. Could it be, for example, that *Hw* not only adds sensilla to both compartments but also shifts or destroys the boundary between them?

To test this possibility we have produced clones of *mwh* cells in *Hw* flies by the procedures described in Section 2.2.2.c, taking advantage of the *Minute* technique to make them very large. These clones grow up to a border, a line of clonal restriction, just as do similar clones in wild-type flies; the border is located, as usual, a few cells anterior to L4. Thus, compartmentalization appears to operate in *Hw* flies just as it does in wild-type flies, and the lack of effect of the compartment boundary on axon growth appears to be genuine.

4.5. *The Next Hypothesis—Pupal Nerves Guide Adult Axons*

Demonstrating that the A–P boundary does not constitute a barrier to axon growth does not explain why axons grow out of their own veins into L3 if the physical opportunity for them to do so exists (Section 4.3). We suggest that this happens because L3 contains a preexisting nerve bundle which acts as a guide for the newly formed axons.

Pupal nerves (or pioneer fibers in insects without a major metamorphosis) have been described in every insect appendage in which they have been looked for (see Chapter 7). Eliminating them experimentally leads to aberrant bundling of peripheral axons,[59] so they are not only present but functionally important. Axons have been seen in leg discs of *Drosophila* prior to metamorphosis.[60] Finally, Waddington[61] described nerve bundles in appropriate locations in developing wings on the basis of light-microscopic evidence. We are currently searching for such pupal nerves with transmission electron microscopy.

We suppose that as the axons of sensory neurons differentiating in normal locations start to grow, they encounter a pupal nerve in their immediate vicinity and follow it to the CNS. If the sensory neurons differentiate in an ectopic location they may grow in any direction. If their initial, undirected growth leads them to a pupal nerve, they too will follow this nerve to the CNS. The adult axon pattern in the wings of *Hw* flies thus leads us to two inferences: (1) compartment boundaries do not restrict the growth of sensory axons, and (2) pupal nerves provide preferred paths into the CNS. Some of the strong evidence for (1) has been summarized here. Hypothesis (2) leads to a study of axons as they are developing, a project we are undertaking at the present time.

4.6. *Evaluation*

This analysis was motivated by a question stemming directly from the developmental genetic framework established in Section 3. We wanted to test the hypothesis that the axons of peripheral sensory neurons remain confined to a single compartment as do the epidermal cells which secrete cuticle. The evidence is clearly against this hypothesis.

The observations, then, contribute to general developmental biology by helping to define the role of compartments, albeit in a negative way. We see that the defining property of compartments, that populations of cells which border on each other do not intermingle across a well defined boundary, is not recognizable in the growth pattern of sensory axons. This is true even though the sensory cells are derived from the same epidermal cell population as are the cuticle-secreting cells whose behavior is the basis of the whole idea of compartments.

Seen from a neurobiological perspective, the observations lead straight to an area of study being pursued actively in other neural subsystems: the search for the very earliest axons in a given area, their role as guides for subsequently formed axons, and the question of why the first axons grow where they do over the nonneural substrate and not somewhere else. Whether a genetic mode of analysis will contribute to a solution of this last question remains to be seen.

5. CENTRAL PROJECTIONS IN MUTANTS OF THE ANTENNAPEDIA COMPLEX

5.1. *Antennapedia*

If a leg grows in place of an antenna (Fig. 2), will its sensory axons terminate in the CNS as if they came from a leg, from an antenna, or neither? This purely empirical question piqued my curiosity around seven years ago when I first heard my colleague Gerold Schubiger, a *Drosophila* developmentalist, describe homeotic mutants to our faintly disbelieving group of neurobiologists. Who would have thought that a casual lunchtime discussion would inspire a new course of investigation for years to come?

It took some time to obtain the answer to this simple question, especially using the method of experimental degeneration[62] which required preparing 1 μm serial sections of the brains, subesophageal ganglia, and thoracico-abdominal nerve masses of many flies. The answer was startling to us[63]: the regions of termination of axons from the homeotic appendages were identical with those in which normal antennal fibers terminate. The axons from the head legs did not pass down to the thoracico-abdominal nerve mass where axons from thoracic legs terminate. They also did not wander in the brain as if lost. Rather, they clearly terminated in regions appropriate to antennal fibers, both chemosensory and mechanosensory. This work has since been extended and refined by Stocker and Lawrence[64] using cobalt fills, but the answer is the same (Fig. 11): homeotic leg fibers in *Antennapedia* project to antennal centers in the brain. In addition, a tract passing into the subesophageal ganglion is often found; this is not present in the projection of the antennae in wild-type flies.

When mitotic recombination clones are generated in animals heterozygous for *spineless-aristapedia*, a related recessive mutation with a similar phenotype, the axons of their sensory neurons project into a CNS whose cells are genotypically wild type. The projection patterns are virtually the same as in mutant flies. In other words, the genotype of the brain does not seriously affect the projection. Therefore, even if a homeotic transformation of the brain occurs, concurrent with the transformation of the antenna into a leg, it must not be a major influence on the projection of axons in mutant flies.

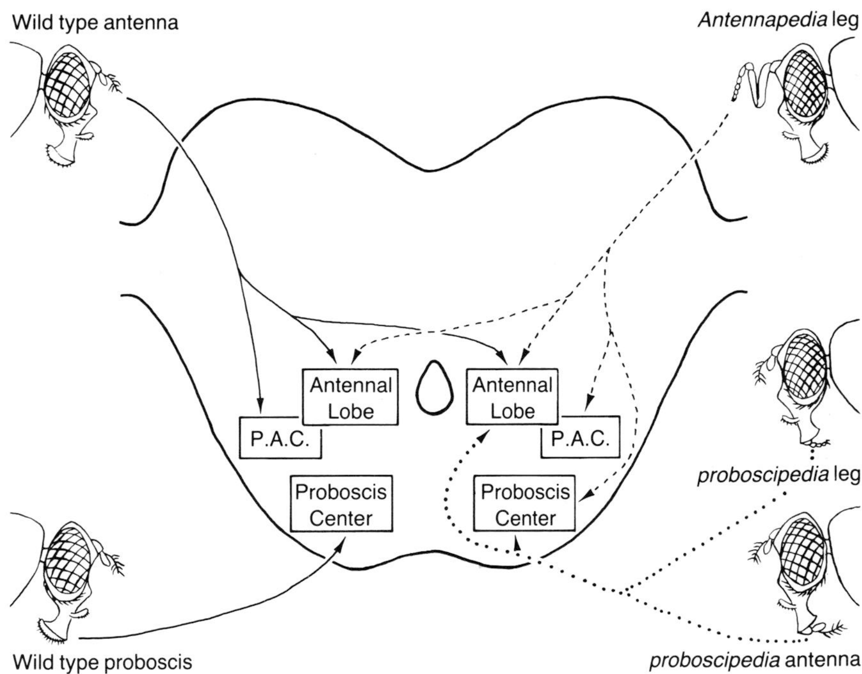

Figure 11. Central projections in mutants of the ANT-C. In wild-type flies (left), the antennal receptors project to both ipsilateral and contralateral antennal lobes, and to the ipsilateral posterior antennal center (P.A.C.); proboscis receptors project to the proboscis center. In the mutants the same target areas are reached even though the appendages assume different morphologies; some novel interconnections appear, and some expected ones do not.

5.2. *Proboscipedia*

Proboscipedia (*pb*) is a particularly intriguing mutation because its effect is temperature-sensitive in an unusual way. Most TS mutants show a wild-type phenotype if they undergo development at some particular range of temperatures, and the mutant phenotype if they develop at some other range of temperatures. In *proboscipedia*, by contrast, a mutant effect is seen at all temperatures; its nature, however, switches. Temperatures around 17°C result in the formation of antennal structures in place of mouth parts. Higher temperatures, around 28°C, lead to the development of legs instead of mouthparts. Thus, in one and the same location on different flies the cuticle may take the form of a proboscis, an antenna, or a leg. What about the neurons?

Stocker[65] has examined this intriguing situation and finds the following (Fig. 11). The sensory axons from normal mouthparts travel to the CNS through a single nerve and have well-defined projection areas, mainly in the subesophageal ganglion where they are called the proboscis center. Axons coming from homeotic *pb*-antennal structures may use an additional route to reach the CNS, and axons from *pb*-leg structures may use any one or several of four nerves. Once in the subesophageal ganglion the axons of all three kinds of appendages converge on the same projection area, even though they have entered the CNS by a variety of nerves and may have to take different routes through the ganglion to reach this target. In addition, mutant flies show a tract of fibers passing dorsally into the antennal lobes, irrespective of whether they originate in antennal or leg structures. This tract is not found in the proboscis projection of wild-type flies.

As was the case in *spineless-aristapedia*, projections from mitotic recombination clones of pb^{-}/pb^{-} into a wild type (pb^{-}/pb^{+})CNS showed much the same patterns as projections in mutant flies in which the CNS as well as the appendage was mutant. Some minor differences were observed, but again the main features were the same in both cases and a direct influence of the *proboscipedia* mutation upon the CNS was not indicated.

5.3. *Interpretation*

5.3.1. Specific Inferences. Several specific points emerge from these studies on mutants of the ANT-C. Among them are the following.

1. The ability of axons to reach a specific target area does not necessarily depend on their following a particular route to that area. For

example, axons from *pb*-legs reach the proboscis center by a variety of intraganglionic routes, depending on which particular nerve carries them to the CNS.

2. The projection patterns from homeotic appendages are very orderly and specific. There is no indication of wandering or of random projections.

3. The dominant projection from these homeotic appendages is to the area(s) in which the axons of the normal appendage developing in the same location would have terminated.

4. The details of the axon terminal distribution within a given projection area are different for wild-type flies and for the various mutants. I have not reviewed the data here; for details, see the papers of Stocker and collaborators.[63–65]

5. The paths taken and targets reached within the CNS cannot be predicted from the morphology of a homeotic appendage. A small set of target areas in the CNS receives fibers from both normal and homeotic appendages, but the combinations are varied and still to be explained. For example, normal antennal fibers reach the antennal lobes and posterior antennal center; *pb*-antennal fibers reach the antennal lobes, not the posterior antennal center, but do terminate in the proboscis center. Antennal legs reach the posterior antennal center, but *pb*-legs do not, even though both reach the antennal lobes and the proboscis center.

6. Whether the CNS is mutant or wild type is in most respects not important to the establishment of the projection pattern.

5.3.2. General Interpretation. The full meaning of this simple yet complex set of peripheral–central relationships has yet to be understood. The most striking single feature is orderliness. For any appendage, normal or homeotic, there is a limited set of target areas and of preferred though not unique paths by which they are reached.

Prime among the targets are those of the appendage which normally develops in a given location. This cannot be due to simple mechanical factors [inference 1 above], since axons can follow different routes to a single target area. It seems economical to suppose that the sensory neurons of all the various appendages that can develop on the head have in common at least many features of the (unknown) mechanisms which govern their choice of target area.

Why should the neurons have target-seeking features in common when the appendages look so different? Possibly because the appendages are all serially homologous, and the neurons within them are more conservative (less differentiated according to appendage type) than are the epidermal cells which secrete the appendage-specific cuticle. However, in the next section I will argue for a different interpretation, namely that *homeotic mutations need not affect sensory neurons* in spite of their profound effects on the cuticle.

The studies on genetic mosaics indicate that mutants in the ANT-C do not (or at least need not) affect the CNS. Neither in the case of an antenna-to-leg transformation[64] nor in the case of proboscis-to-antenna or proboscis-to-leg transformations[65] was there any substantial difference in the projection pattern formed by *mutant axons* in a mutant and in a wild-type CNS. However, the complementary experiment, comparing the projection of *wild-type axons* in a wild type and in a mutant CNS, has not been done in any homeotic system.

6. CENTRAL PROJECTIONS IN MUTANTS OF THE BITHORAX COMPLEX

Three laboratories, those of Ghysen and of Strausfeld as well as my own, have recently published studies on the projections of sensory neurons in wings, halteres, and homeotic appendages in wild-type *Drosophila* and in mutants of the BX-C. Out of the great deal of detail becoming available I will present here only a few points, selected to illustrate a series of inferences about the general organizational features of these pathways and rules of response to perturbations of normal development. Three recent symposium papers provide convenient summaries.[66–68]

6.1. *Different Classes of Receptors Form Different Projections*

The variety of receptors on the wing is astonishing, especially since we most often think of the wing as an organ of locomotion rather than an organ of sensation. We have already encountered the three major classes—bristles, s.c., and chordotonal organs (section 4.2; see Fig. 8).

The bristles are a heterogeneous class of receptors. Three types have been described[69]: thick mechanoreceptors, thin mechanoreceptors (Fig. 8A), and mixed chemomechanoreceptors (Fig. 8B). Each type has a characteristic distribution in the three rows of bristles on the leading edge of the wing. The s.c. can be divided into two subclasses, large s.c. and small s.c., which differ profoundly in the projections they make within the CNS. The large s.c. (Fig. 8C, D) are morphologically a homogeneous group. The small s.c. (Fig. 8E, F) are not—half a dozen different morphological types are aggregated into type-specific clusters which must be presumed to provide the CNS with specific information about mechanical events in the wing. There are striking parallels between the dorsal and ventral clusters on the wing and on the haltere, and between wing and haltere groups.[70–72]

Figure 7 summarizes the known projections of these various classes of sensilla. The axons of the bristle receptors terminate in a discrete ventral region of mesothoracic neuropil near their point of entry. As far as is known, all types of bristles project here. The axons of the large s.c. travel in two ventral tracts and branch elaborately in all three neuromeres (cf. Fig. 12A). The axons of the small s.c. form a bifurcation near their point of entry into the CNS and travel in dorsal tracts to terminate in the metathoracic neuromere and in the subesophageal ganglion; a few strands terminate in the mesothoracic neuromere. No information is available on the relationship of the various morphological subclasses of small s.c. and detailed features of the central pathway. The course followed by axons of the chordotonal organs remains unknown.

6.2. *The Projection of Single Axons Is Not Always Precisely Specified*

The large s.c. all have a similar morphology, are few in number (7 or 8), and occur in fixed locations. The only known variation is whether the dorsal surface of vein L3 bears 3 or 4 such sensilla. As far as is known, all project into one of two bundles in the ventral part of the CNS (Figs. 7 and 12).

Both Ghysen[73] and Burt and Palka[74] have seen that a given sensillum (the most distal on L3) may enter either the lateral or the medial ventral tract. The two tracts join posteriorly, so at least some of the same destinations can be attained by either route. A similar indeterminacy of tract selection apparently does not exist in the case of the unique large s.c., in which there is no variation at all in peripheral location and number.[73]

6.3. *Axons from the Normal Wings of Mutant Flies Branch More*

In the first close examination of the branching patterns of fibers from the normal, mesothoracic wings of four-winged flies (Figs. 4 and 5) we have found that the axons of the large s.c. enter the usual two ventral tracts, but they tend to produce numerous extra branches.[74] This is illustrated in Fig. 12B.

Four-winged flies have a double set of large s.c. axons, one from the normal wings and one from the homeotic wings. Could the extra branching be caused by the simultaneous presence of the homeotic

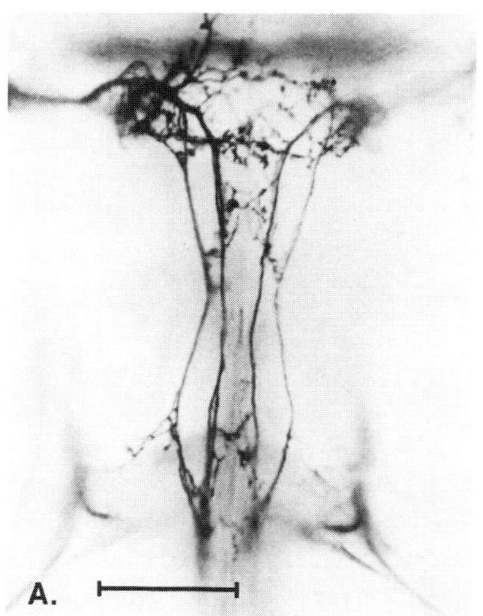

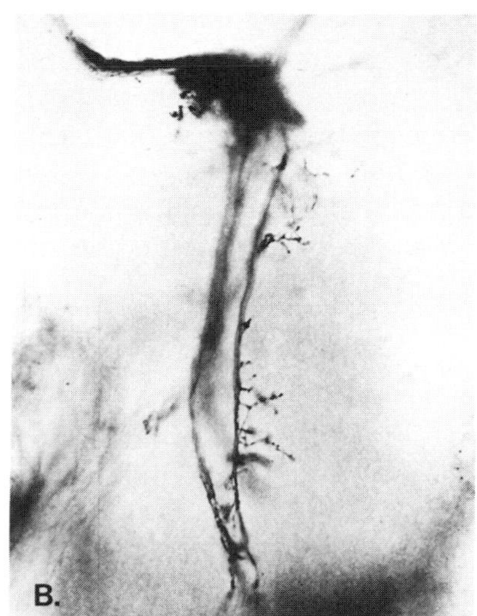

Figure 12. Photomicrographs of the large s.c. projection in (A) a wild-type fly (filled on both sides) and (B) a four-winged fly (filled on the left only). The mutant genotype was *bx*^{3} *pbx*/*Ubx*^{130}, where *Ubx*^{130} acts like a deletion for *bx*^{3} and *pbx* (see Lewis[32]; Morata and Kerridge[93]). Note how few lateral branches are seen along the ventral tracts in the wild-type animal, and how many appear, especially along the medial tract, in the mutant. The bristle axon projection is shown out of focus in (B). Scale, 50μm.

axons? This hypothesis can be tested by producing flies which are genotypically four-winged (*bx pbx*) but lack the homeotic wings because they are also *wingless* (*wg*). The *wingless* mutation causes the dorsal appendages (wings, halteres, or homeotic appendages) to fail to develop, singly or in any combination, so that among *wg; bx pbx* flies there will be some which have front wings but not hind wings. The extra branching persists in such flies, so the presence of homeotic axons appears not to be a necessary causal factor.

A second argument suggesting that the extra branching is not caused by extra axons is that it fails to appear in *Hairy wing* flies in spite of the fact that they have many additional large s.c. on their wings (Fig. 9B) and their ventral tracts are noticeably thicker, presumably due to the presence of the additional axons.

Since we have been unable to account for the extra branching by either adding or removing other, potentially interacting sensory fibers, we have been forced to consider two hypotheses relating to the action of the BX-C mutations: (1) they may have some previously unknown effect on the mesothoracic wings, even though these look perfectly normal, or (2) they may have some effect on the CNS. Both of these hypotheses are potentially testable through the use of genetic mosaics.

In addition to generating new hypotheses about the role of BX-C genes in the specification of segments, these results reinforce my earlier comment about the need for caution in studying mutants. No part of a mutant fly can be considered unaltered unless it is demonstrated to be so by direct examination or experiment. Nothing can be taken for granted.

6.4. *Some Axons from Homeotic Wings Follow Normal Wing Tracts*

The axons from the large s.c. on homeotic wings enter the same lateral and medial ventral tracts as those from the normal, mesothoracic wings. As Ghysen[75] was the first to point out in this system, this suggests that incoming axons follow a preexisting "trail" or substrate pathway in the CNS and that this pathway is not polarized—i.e., that it can be followed in both directions. Note how different this result is from the predominant behavior of axons in ANT-C mutants, described in Section 5. The axons from *Antennapedia* and *proboscipedia* homeotic legs terminate in antennal and proboscis centers, not in leg centers. The large s.c. axons of these *bithorax* homeotic wings, by contrast, follow the same course and terminate in the same regions as the corresponding axons from the normal wings.

One suggestion about the possible nature of the path followed by the homeotic large s.c. axons is simply that it consists of the coexisting normal axons.[69] This hypothesis has been tested and rejected.[66] In *bx pbx* flies whose normal wings are lacking because of the action of *wingless* (see section 6.3 above), the homeotic large s.c. continue to use the usual lateral and medial ventral tracts. Other axons (or possibly glial cells) already present in the CNS at the time the adult sensory fibers grow in must provide the required, labeled cellular substrate for axonal growth along particular paths.

6.5. *Some Axons from Homeotic Wings Follow Haltere Tracts*

I have been struck for a long time by the observation that axons from the small s.c. of *bithorax* homeotic wings form a projection virtually indistinguishable from that of a normal haltere (Fig. 13). This class of fibers, then, follows the rule we have seen in *Antennapedia* and *proboscipedia*, and not the rule described in the previous section for the axons of homeotic large s.c.

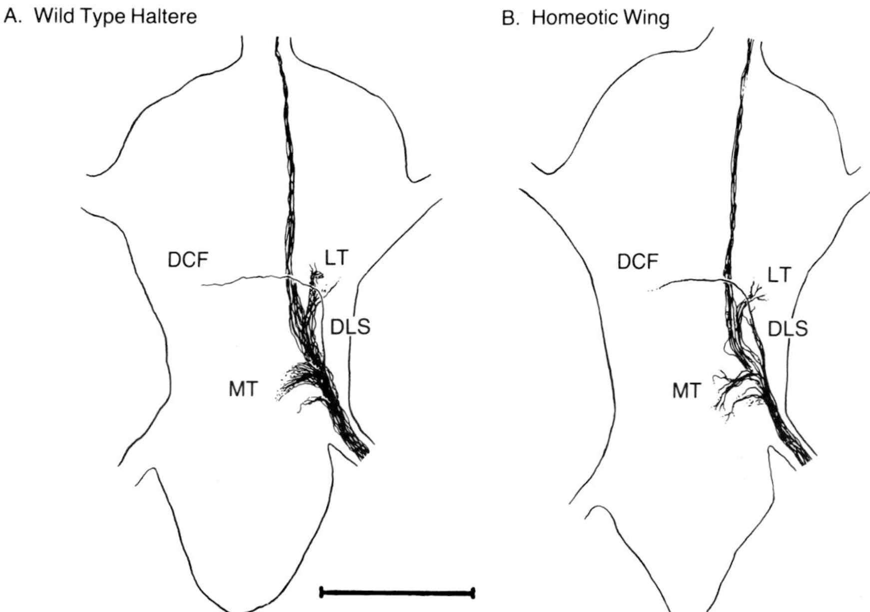

Figure 13. Thoracic projections of small s.c. from (A) the haltere of a wild-type fly and (B) the homeotic wing of a *bithorax* fly (bx^3/Ubx^{130}). Several components are labeled: medial tuft (MT), lateral tuft (LT), dorsolateral strand (DLS), and dorsal crossing fibers (DCF). The functional significance of the various components is not known. For details, see Palka *et al.*,[69] from which this figure is adapted; Ghysen[75]; Strausfeld and Singh.[68] Scale, 100μm.

6.5.1. Removal of Potentially Competing Wing Axons Has No Effect. The fibers of the wing small s.c. and of the haltere receptors, most of which are also small s.c. (described in detail by Cole *et al.*[71]), travel very close together in the CNS though the projections are clearly distinguishable at a number of points. Would the fibers coming from homeotic wing s.c. travel along the wing rather than the haltere pathway if the axons coming from the normal wings were eliminated? This can be done both surgically, by removing most of a wing imaginal disc late in larval life before the adult receptors differentiate, or genetically by using the *wingless* mutation. Neither method, however, produces any recognizable alteration in the halterelike course of the homeotic small s.c. axons.[67] Their choice of pathway, therefore, cannot be attributed to some selective advantage possessed by the normal wing small s.c. for a limited substrate; rather, it appears to reflect a genuine cellular choice.

I take it to be significant that removal of potentially interacting fibers, most conveniently by the *wingless* mutation, has no effect on three independent cellular behaviors: (1) the extra branching of large s.c. axons from the normal wings of *bx pbx* flies; (2) the path followed by the large s.c. axons from the homeotic wings of *bx pbx* flies; and (3) the path followed by small s.c. axons from the homeotic wings of bithorax flies of a variety of genotypes. Deafferentation has been shown to have powerful effects on postsynaptic neurons in a variety of other insects,[76,67] but thus far no effects have been shown on the paths of the remaining primary sensory axons, either in *Drosophila* or in other species.

6.5.2. Rerouting Homeotic Sensory Axons to Normal Wing Entry Points. In about 10% of genetically *wingless* flies lacking the anterior mesothoracic wings, the metathoracic nerve is rerouted along the thoracic musculature and enters the CNS in the mesothorax, usually with the mixed nerve in which wing sensory axons normally travel. (For a possible explanation of this phenomenon, see Ghysen and Janson.[66]) Thus, wing deafferentation experiments using *wingless* automatically produce individuals in which haltere or homeotic axons are made to enter the CNS where wing axons should have entered.

The consequences of such rerouting for homeotic small s.c. axons are quite striking. Instead of forming a compact and orderly bifurcation as normal wing small s.c. axons do, multiple, sometimes interlacing strands are produced (Fig. 14). Some of them generally do end up in the normal wing ascending and descending tracts. Thus, these supposedly wing-quality axons form a normal haltere projection when they enter the metathorax, whose normal appendage is the haltere, but they seem unable to form a normal wing projection when they enter the wing-bearing segment, the mesothorax. A hypothesis to account for these findings is presented in Section 7.2.2.

This description does not apply to the large s.c. Their axons not only follow the usual lateral and medial ventral tracts when they enter the metathorax, but they enter the same tracts (normally used by wing axons) when they enter the mesothorax as a result of rerouting.[66] Thus, the large and small s.c. axons follow very different rules of pathfinding in the homeotic situation.

6.5.3. Bithorax and Anterobithorax Projections Compared. The effects of the *wingless* mutation in the present context are probably rather like those of surgical removal. Thus far we have not seen any indication that the mutation has any effect on the projections we have studied other than producing deafferentation in one or another segment. These surgery-like perturbations have been conspicuously ineffective in altering neural pathways.

However, the projection pattern of the homeotic small s.c. can be altered—it can be caused to become very winglike—by genetic means. Our work on this point is still preliminary, but sufficiently convincing to warrant presentation here.

The mutation *anterobithorax*, located adjacent to *bithorax* in the BX-C,[33] produces a transformation of anterior haltere to anterior wing, much like *bithorax* does. The triple mutant *abx bx pbx/abx bx pbx* produces the most perfect set of metathoracic wings known (Lewis, personal communication), a description amply borne out by analysis with the SEM (Fig. 5; Cole *et al.*[71,72]). The projection of the small s.c. from these homeotic wings is distinctly winglike, particularly in the subesophageal ganglion (Schubiger and Palka, unpublished). In fact, even the projection from *abx/abx* homozygotes, whose homeotic wings are far from perfect, has many winglike features which are not seen, for example, in *bx/bx* (A. Ghysen, personal comm.; Ghysen *et al.*[77]). It then becomes necessary to ask not only why *bithorax* does not lead to a winglike neural projection for the small s.c., but also why *anterobithorax* does so. Several hypotheses bearing on this point are discussed in Section 7.

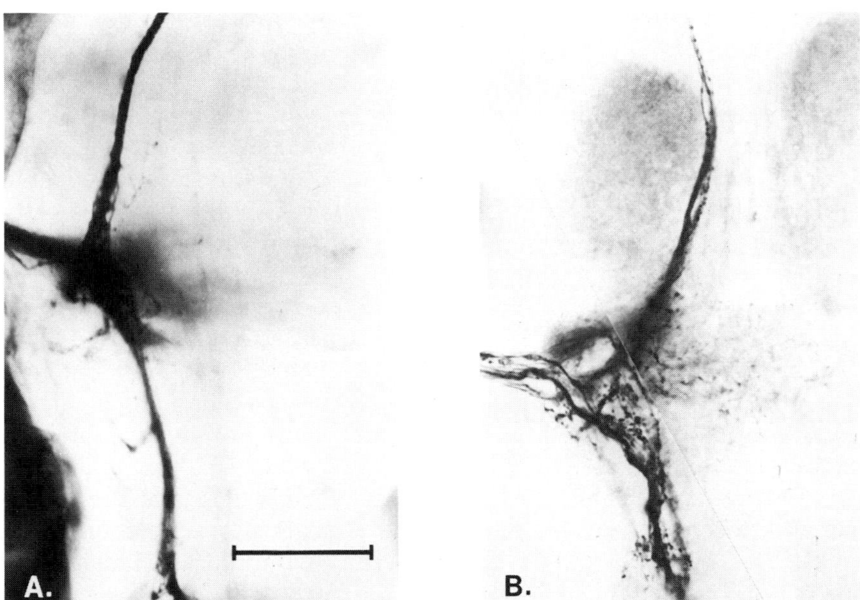

Figure 14. Projection of small s.c. in (A) a wild-type fly, and (B) a *bithorax* mutant (bx^3/Ubx^{130}) which was also genetically *wingless* and lacked both wings. The nerve from the homeotic appendage was rerouted to the mesothorax and, after entering the CNS where wing fibers should have entered, produced a disordered small s.c. projection. Photograph (B) is a montage of two focal planes from the same specimen. Scale, 40 μm.

6.6. *Some Axons from Homeotic Wings Find an Adequate Home in the Metathorax*

The bristle axons from homeotic wings form a complex ventral projection. Part of this projection can have the appearance of a metathoracic replication of the normal mesothoracic bristle projection. We have interpreted this to indicate substantial serial homology between the meso- and metathoracic neuromeres of the CNS. The projections, however, are not only complex but also variable, and I will not discuss them further here. For details, see the summary papers of Palka and Schubiger[67] and Strausfeld and Singh,[68] and the original references cited therein.

6.7. *Is the CNS Directly Affected by BX-C Mutations?*

There is conflicting evidence on this very important point. The only mosaic study[69] found that the sensory projections from homeotic appendages into a wild-type CNS were largely like those into a mutant CNS, but some differences were observed which we attributed to minor direct effects of the mutations on the CNS. Strausfeld and Singh[68] compared the branching patterns of neurons originating in the brain once they entered the metathoracic neuromere in wild-type and mutant flies. Some neurons looked the same, but some branched more in the mutants. If one assumes that the mutations had no effect on the cell bodies in the brain, this finding could be interpreted to hint at a mutation-associated change in the metathoracic neuromere. However, no experiment yet performed separates direct mutational effects on the CNS from secondary effects consequent upon the altered sensory input resulting from the presence of a homeotic appendage (see section 7.3 below). Furthermore, the observed indications of central changes are minor at best. Therefore Ghysen, for example, has argued that this potential complication in the interpretation of sensory projection patterns can safely be ignored.

On the other hand, Lewis[32] has observed a failure of the central ganglia to condense in the embryos homozygous for a deletion of the entire BX-C (section 3.2.1). Is this associated with internal changes? We do not yet know, and the answer is difficult to obtain because unambiguous internal markers on the basis of which one segmental ganglion could be distinguished from another have not been discovered.

The most suggestive evidence favoring a central homeotic change comes from Green.[78] He has back-filled leg motor neurons with horseradish peroxidase and observed characteristic differences between meso- and metathoracic cells. The most conspicuous difference is in the location of the cell bodies within the neuromeres: mesothoracic motor neurons lie anteriorly and their axons pass rather straight through the neuropil to exit via a posterior nerve. In the metathorax the somata lie posteriorly and the axons loop forward before exiting through a posterior nerve. In *abx bx pbx/abx bx pbx* triple mutants, the cell bodies in the metathorax tend to assume the mesothoracic configuration: anterior cell bodies with axons passing straight back to the posterior motor nerve.

How strong is this evidence? The events which determine soma position within a ganglion are not known, and it is possible that a change in position is an epiphenomenon of some factor associated with the homeotically transformed periphery of the fly (C. S. Goodman, personal communication). But the effect is there, and at the very least caution is indicated in making the assumption that the CNS is completely spared by mutations of the BX-C.

7. ANALYSIS

7.1. *Transplantation by Mutation*

We originally viewed homeotic mutants simply as constituting cases of nontraumatic transplantation. They would permit us to study the course of axons from a leg on the head or a wing on the haltere segment without performing any surgery, cutting any axons (including the presumptive early-formed pioneers), or worrying about tracks left behind as cut axons degenerated. Likewise, we could ignore possible differences between regeneration and undisturbed development.

7.1.1. *Summary of Results.* A number of results in homeotic mutants do appear to be fairly interpreted on this assumption. Let me summarize some of these: (1) Sensory axons follow specific central pathways, both in wild-type and in mutant animals. (2) They terminate in defined areas of the CNS. (3) While the pathways and termination areas are well defined, they are not necessarily unique. There can be more than one path to a given destination, and axons in mutant animals may reach areas which the normal appendages do not. (4) In some mutants there is considerable variability in the projection of some, though not necessarily all, types of sensilla. (5) The substrate pathways are not polarized, and can be followed in either direction.

7.1.2. *Parallels with Grafting Experiments.* If it is reasonable to view homeosis as a transplantation by mutation, we should find parallels to these results in data from surgical transplantation experiments. To make such a comparison we consider the extensive work on the grafting of sensory structures to ectopic locations done by Anderson[79–81] and Bacon and Anderson[82] (reviewed by Anderson[83]).

The basic experiment has been to graft pieces of receptor-bearing cuticle from the heads of grasshoppers to a series of sites, both on the head and on the thorax. The results are indeed strikingly similar to those I have just summarized for mutant flies: axons from both normally situated and ectopic receptors follow particular tracts in the CNS. They can follow these tracts in either direction for at least part of their length. The areas of termination are appropriate to the original tissue in which the cell bodies are embedded, no matter to what ectopic site that tissue may have been grafted. The pathways and termination areas are well defined, but the choices made by particular axons can be variable.

7.2. *Special Contributions of Genetic Studies*

The results just reviewed reveal great similarities between homeosis and surgical transplantation. However, many of the details require additional analysis.

7.2.1. Novel Findings We were forced to start asking questions about the effects of homeotic mutations on neural assembly as soon as the first results were obtained: homeotic leg axons in *Antennapedia* were shown to terminate selectively in antennal areas, and at least five different hypotheses were proposed to account for this finding.[63] The results have continued to be surprising. Who would have thought in advance that the axons of *proboscipedia* homeotic legs and homeotic antennae would project to exactly the same places (section 5.2)? Who would have expected that the axons of the large and the small s.c. of *bithorax* homeotic wings would behave so differently, both when they enter the metathoracic neuromere and when they are rerouted to the mesothoracic one (sections 6.4, 6.5 and 6.5.2)? Who would have thought that when the anterior compartment is transformed in an apparently similar way by *bithorax* and *anterobithorax*, different central projections would be observed (section 6.5.3)?

7.2.2. A Hypothesis—You Can't Tell a Book by Its Cover. We have proposed the following simple hypothesis to account for these findings in BX-C mutants: the cuticle of *bithorax* homeotic appendages expresses the homeotic transformation and shows wing morphology, but the sensory cells of the small s.c. are not transformed and retain a haltere identify.[67] This is why they project as if they were coming from a haltere (section 6.5) and continue to do so when potentially competing wing axons are eliminated (section 6.5.1), but are significantly disarrayed when they are rerouted to enter the CNS in the wing segment (section 6.5.2). The same inference has been drawn by Ghysen *et al.*,[77] partly from independently obtained evidence parallel to ours and partly from a much more extensive genetic analysis.

7.2.3. *Why Such a Difference?* How might a discrepancy between the external morphology of a sensillum and the behavior of its axon be brought about? We consider four hypotheses:

7.2.3.a. A mixed population of sensilla. In the genotypes first used in these experiments (e.g., Figs. 13 and 14), some small s.c. with unmistakably haltere morphology occur on the homeotic wing, in addition to the nearly complete complement of wing sensilla.[69–72,84] Perhaps this heterogeneity is brought to prominence in rerouting experiments and accounts for the disorganization which these produce. The coherent behavior of the mixed population when the axons enter the metathorax would then reflect additional and unknown factors, such as the affinity of similar axons for each other. On this hypothesis the apparent discrepancy between morphology and projection would be an artifact.

7.3.2.b. Differential thresholds to gene products. Suppose that the sensory neurons have a lower threshold to the *bithorax* substance (section 3.2.3) than do cuticle-secreting cells. Then in a mutant the amount and/or activity of the substance might be sufficient to keep the neurons metathoracic, but be insufficient for the epidermal cells, which would therefore revert to the mesothoracic state and produce wing structures including sensilla. This kind of model was proposed by Morata[85] to account for a mixed meso–metathoracic phenotype in the cuticle of *Contrabithorax* (cf. Fig. 4).

7.2.3.c. Neuron-specific genes. The genetic analysis of Ghysen *et al.*[77] suggests that the genes whose on/off state controls the activity of cuticle-secreting epidermal cells are different from those which control the segmental identity of neurons. The evidence is based on mutants of the BX-C which I have not discussed here, on mutants of a possible regulatory gene for the BX-C, and on ether-induced phenocopies. This hypothesis is the newest candidate for explaining the disparity between sensillar morphology and projection, and accounts for the widest range of phenomena. For details the reader is referred to the original publication, which also contains a genetic argument against the differential threshold hypothesis.

7.2.3.d. Genes with restricted roles. The novel idea introduced by Ghysen *et al.*[77] is that some genes, such as *bx*, control cuticle-secreting cells but not the associated nerve cells. In their words, "the segmental identities of epidermis and neurones are under distinct control", and they suggest a search for hypothetical neuron-specific genes. However, there is no reason why some genes might not affect both epidermal cells and nerve cells, while others affect one class and not the other. Indeed, the mutant *abx* produces both a bithorax phenotype in the periphery and a winglike projection of the small s.c. axons (section 6.5.3). Furthermore, it is present in the genotype which Green describes as producing an altered motor neuron morphology in the CNS (section 6.7). Since the mutation appears to affect at least three classes of cells—cuticle-secreting epidermal cells, peripheral sensory cells, and central motor neurons—the *abx* gene can hardly be described as neuron-specific. However, the *bx* gene may not affect neurons, and that is the important point.

7.2.4. BX-C and ANT-C Compared. I have repeatedly emphasized the general similarity between *bithorax* small s.c. projections and *Antennapedia* and *proboscipedia* projections. Do any of the foregoing hypotheses developed for BX-C mutants help to explain the phenomenology seen in ANT-C mutants? For example, do *Antennapedia* homeotic leg axons project to antennal centers because the mutation affects only the cuticle and not the neurons? This is unlikely to be the whole story, since within the antennal centers the distribution of endings is quite different in wild-type flies and in *Antennapedia* mutants. Nevertheless, the basic idea that epidermal cells and neurons may be differentially affected by a given mutation (and by inference also by its normally functioning wild-type allele) may well be widely applicable.

7.3. The Strengths and Limitations of Mosaic Studies

In most respects, the projections of mutant sensory neurons into wild-type central nervous systems (in mosaic animals) have turned out to look much like their projections into mutant nervous systems. What, then, is the point of painstakingly making mosaics?

In the first place, of course, we could not know that this would be the case until the mosaic experiments were done. Secondly, mutations in both the ANT-C (*spineless-aristapedia, proboscipedia*) and the BX-C (*bithorax*) have been studied in mosaic animals and yielded the same result: little or no difference between projections into mutant and into wild-type CNS. Therefore, the result has considerable generality. We can conclude that the CNS need not be transformed by a homeotic mutation in order for the major features of the projection pattern to be established.

Can we draw the wider inference that these mutations have no direct effect at all on the CNS? I believe not. Section 6.7 summarizes some of the evidence that changes do occur in the CNS of BX-C mutants.

The strongest evidence, that of Green,[78] is based on the location and morphology of motor neurons, whereas we and most other workers have studied sensory projections. It is quite conceivable that a particular homeotic mutation might affect motor neurons either with (*abx*) or without (*bx*) noticeably affecting the branching patterns of primary sensory axons. But it is equally conceivable that the effect upon the motor neurons is the indirect consequence of changes in the complement of sensory axons entering the same neuromere. A mosaic experiment, producing flies with a mutant CNS but a normal periphery, would help to settle the point.

Mosaic analyses, however, do not solve all problems. Suppose that we obtained the result that is the opposite of what has actually been found—that in a particular case the projection from a homeotic appendage in a wild-type CNS looked very different than in a mutant CNS. This certainly could be due to a direct effect of the mutation on the CNS. But target cells in the CNS might have differential responses to the presence of homeotic axons, or to the absence of normal axons, or to different numbers of axons, and these in turn might affect the paths of incoming axons. In no animal do we know the full range of cellular interactions that occur during neural development, and possible interactions need to be tested by experiments designed to suit particular cases. Genetic mosaics are one of the most powerful tools in this process, but no single experimental design is likely to test adequately for all possible explanations of a given phenomenon.

7.4. *The Role of Compartments*

The role of compartments in neural development remains enigmatic, and may be different in different locations.

7.4.1. Compartments and Peripheral Axon Paths. In sections 4.3 and 4.4 I showed that sensory axons do not remain confined to a single compartment but can cross even the best-defined compartment boundaries freely. Thus, a test which could have shown a direct effect of compartmentalization upon peripheral axon paths failed to do so. Instead, we were led to conclude that the dominant immediate factor in establishing the paths of sensory axons is one familiar from other insect systems, preexisting nerves with a guiding function. Whether compartmentalization affects the placement of the guiding nerves has not yet been examined.

7.4.2. Compartments and Central Projections. Does the location of a peripheral sensory cell body in one or another compartment govern (or at least allow the experimenter to predict) the choice of paths which its axon will take in the CNS? Evidence in the affirmative, and a strong defense of the idea, has been provided by Ghysen and his collaborators.[66,73,77,86]

The idea is attractive. It links neural development and body surface development, and provides simple rules for pathway selection. Still, I wish to insert a note of caution about it: it is essential to distinguish clearly whether axons project along the same path within the CNS because they originate in the same compartment, or merely because they originate close together. Topographic representation need not have anything to do with compartments. A critical test is difficult to make because of the actual distribution of receptors relative to well-mapped compartment boundaries, and the best we can do at the moment is to keep the question in mind when evaluating the available data.

There is no particular discrepancy between data indicating a lack of effect of compartments on peripheral pathways and a strong effect on central pathways. For example, in orthopteran insects such as crickets and grasshoppers, all the sensory fibers in a given appendage follow the peripheral pioneer fibers to the CNS (see Chapter 7). Once within the CNS, however, they quickly diverge, presumably following other cues (M. Shankland). The dominant guiding factors in the periphery and the CNS seem to be different. By analogy, it is entirely reasonable to suppose that sensory fibers in *Drosophila* might be guided by preexisting pupal nerves in the periphery quite independently of compartment boundaries, but within the CNS their compartment of origin would be reflected in their choice of tracts and termination areas.

7.4.3. Compartments within the CNS. The first systematic search for compartments within the CNS and other internal tissues, based on the behavior of clones detected with histochemical techniques, has yielded negative results. No compartments could be clearly demonstrated.[91] Thus, we see the somewhat peculiar situation that compartments seem not to matter in making peripheral sensory nerves or central nervous systems, but may play a role in the behavior of sensory axons within the CNS. Surely more remains to be learned!

7.5. Evaluation and Prognosis

The study of genetic influences on the development of neural pathways in *Drosophila* is just beginning (for extensive reviews, see Hall and Greenspan[3]; Hall *et al.*[4]). Still, enough data have been obtained to give reasonable support to a Waddingtonian view: the hypotheses of experimental embryology, such as guidance by contact between cells, are an essential part of our thinking. However, experiments using mutants, particularly homeotic mutants, yield data inviting interpretation not only in cellular terms but also in genetic terms.[87] The resulting hypotheses are different in kind from those generated by surgical and other nongenetic experiments. Furthermore, they are detailed, explicit, and testable.

The immediate future of this work includes studies at all three levels of analysis: description, formulation of rules, and a search for molecular mechanisms. For instance, in my lab I want to investigate axons growing in the wing and describe their behavior at interesting choice points. The first mosaic study based on clones of homeotic cells in the CNS is now in progress (S. Green, personal communication)—this, like most of the work described in the present chapter, is analysis at the level of rules. A search for molecular mechanisms involved in compartmentalization utilizing monoclonal antibodies has begun,[88,89] and an extension of this approach to the nervous system would be logical (see Chapter 3).

Thus, studying the neurobiology of mutants in *Drosophila* has led to surprising observations and to ideas which could not have been derived from nongenetic studies. We have been through an initial phase of rapid exploration and are now in a strong position to pursue more rigorous studies, utilizing but by no means limited to genetic materials and techniques.

ACKNOWLEDGMENTS

My interest in *Drosophila* neurobiology has been nurtured by my long-time collaborator Margrit Schubiger, who commented thoughtfully on this manuscript as she has on my other endeavors. Steve Hart rejoined the lab at just the right time to apply his talents to the figures (both the line drawings and the SEM's) and his mind to the problems. The ideas in this paper owe much to extensive discussions with Alain Ghysen and Gunther Stent, especially during their visits to Seattle during 1980–81. I want finally to thank Prof. E. B. Lewis, who has so generously provided stocks and advice to our lab as he has to many others. Our work has been supported by grants NS-07778 from the NIH and BNS-7914111 from the NSF.

8. REFERENCES

1. Ramón y Cajal, S., 1909, *Histologie du Système Nerveux de l'Homme et des Vertébrés*, vols. I and II, Reprinted by Instituto Ramón y Cajal del C. S. I. C., Madrid, 1952–1955.
2. Ward, S., 1977, Invertebrate neurogenetics, *Ann. Rev. Genet.* **11**:415.

3. Hall, J. C., and Greenspan, R., 1980, Genetic analysis of *Drosophila* neurobiology, *Ann. Rev. Genet.* **13**:127.
4. Hall, J. C., Greenspan, R. J., and Harris, W. A., 1981, *Neurogenetics*, Neuroscience Research Program, MIT Press, Cambridge, in press.
5. Lewis, E. B., 1963, Genes and developmental pathways, *Am. Zool.* **3**:33.
6. Stent, G. S., 1980, The genetic approach to developmental neurobiology, *Trends Neurosci.* **3**:49.
7. Stent, G. S., 1981, Strength and weakness of the genetic approach to the development of the nervous system, *Ann. Rev. Neurosci.* **4**:163.
8. Waddington, C. H., 1956, *Principles of Embryology*, George Allen & Unwin, London.
9. Judd, B. H., 1976, Genetic units of *Drosophila*—Complex loci, in: *The Genetics and Biology of Drosophila*, vol. 1b (M. Ashburner and E. Novitski, eds.), pp. 767–799, Academic Press, London.
10. Lindsley, D. L., and Grell, E. H., 1968, Genetic variations of *Drosophila melanogaster*, *Carnegie Inst. Washington Publ.* 627.
11. García-Bellido, A., 1975, Genetic control of wing disc development in *Drosophila*, in: *Cell Patterning*, Ciba Foundation Symposium 29 (new series), pp. 161–178, Elsevier-Excertpa Medica-North Holland, Amsterdam.
12. Postlethwait, J. H., and Schneiderman, H. A., 1973, Developmental Genetics of *Drosophila* imaginal discs, *Ann. Rev. Genet.* **7**:381.
13. Ouweneel, W. J., 1975, Developmental genetics of homeosis, *Adv. Genet.* **18**:1.
14. Stern, C., 1968, *Genetic Mosaics and Other Essays*, Harvard University Press, Cambridge, MA.
15. Palka, J., 1979*a*, Mutants and mosaics, tools in insect developmental neurobiology, *Symp. Soc. Neurosci.* **4**:209.
16. Hall, J. C., Gelbart, W. M., and Kankel, D. R., 1976, Mosaic systems, in: *The Genetics and Biology of Drosophila*, vol. 1a (M. Ashburner and E. Novitski, eds.), pp. 265–314, Academic Press, London.
17. Hall, J. C., Tompkins, L., Kyriacou, C. P., Siegel, R. W., Schilcher, F. von, and Greenspan, R. J., 1980, Higher behavior in *Drosophila* analyzed with mutations that disrupt the structure and function of the nervous system, in: *Development and Neurobiology of Drosophila* (O. Siddiqi, P. Babu, L. M. Hall, and J. C. Hall, eds.), pp. 425–454, Plenum Press, New York.
18. Bhaskaran, G., and Sivasubramanian, P., 1969, Metamorphosis of imaginal disks of the housefly: Evagination of transplanted disks, *J. Exp. Zool.* **171**:385.
19. Becker, H. J., 1976, Mitotic recombination, in: *The Genetics and Biology of Drosophila*, vol. 1c (M. Ashburner and E. Novitski, eds.), pp. 1020–1087, Academic Press, London.
20. Morata, G., and Ripoll, P., 1975, Minutes: Mutants of *Drosophila* autonomously affecting cell division rate, *Dev. Biol*, **42**:211.
21. Suzuki, D. T., Kaufman, T., Falk, D., and the U.B.C. Drosophila Research Group, 1976, Conditionally expressed mutations in *Drosophila melanogaster*, in: *The Genetics and Biology of Drosophila*, vol. 1a (M. Ashburner and E. Novitski, eds.), pp. 207–263, Academic Press, London.
22. Kauffman, S. A., 1973, Control circuits for determination and transdetermination, *Science* **181**:310.
23. Hadorn, E., 1978, Transdetermination, in: *The Genetics and Biology of Drosophila*, vol. 2c (M. Ashburner and T. R. F. Wright, eds.), pp. 555–617, Academic Press, London.
24. Kauffman, S. A., Shymko, R. M., and Trabert, K., 1978, Control of sequential compartment formation in *Drosophila*, *Science* **199**:259.

25. Lewis, E. B., 1951, Pseudoallelism and gene evolution, *Cold Spring Harbor Symp. Quant. Biol.* **16:**159.
26. Lewis, E. B., 1954, Pseudoallelism and the gene concept, *Caryologia Suppl.* **6:**100.
27. Lewis, E. B., 1955, Some aspects of position pseudoallelism, *Am. Nat.* **89:**73.
28. Lewis, E. B., 1964*a*, Genetic control and regulation of pathways, in: *The Role of Chromosomes in Development* (M. Locke, ed.), pp. 231–252, Academic Press, New York.
29. Lewis, E. B., 1964*b*, Genetic control and regulation of developmental pathways, *Symp. Soc. Dev. Biol.* **23:**231.
30. Lewis, E. B., 1967, Genes and gene complexes, in: *Heritage from Mendel* (R. A. Brink and E. D. Styles, eds.), pp. 17–47, University Wisconsin Press, Madison, WI.
31. Lewis, E. B., 1968, Genetic control of developmental pathways, *Proc. Int. Congr. Genet.* **2:**96.
32. Lewis, E. B., 1978, A gene complex controlling segmentation in *Drosophila, Nature* (London) **276:**565.
33. Lewis, E. B., 1981, Developmental genetics of the bithorax complex in *Drosophila,* in: *ICN-UCLA Symposia on Molecular and Cellular Biology,* vol. XXIII (D. D. Brown and C. F. Fox, eds.), Academic Press, New York, in press.
34. García-Bellido, A., 1977, Homeotic and atavic mutations in insects, *Am. Zool.* **17:**613.
35. Shearn, A., 1980, What is the normal function of genes which give rise to homeotic mutations? in: *Development and Neurobiology of Drosophila* (O. Siddiqi, P. Babu, L. M. Hall, and J. C. Hall, eds.), pp. 155–162. Plenum Press, New York.
36. Schubiger, G., and Newman, S. M., 1981, Determination in *Drosophila* embryos, *Am. Zool.*, in press.
37. Kaufman, T. C., Lewis, R., and Wakimoto, B., 1980, Cytogenetic analysis of chromosome 3 in *Drosophila melanogaster*: The homeotic gene complex in polytene chromosome interval 84A-B, *Genetics* **94:**115.
38. Lewis, R. A., Wakimoto, B. T., Denell, R. E., and Kaufman, T. C., 1980, Genetic analysis of the antennapedia gene complex (ANT-C) and adjacent chromosomal regions of *Drosophila melanogaster*. II. Polytene chromosome segments 84A-84B1,2, *Genetics* **95:**383.
39. García-Bellido, A., Ripoll, P., and Morata, G., 1973, Developmental compartmentalization of the wing disk of *Drosophila, Nature New Biol.* **245:**251.
40. García-Bellido, A., Ripoll, P., and Morata, G., 1976, Developmental compartmentalization in the dorsal mesothoracic disc of *Drosophila, Dev. Biol.* **48:**132.
41. Crick, F. H. C., and Lawrence, P. A., 1975, Compartments and polyclones in insect development, *Science* **189:**340.
42. Morata, G., and Lawrence, P. A., 1977, Homeotic genes, compartments and cell determination in *Drosophila, Nature* (London) **265:**211.
43. Steiner, E., 1976, Establishment of compartments in the developing leg imaginal discs of *Drosophila melanogaster, Wilhelm Roux Arch. Entwicklungsmech. Org.* **180:**9.
44. Morata, G., and Lawrence, P. A., 1975, Control of compartment development by the *engrailed* gene in *Drosophila, Nature* (London) **255:**614.
45. Lawrence, P. A., and Morata, G., 1976, Compartments in the wing of *Drosophila*: A study of the *engrailed* gene, *Dev. Biol.* **50:**321.
46. Morata, G., and Lawrence, P. A., 1977, The development of *wingless,* a homeotic mutation of *Drosophila, Dev. Biol.* **56:**227.
47. Sharma, R. P., and Chopra, V. L., 1976, Effect of *wingless* (*wg*) mutation on wing and haltere development in *Drosophila melanogaster, Dev. Biol.* **48:**461.
48. Deak, I. I., 1978, Thoracic duplications in the mutant *wingless* of *Drosophila* and their effect on muscles and nerves, *Dev. Biol.* **66:**422.

49. Hayes, P. H., Girton, J. R., and Russell, M. A., 1979, Positional information and the bithorax complex, *J. Theor. Biol.* **79:**1.
50. Karlsson, J., 1982, Homeotic genes and the function of compartments in *Drosophila*, submitted for publication.
51. Power, M. E., 1943, The brain of *Drosophila melanogaster*, *J. Morphol.* **72:**517.
52. Power, M. E., 1946, The antennal centers and their connections with the brain of *Drosophila melanogaster*, *J. Comp. Neurol.* **85:**485.
53. Power, M. E., 1948, The thoraco-abdominal nervous system of an adult insect, *Drosophila melanogaster*, *J. Comp. Neurol.* **88:**347.
54. Kankel, D. R., Ferrus, A., Garen, S. H., Harte, P. J., and Lewis, P. E., 1980, The structure and development of the nervous system, in: *The Genetics and Biology of Drosophila*, vol. 2d (M. Ashburner and T. R. F. Wright, eds.), pp. 295–368, Academic Press, London.
55. Hertweck, H., 1931, Anatomie und Variabilität des Nervensystems und der Sinnesorgane von *Drosophila melanogaster* (Meigen), *Z. Wiss. Zool. Abt. A* **139:**559.
56. White, K., and Kankel, D. R., 1978, Patterns of cell division and cell movement in the formation of the imaginal nervous system in *Drosophila melanogaster*, *Dev. Biol.* **65:**296.
57. Lawrence, P. A., 1975, The structure and properties of a compartment border: The intersegmental boundary in *Oncopeltus*, in *Cell Patterning*, Ciba Foundation Symposium 29 (new series), pp. 3–16. Elsevier-Excerpta Medica-North Holland, Amsterdam.
58. Palka, J., Schubiger, M., and Hart, H. S., 1981, The path of axons in the wing of *Drosophila* in relation to compartment boundaries, *Nature*, **294:**447.
59. Edwards, J. S., Chen, S.-W., and Berns, M. W., 1981, Cercal sensory development following laser microlesions of embryonic apical cells in *Acheta domesticus*, *J. Neurosci.* **1:**250.
60. Reed, C. T., Murphy, C., and Fristrom, D., 1975, The ultrastructure of the differentiating pupal leg of *Drosophila melanogaster*, *Wilhelm Roux Arch. Entwicklungsmech. Org.* **178:**285.
61. Waddington, C. H., 1940, The genetic control of wing development in *Drosophila*, *J. Genet.* **14:**75.
62. Lamparter, H. E., Akert, K., and Sandri, C., 1967, Wallersche Degeneration im Zentralnervensystem der Ameise, *Schweiz. Arch. Neurol. Neurochir. Psychiatr.* **100:**337.
63. Stocker, R. F., Edwards, J. S., Palka, J., Schubiger, G., 1976, Projection of sensory neurons from a homeotic mutant appendage, *Antennapedia*, in *Drosophila melanogaster*, *Dev. Biol.* **52:**210.
64. Stocker, R. F., and Lawrence, P. A., 1981, Sensory projections from normal and homeotically transformed antennae in *Drosophila*, *Dev. Biol.*, **82:**224–237.
65. Stocker, R., 1981, Homeotically displaced sensory neurons in the proboscis and antenna of *Drosophila* project into the same identified brain regions though by different pathways, in preparation.
66. Ghysen, A., and Janson, R., 1980, Sensory pathways in *Drosophila* central nervous system, in: *Development and Neurobiology of Drosophila* (O. Siddiqi, P. Babu, L. M. Hall, and J. C. Hall, eds.), pp. 247–265, Plenum Press, New York.
67. Palka, J., and Schubiger, M., 1980, Formation of central patterns by receptor cell axons in *Drosophila*, in: *Development and Neurobiology of Drosophila* (O. Siddiqi, P. Babu, L. M. Hall, and J. C. Hall, eds.), pp. 223–246, Plenum Press, New York.
68. Strausfeld, N. J., and Singh, R. N., 1980, Peripheral and central nervous system projections in normal and mutant (bithorax) *Drosophila melanogaster*, in: *Development*

and Neurobiology of Drosophila (O. Siddiqi, P. Babu, L. M. Hall, and J. C. Hall, eds.), pp. 267–290, Plenum Press, New York.
69. Palka, J., Lawrence, P. A., and Hart, H. S., 1979, Neural projection patterns from homeotic tissue of *Drosophila* studied in *bithorax* mutants and mosaics, *Dev. Biol.* **69:**549.
70. Cole, E. S., and Palka, J., 1980, Sensilla on normal and homeotic wings of *Drosophila, Am. Zool.* **20:**740.
71. Cole, E. S., Hart, H. S., and Palka, J., 1981, Patterns of sensilla on the wing and haltere of *Drosophila* analyzed with scanning electron microscopy, in preparation, see reference 92.
72. Cole, E. S., Hart, H. S., and Palka, J., 1981, Sensilla on normal and homeotic wings of *Drosophila* analyzed with scanning electron microscopy, in preparation, see reference 92.
73. Ghysen, A., 1980, The projection of sensory neurons in the central nervous system of *Drosophila*: Choice of the appropriate pathway, *Dev. Biol.* **78:**521.
74. Burt, R., and Palka, J., 1981, The central projections of mesothoracic sensory neurons in wild type *Drosophila* and *bithorax* mutants, *Develop. Biol.*, in press.
75. Ghysen, A., 1978, Sensory neurons recognize defined pathways in *Drosophila* central nervous system, *Nature (London)* **274:**869.
76. Anderson, H., Edwards, J. S., and Palka, J., 1980, Developmental neurobiology of invertebrates, *Ann. Rev. Neurosci.* **3:**97.
77. Ghysen, A., Janson, R., and Santamaria, P., 1982, Genetic control of neuronal pathways in *Drosophila,* submitted for publication.
78. Green, S. H., 1981, Segment-specific organization of leg motoneurones is transformed in bithorax mutants of *Drosophila, Nature (London)* **292:**152.
79. Anderson, H., Bacon, J., 1979, Developmental determination of neuronal projection patterns from wind-sensitive hairs in the locust, *Schistocerca gregaria, Dev. Biol.* **72:**364.
80. Anderson, H., 1981*a*, Development of a sensory system: The formation of central projections and connections by ectopic wind-sensitive hairs in the locust *Schistocerca gregaria,* in preparation.
81. Anderson, H., 1981*b*, Projections from sensory neurons developing at ectopic sites in insects, *J. Embryol. Exp. Morphol.* **65**(Suppl.):209.
82. Bacon, J., and Anderson, H., 1981, Developmental determination of central connections from wind-sensitive hairs in the locust *Schistocerca gregaria,* in preparation.
83. Anderson, H., 1981*c*, The organization of mechanosensory inputs within the locust central nervous system, in preparation.
84. Adler, P. N., 1978, Mutants of the bithorax complex and determinative states in the thorax of *Drosophila melanogaster, Dev. Biol.* **65:**447.
85. Morata, G., 1975, Analysis of gene expression during development in the homeotic mutant *Contrabithorax* of *Drosophila melanogaster, J. Embryol. Exp. Morphol.* **34:**19.
86. Vandervorst, Ph., and Ghysen, A., 1980, Genetic control of sensory projections in *Drosophila, Nature (London)* **286:**65.
87. Palka, J., 1979*b*, Theories of pattern formation in insect neural development, *Adv. Insect Physiol.* **14:**256.
88. Wilcox, M., Brower, D., and Smith, R. J., 1980, Monoclonal antibodies in the analysis of *Drosophila* development, in: *Development and Neurobiology of Drosophila* (O. Siddiqi, P. Babu, L. M. Hall, and J. C. Hall, eds.), pp. 193–199, Plenum Press, New York.
89. Brower, D. L., Smith, R. J., and Wilcox, M., 1980, A monoclonal antibody specific for diploid epithelial cells in *Drosophila, Nature (London)* **285:**403.
90. Shankland, M., 1981, Development of a sensory afferent projection in the grasshopper

embryo. II. Growth and branching of peripheral sensory axons within the central nervous system, *J. Embryol. Exp. Morphol.* **64**:187.

91. Ferrus, A., and Kankel, D. R., 1981, Cell lineage relationships in *Drosophila melanogaster*: The relationships of cuticular to internal tissues, *Develop. Biol.* **85**:485.
92. Cole, E. S., and Palka, J., 1982, The pattern of campaniform sensilla on the wing and haltere of *Drosophila melanogaster* and several of its homeotic mutants, submitted for publication.
93. Morata, G., and Kerridge, S., 1980, An analysis of the expressivity of some bithorax transformations, in: *Development and Neurobiology of Drosophila* (O. Siddiqi, P. Babu, L. M. Hall and J. C. Hall, eds.), Plenum Press, New York, pp. 141–154.

5

Embryonic Development of Identified Neurons in the Grasshopper

COREY S. GOODMAN

1. INTRODUCTION

Several years ago we began to examine the embryonic development of the grasshopper nervous system. We hope that by someday understanding the cellular and molecular mechanisms underlying the development of this relatively simple and highly accessible nervous system, we will help answer some of the fundamental questions common to the development of all nervous systems. This chapter describes the beginning of such an approach. In particular, the chapter will examine the progeny of two different neuronal precursor cells (called the median neuroblast or MNB, and midline precursor 3 or MP3), and will describe the differentiation from birth to maturation of identified neurons that arise from specific cell divisions of these two precursors. After examining the lineage and differentiation of the progeny of these two precursors in a single segment, the development of these cells in other segments will be examined. Our results demonstrate how segmental specializations in the nervous system can arise by segment-specific differentiation and segment-specific cell death of identified neurons of known lineage.

COREY S. GOODMAN · Department of Biological Sciences, Stanford University, Stanford, CA 94305.

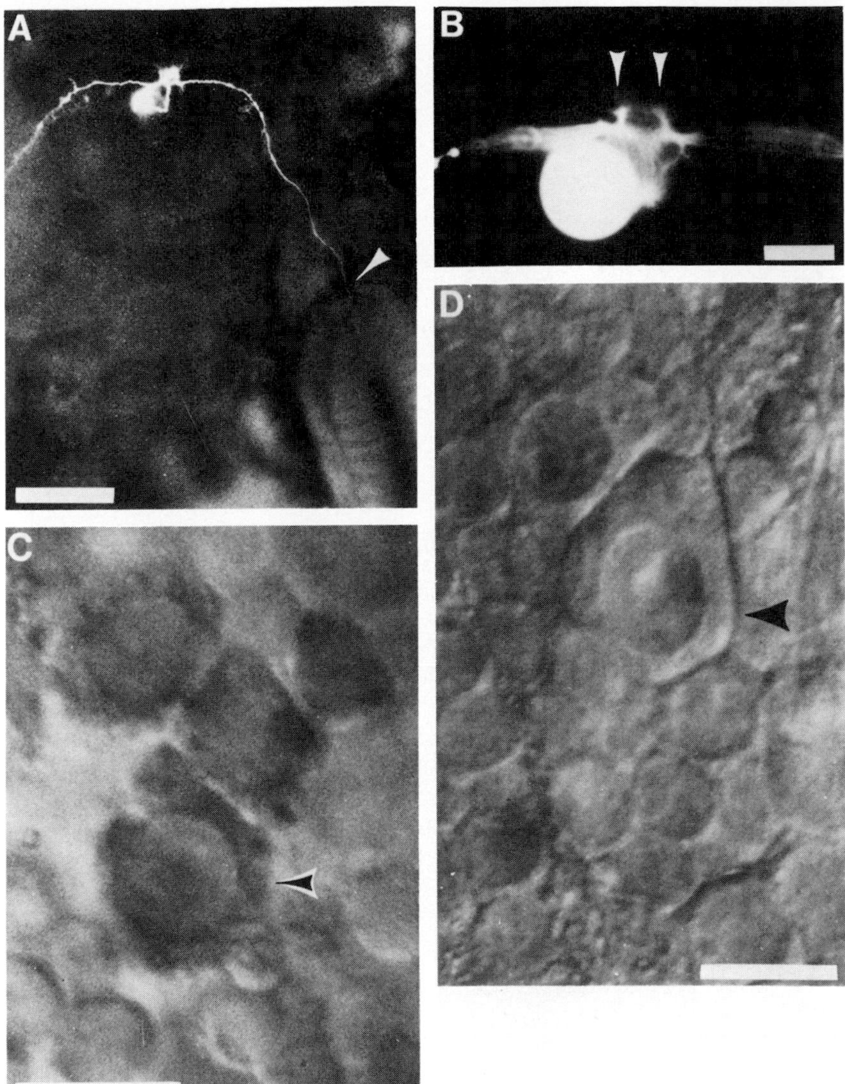

Figure 1. Morphology of DUM 5 (DUMETi), one of the oldest progeny of the MNB, in the metathoracic (T3) ganglion at several stages of grasshopper embryogenesis. (A) Peripheral morphology of DUM 5 in a 13-day embryo, revealed by fluorescence of the intracellularly injected dye Lucifer Yellow. Arrow marks axon of DUM 5 coursing over extensor tibiae muscle (the cross-striations of the muscle are visible). The shallow depth of focal plane prevents visualization of the axon over the entire length of muscle. (B) Central morphology of DUM 5 in a different 13-day embryo, stained as in (A). The cell body appears unusually large because of the intense fluorescence. Arrows mark initial outgrowth of central arborizations. (C) Neutral red staining of the soma of DUM 5 (arrow)

Much of the work on the MNB and MP3 progeny was done in collaboration with Nicholas Spitzer (Biology Department, U.C. San Diego) and Michael Bate (Zoology Department, Cambridge University).

Our reasons for turning to the grasshopper embryo are much the same as William Morton Wheeler's when, in 1893, he published his classic monograph on the grasshopper embryo entitled simply "A contribution to insect embryology."[1] The early embryos are large and made up of large, accessible cells, particularly in the nervous system. In 1976 Michael Bate rekindled interest in the grasshopper embryo when he published the first of two papers[2,3] showing the stereotyped pattern of neuronal precursor cells. In particular, the precursors are large, highly accessible, and reproducible in number and pattern from embryo to embryo. Whereas Wheeler was limited to fixed and sectioned material, today we can view the dissected embryo with Normarski interference contrast optics and impale cells with microelectrodes for dye injections or physiological recordings (Fig. 1). Not only are the individual cell bodies and early fiber pathways visible, but with the appropriate optics the individual axons and in some cases the growth cones are visible and can be penetrated with microelectrodes.

2. THE GRASSHOPPER NERVOUS SYSTEM

Before describing its development, we first need a short description of the final differentiated form: the adult grasshopper nervous system. A grasshopper's central nervous system (CNS), like that of most metazoan animals, is bilaterally symmetrical and metamerically arranged to correspond to the basic segmental body plan (Fig. 2). The sensory neurons have their cell bodies in the periphery and send their axons into the CNS. Within the CNS are several hundred thousand neurons, most located in the brain and optic lobes. Fortunately, the chain of segmental ganglia is much simpler and contains at most a few thousand neurons per segment. Early in embryogenesis each body segment has a segmental ganglion, but as development proceeds, some fusion of ganglia takes place leading to the final adult form. In the adult, the

---

and two other identified MNB progeny (DUM 3, 4, 5 and DUM 4, 5) in a desheathed preparation of a 15-day embryo. A fourth and smaller soma is also stained at this stage. (D) Interference contrast view of the dorsal surface of the ganglion in an 18-day embryo; the soma of DUM 5 is marked with an arrow. The volume of DUM 5 (mostly cytoplasmic) is large as compared with other MNB progeny. Calibration bars: (A) 200 μm; (B) 50 μm; (C and D) 25 μm. (From Goodman *et al.*[11])

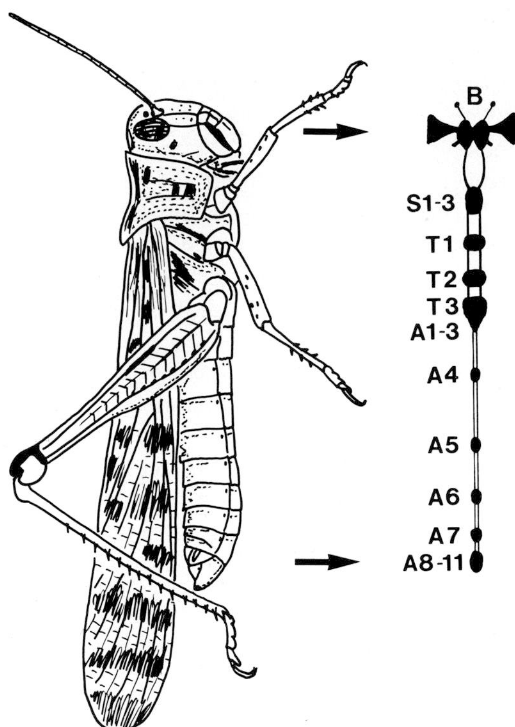

Figure 2. (Left) Schematic diagram of an adult grasshopper (*Schistocerca americana*) showing its basic segmental body plan, consisting of a head (including an unknown number of brain segments and segments S1–3 which control the mouth parts), thorax (segments T1–3, with three pairs of legs and two pairs of wings), and abdomen (segments A1–11). (Right) Schematic diagram of the grasshopper CNS showing the brain (B) and optic lobes, and the chain of unfused and fused segmental ganglia (S1–3, T1–3, A1–11). (The ganglia are a bit larger than in the animal.) Each thoracic ganglion contains about 3000 neurons; each abdominal ganglion contains about 500 neurons.

subesophogeal ganglion consists of three fused embryonic ganglia (S1–S3) and contains about 5000 neurons. This fused ganglion innervates the mouth parts and other structures of the head. The three thoracic ganglia (T1, pro-; T2, meso-; and T3, metathoracic) innervate the three pairs of legs and two pairs of wings. Each contains about 3000 neurons, the most for any single segment. The 11 abdominal segments do not have appendages but rather have other specializations. Each has a ganglion (A1–A11) with about 500 neurons. The first three abdominal ganglia (A1–A3) fuse with the T3 ganglion, the next four remain unfused (A4–A7), and the last four (A8–A11) fuse to form the terminal abdominal ganglion. Thus, the thoracic and abdominal ganglia are associated with different segmental appendages and/or structures, with different behaviors, and contain different numbers of neurons (3000 vs. 500).

It is likely that most of the neurons in the segmental ganglia can be described as individually unique cells (identified neurons) or at least as parts of small clusters of equivalent neurons. Our knowledge about the morphology of individual identified neurons is greatest for the T2 and T3 ganglia and is due largely to work in the laboratories of Malcolm Burrows at Cambridge University and Keir Pearson at the University of Alberta. Several points are clear from their studies. First, most identified neurons have complex morphologies that are reproducible in basic structure from animal to animal. Second, many identified neurons are specialized for, and only found in, one or a few segmental ganglia (i.e., neurons with that particular morphology are not found in the other ganglia).

3. GRASSHOPPER EMBRYOLOGY

The eggs of the grasshopper *Schistocerca americana* are oval in shape (8 mm by 2 mm) and enclosed in a tough protective eggshell; clusters of 80–100 are laid in moist sand or soil. The timing of embryogenesis is highly dependent upon temperature. For example, at 33°C (the temperature used in our studies), the juveniles of *S. americana* hatch out of the egg case 20 days after fertilization. Thus, when we speak of days of development, we mean out of the 20 days at 33°C. Each day at 33°C is 5% of development (1% = 4.8 hr). The relative age of embryos raised at different temperatures can be conveniently compared on the basis of morphological criteria for 5%[4] and in some cases 1–2% stages.

The initial female pronucleus sits in a bit of cytoplasm within the yolky egg. After fertilization, the nucleus divides into several thousand cleavage nuclei, or energids, each surrounded by a bit of cytoplasm and each lacking a cell membrane. These nuclei migrate to the outside of the egg to the periplasm, where they form a syncitial blastoderm. Cell membranes form around the nuclei, leading to the cellular blastoderm. One part of this blastoderm thickens and becomes the germ band; the rest becomes the serosa, a cellular membrane surrounding the yolk. The blastoderm undergoes gastrulation, leading to the three basic cell layers: an outer (ventral) layer of ectoderm, a middle layer of mesoderm, and an inner (dorsal) layer of endoderm. The germ band then elongates giving rise to a segmental band of cells representing the basic body plan of cephalic, thoracic, and abdominal segments.

4. NEURONAL PRECURSOR CELLS

The nervous system forms from the ectoderm. The ectodermal epithelium that generates the nervous system runs down the middle of the embryo from head to tail as a strip of contiguous segmental plates of cells (Fig. 3). The dorsal surface of the neural epithelium is covered by a conspicuous noncellular basement membrane which separates it from the mesoderm; this basement membrane is probably secreted by

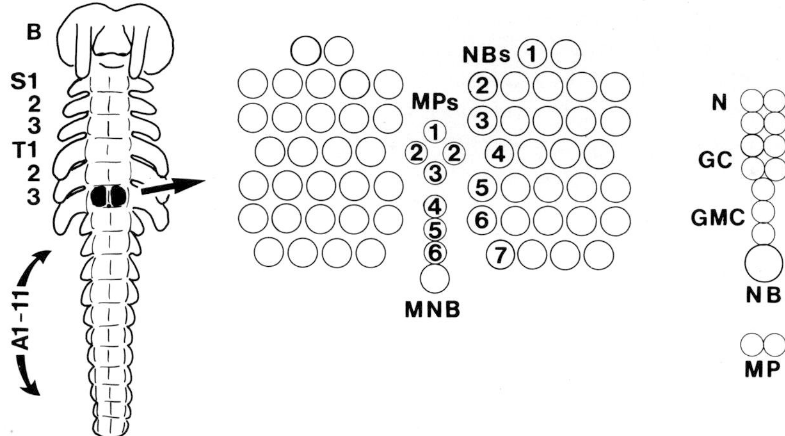

Figure 3. (Left) Schematic diagram of a 30% embryo[8] showing the segmental structure of the ectoderm (embryo is about 3 mm long). The middle of the ectoderm is a longitudinal strip of neuroepithelium which gives rise to the CNS. The location of the neuronal precursors for a single segment (T3) are drawn in black. (Middle) Pattern of neuronal precursors for a single segment (T3) include two plates of 30 NBs arranged in a precise pattern of seven rows, and one MNB making a total of 61 NBs. Anterior to the MNB along the dorsal midline are seven other cells called MPs. (Right) Pattern of cell division of the neuronal precursors. The MPs divide only once and give rise to two progeny. The NBs maintain their large size as stem cells and divide repeatedly to give rise to a chain of ganglion mother cells (GMC). As each GMC gets about three cells away from the NB, it divides one final time into two ganglion cells (GC) making a chain of doublets, which then differentiate into neurons (N). NBs generate from 10–100 progeny in a reproducible pattern; all NBs finally die and degenerate.

the ectoderm at an early stage. Within the neural epithelium, certain cells specialize as neuronal precursors, rounding up and generally enlarging relative to the cells around them. There are two types of neuronal precursors for the segmental ganglia (Fig. 3): neuroblasts (NBs)[2] and midline precursors (MPs).[3] Both types of precursors are large and conspicuous and can be easily counted from segment to segment within the same embryo, or from embryo to embryo for the same segment. A remarkable observation is that the pattern and number of precursor cells is repeatable in both cases (with minor changes at the anterior and posterior ends of the chain). There are two plates of 30 NBs each, arranged in seven rows of from two to five cells per row, and 1 MNB, making a total of 61 NBs. There are also seven MPs precisely arranged along the dorsal midline. After brief discussions of MP1 and MP2, we will examine in detail the MNB and MP3 and their progeny.

Each MP divides only once to produce two cells (Fig. 4). Each NB

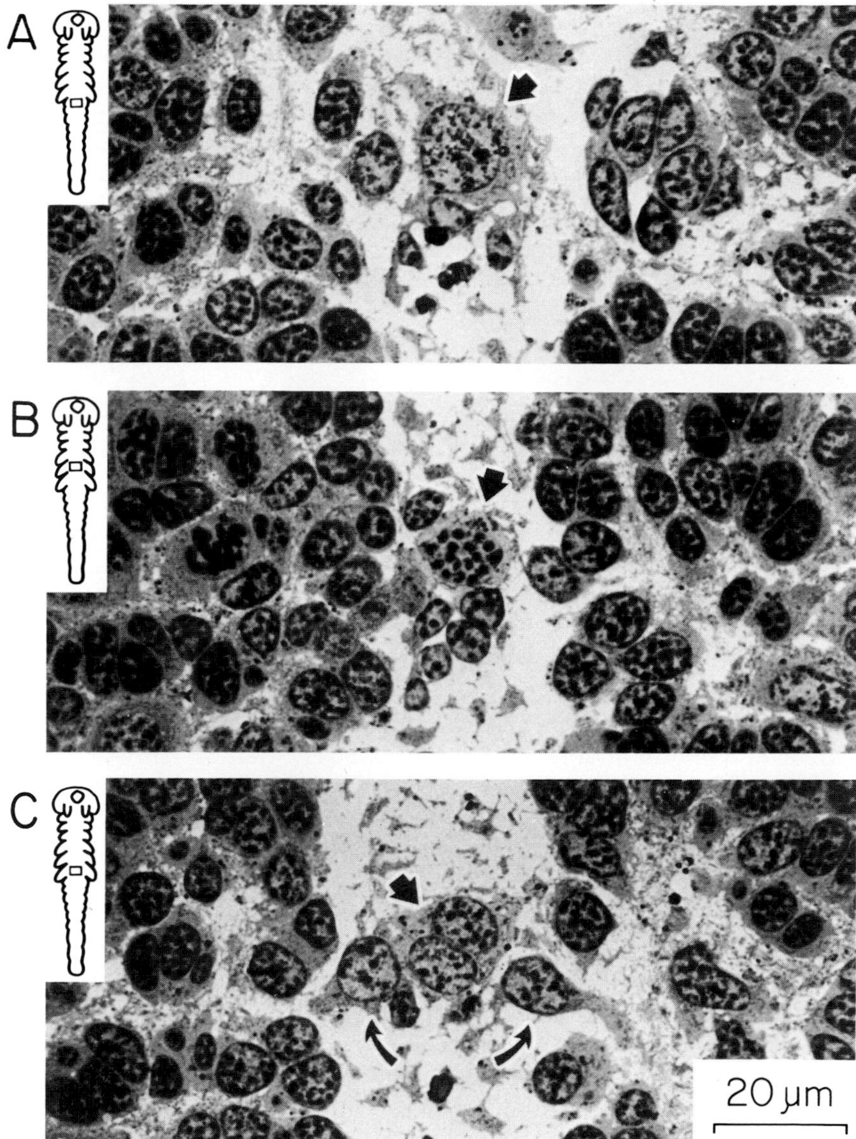

Figure 4. Photomicrographs of horizontal sections through the A1 (A), T2 (B), and T3 (C) segments of a 30% embryo showing the MP3 in (A), undergoing its single cell division in (B), and its two progeny in (C). Large arrows indicate MP3 and/or progeny; small arrows indicate progeny from either MP1 or MP2. (From Goodman *et al.*[9])

maintains its large size as a stem cell while it divides repeatedly to give rise to a chain of smaller cells (ganglion mother cells, GMC) each of which divides once more to generate a chain of doublets (ganglion cells, GC), which then differentiate into neurons. Thus, each NB contributes a clone of prospective neurons to the developing nervous system. Eventually the NBs die and degenerate, with some having produced as few as 10 neuronal progeny and others as many as 100.

5. EARLY AXONAL PATHWAYS

The first growth cones to navigate do so without having an existing nerve to follow. In the grasshopper, the cells subserving this pathfinding or pioneering role are large and conspicuous in both the periphery and CNS.[3,5,6] In the periphery, for example, cells called peripheral pioneers establish certain pathways and the axons of sensory neurons follow them. Early in embryogenesis, when the distances from periphery to center are short, a single cell moves just to the inside of the limb bud epithelium, divides into two cells, and both send growth cones toward the CNS along a stereotyped path (Fig. 5). There are no axons to follow, but rather each grows along the basement membrane on the inside of the ectodermal epithelium, their pattern of growth revealing a system of unknown cues within the limb bud to which they are responding. It has recently been shown that if the peripheral pioneer cells in the cercus of a cricket are eliminated with a laser, then the growth of later axons is disorganized and the normal pattern of peripheral nerves does not properly develop[7] (see Chapter 7).

A similar sequence of events occurs in the CNS; large and conspicuous cells send out growth cones that establish the early fiber pathways. Each segment develops a stereotyped pattern of nerve pathways in the form of longitudinal, commissural, and lateral fiber tracts. The very first pathways are again made by neurons whose growth cones navigate upon the ventral surface of the basement membrane that lies on the dorsal surface of the neural epithelium. These first growth cones come from the progeny of midline precursors 1, 2_L, and 2_R (MP1, $MP2_L$, and $MP2_R$).[3] Each MP2 divides once with its two progeny arranged dorsoventrally (vertically). The MP1 divides once with its two progeny arranged mediolaterally (horizontally); each MP1 progeny soon comes to lie over a pair of MP2 progeny. Thus a trio of cells sits on each side of the midline with, from dorsal to ventral, a MP1 progeny, the dorsal MP2 progeny, and the ventral MP2 progeny. Invariably, all three cells on each side send growth cones up to the dorsal basement membrane.

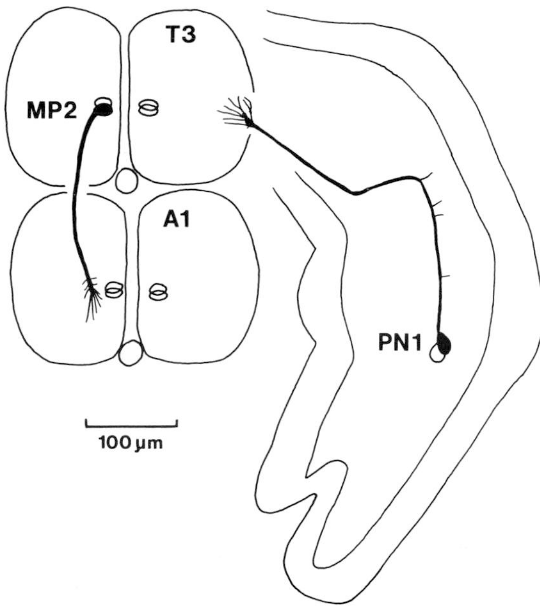

Figure 5. The early axonal pathways in the CNS and periphery are laid down by large and conspicuous "pioneer" cells. The morphology of the cells is revealed by intracellular injection of the fluorescent dye Lucifer Yellow; cells are drawn using a camera lucida. In the CNS, the two progeny of MP2 establish the first longitudinal axonal pathway linking the segments. In the periphery, the two progeny of pioneer neuron 1 (PN1) establish the first pathway linking the limb bud and the CNS. In this 36% embryo, the growth cones of the peripheral pioneers were just entering the CNS.

The growth cone of the ventral MP2 turns anteriorly, the growth cone of the dorsal MP2 turns posteriorly (Fig. 5), and the growth cone of the MP1 turns posteriorly with the dorsal MP2. In this way, the first longitudinal axonal pathways are generated on either side of the midline (Fig. 6A). An important point is that the same pathways typically are laid down in every segment of the nervous system. Other cells complete the ladderlike pattern of axonal pathways by forming commissures across the midline, other longitudinal pathways, and lateral pathways to the peripheral nerves. Not all pathways are laid down by specialized peripheral pioneers or central midline precursor cells; rather, some pathways are generated by these cells, and others in both the CNS and periphery by the progeny of NBs. Thus, the periodic organization of the neuroectoderm produces not only a repeated pattern of precursor cells, but also a repeated pattern of growth cones and axonal pathways. This pattern is expressed as a framework of axonal pathways within which

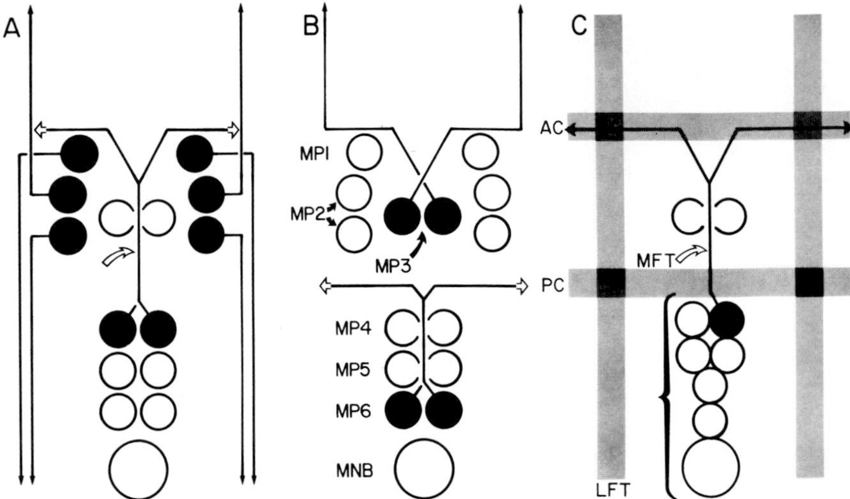

Figure 6. Schematic diagrams of the position and processes of the 14 progeny of the seven MPs and the early progeny of the MNB. (A) The processes of the progeny of MP1, $MP2_L$, and $MP2_R$ establish the longitudinal fiber tracts (LFT). The processes of the MP4 progeny establish the median fiber tract (MFT) and bifurcate before the anterior commissure (AC). (B) The MP3 progeny decussate and send processes out the contralateral sides of the AC and then anteriorly in the LFT. The MP6 progeny extend processes anteriorly that bifurcate in posterior commissure (PC). The terminations of the processes of the MP4 and MP6 progeny are presently unknown (open arrows). (C) The early progeny of the MNB (e.g., black cell) extend processes that follow the MFT established by the MP4 progeny. (From Goodman *et al.*[9])

later neurons in each segment differentiate as their growth cones navigate along the pathways and choose which way to go (see also Chapter 8).

6. CELL LINEAGE OF THE MEDIAN NEUROBLAST

Each segmental array of neuroblasts contains a single unpaired neuroblast, MNB, at the posterior end of the segment and near the dorsal surface of the neuroepithelium. (Two segments, T1 and A10, also have an extra anterior MNB.) Just anterior to the MNB are three MPs: MP4, MP5, and MP6. Whereas the MNB is about 30 μm in diameter and divides as a stem cell, each of the MPs in front of it is about 20 μm in diameter and divides only once. The six progeny of MP4–6 lie on top of each other with the two progeny of MP4 most dorsal, the two progeny of MP5 in the middle, and the two progeny of MP6 most ventral. Between 30–35% of embryonic development, the two progeny of MP4 send growth cones in the anterior direction along the midline, crossing the posterior commissure and extending over the top of the two progeny of MP3 (Fig. 6). Just anterior to the MP3 progeny, and just posterior to the anterior commissure, the growth cones of the MP4 progeny bifurcate and then extend laterally in a posterior pathway within the anterior commissure. Thus, the MP4 progeny are the "pioneers" for the dorsal median fiber tract (MFT), a pathway later followed by many of the progeny of the MNB. The processes of the MP5 progeny also appear to grow anteriorly and bifurcate in the anterior commissure. These two axons, however, are located just under (ventral to) the axons of the MP4 progeny and appear to form a separate axonal pathway followed by other progeny of the MNB. The processes of the MP6 progeny grow anteriorly and bifurcate in the posterior commissure. Still other progeny of the MNB follow this third pathway. These cells are shown diagrammatically in Fig. 6. Thus, the progeny of MP4–MP6 form three different medial axonal pathways: two extending anteriorly to the anterior commissure (from MP4 and MP5) and one extending anteriorly to the posterior commissure (from MP6).

In the metathoracic ganglion (T3), the MNB begins dividing shortly after 30% of development; it stops dividing and degenerates at about 80% of development. During this 50% period (or 10 days at 33°C) the MNB divides roughly 50 times and produces about 100 neuronal progeny. Thus the MNB divides about once every 5 h at 33°C.

Neuronal differentiation in this lineage is viewed by removing the embryo from the egg at different stages of development (see Chapters 1, 2, and 3 for other approaches to the analysis of lineage). The metathoracic ganglion is viewed under a water immersion lens of a compound microscope with Nomarski interference contrast optics. We follow the fate of cells that arise from specific cell divisions of the MNB by examining living embryos at intervals of less than 1% of development. Similarly we follow the cells in fixed embryos by examining 1-μm serial sections of the metathoracic ganglion at intervals of 1–2% of development. The first three progeny of the MNB were described by Goodman and Spitzer.[8] The lineage of the first 12 progeny has been described by Goodman and Bate (in preparation) as shown in Fig. 7.

The MNB divides initially in the dorsoventral plane, with the daughter cell sitting dorsal and the stem cell ventral. As cell divisions continue, the chain of progeny is pushed anteriorly over the dorsal surface of the MP4 progeny. As each ganglion mother cell gets about

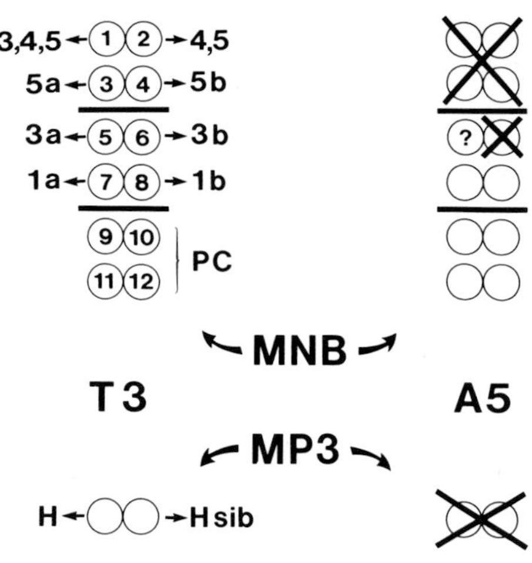

Figure 7. (Left) Cell lineage of the MNB and MP3 in the metathoracic (T3) segment, showing the identities of the first 12 progeny of the MNB and the 2 progeny of MP3 (the H cell and H-cell sib). DUM 3, 4, 5 and DUM 4, 5 arise from the first cell division of the MNB (3, 4, 5 is marked "1" because its growth cone comes out first); DUM 5a (DUMETi) and DUM 5b arise from its second cell division. Groups of four cells are separated by heavy lines because the growth cones from these quartets of cells initially follow the same pathway. Of the second quartet of cells, two send axons out nerve 3 and the next two send axons out nerve 1. In the third quartet, the cells all bifurcate in the posterior commissure (PC) (the ones before them bifurcate in the anterior commissure) and do not send axons out the peripheral nerves. (Right) Cell death of the MNB and MP3 progeny in the fifth abdominal (A5) segment. The first 4 progeny of the MNB die, as well as at least 1 of the next 2 (these cells include DUMETi or DUM 5a which normally innervates the extensor tibiae muscle of the leg in T3). Both progeny of MP3 typically die. The progeny of the MNB destined to die send out growth cones prior to their death. (Goodman and Bate, in preparation.)

three cell divisions away from the MNB, it divides once more in the horizontal plane to generate a column of doublets extending anteriorly. Early in embryogenesis, the MNB and its progeny are encased within the processes of epidermal cells. Later, the somata of the MNB progeny are encased in a common glial packet. It is not known whether the early epidermal cells become the glial cells, or whether other cells assume this role. However, this packaging of the MNB progeny throughout embryonic development allows us to follow these cells easily.

The processes of the first four progeny of the MNB follow the pathway established by the MP4 progeny (Fig. 6C). The first division of the MNB produces a ganglion mother cell that divides into two sibling cells. The cell that sends out its growth cone first becomes an identified neuron called DUM 3, 4, 5 (dorsal unpaired median neuron 3, 4, 5). Its axon follows the MP4 pathway, bifurcates at the anterior commissure, extends to the lateral edge of the ganglion on both sides, and sends axons out peripheral nerves 3, 4, and 5. The sibling of the cell sends its growth cone out a few hours later. The sibling's growth cone follows along on the axon of the first cell, with the exception that when it gets to the lateral edge of the ganglion, it sends axons out peripheral nerves 4 and 5 (but not out nerve 3); this cell is called DUM 4, 5. Thus, these two sibling neurons have certain similarities, yet they can be uniquely identified on the basis of whether they have an axon in nerve 3, and this correlates precisely with whose growth cone was sent out first. The two sibling cells from the second cell division extend processes along the same axonal pathway established by the MP4 progeny and followed by the first pair. They too bifurcate at the anterior commissure and extend laterally. Both of these cells send axons out only nerve 5 on both sides. There is, however, an important difference between these two cells. The first one to send out its growth cone takes a specific pathway via nerve branch 5bld that takes it to the extensor tibiae muscle of the limb bud; this cell is called DUM 5a (in many figures it is simply called DUM 5; it is also known as DUMETi). Its sibling sends its growth cone out next and does not take nerve branch 5bld but rather goes to some other peripheral target; this cell is called DUM 5b. These first four progeny of the MNB are called the first "quartet" of the MNB because they have certain features in common (Goodman and Bate, in preparation). First, they follow the same axonal pathways within the metathoracic ganglion. Second, they become dye coupled (Lucifer Yellow, mol. wt. 450) to one another after they initiate axons and remain dye coupled for several days, yet they do not couple to later progeny of the MNB. The cell bodies of three of the first four progeny of the MNB enlarge during embryogenesis and become three of the largest cells in the metathoracic ganglion. These three cell bodies (DUM 3, 4, 5; 4, 5; and 5a) are shown in a Nomarski photograph in Fig. 8, and schematically in Fig. 9.

The next four cells (cells 5–8) from the MNB are called the second quartet for the same reasons. All of their processes follow the same axonal pathway, the axons of the MP5 progeny, and they become dye coupled to each other after axonal outgrowth. From the third division of the MNB two cells arise that send axons out nerve 3 on both sides. These two cells, called DUM 3a and DUM 3b, are individually distinguishable because their axons take different branches of nerve 3 once they leave the ganglion. From the fourth division of the MNB two cells arise that send axons out nerve 1 on both sides. These two cells, called DUM 1a and DUM 1b, are also individually distinguishable on the same criteria; their axons take different branches of nerve 1 once they leave the ganglion.

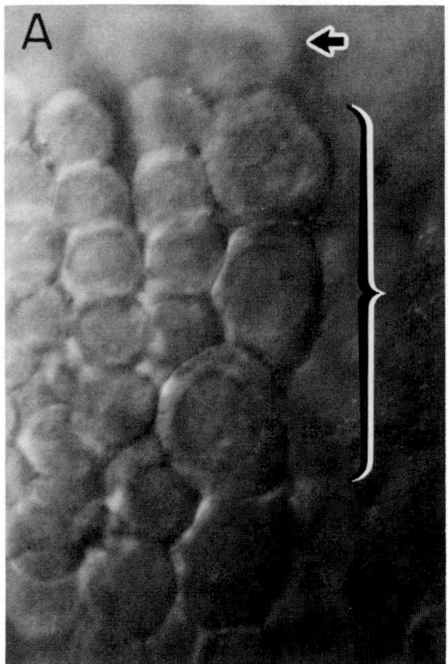

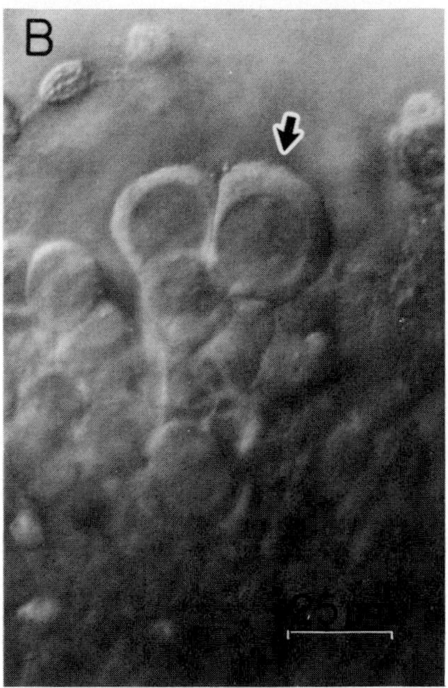

Figure 8. Photomicrographs of the dorsal surface (desheathed) of the metathoracic (T3) ganglion of a 90% embryo visualized with Nomarski interference contrast optics, showing some of the progeny of the MNB (A) and the two progeny of MP3 (B). The plane of focus in A is dorsal to that in B. In A the three oldest progeny of the MNB (from top to bottom: DUM 3, 4, 5; DUM 4, 5; and DUM 5a) are indicated by the bracket. The MP3 progeny lie deep to the focal plane (arrow) and anterior to the MNB progeny. In B, the H cell is indicated by the arrow. (From Goodman *et al.*[9])

The third set of cells (cells 9–12) from the MNB is called the third quartet for the same reasons. The axons of all four cells follow the pathway established by the MP6 progeny and bifurcate in the posterior commissure. The axons of these cells do not leave the ganglion via the peripheral nerves. Rather, they run in the longitudinal axonal pathways; we have not individually identified these cells. Later progeny of the MNB follow one of these three initial pathways (i.e., the MP4, MP5, or MP6 pathways) or the median nerve pathway which extends posteriorly just dorsal to the cluster of MNB progeny.

There are three important points that can be made concerning the cell lineage of the MNB (Goodman and Bate, in preparation). First, this cell lineage is descriptive and predictive, and thus says nothing about mechanism. Unraveling the relative contributions of ancestry and position will require careful experimentation. Its enormous usefulness to us, however, lies in our ability to predict from the day a cell is born what particular neuron it will become if left undisturbed. Second, the progeny from the same and successive cell divisions share certain morphological features in common. The growth cones of successive groups of four progeny of the MNB follow the same pathway initially and only later diverge. This pattern of fours, along with similar patterns of dye coupling, has led us to the idea that there are quartets of neurons in the grasshopper embryo which are groups of highly related and possibly equivalent cells, an idea, however, which awaits an experimental test. Third, although we can predict from which cell division a given identified neuron will arise, we can not always predict which of the two cells it is (or will be) until the two begin axonogenesis. For example, the first cell division of the MNB gives rise to a ganglion mother cell which divides into two cells: DUM 3, 4, 5 and DUM 4, 5. We cannot predict which cell is which until neurite extension begins; invariably, the cell that puts out the first growth cone becomes 3, 4, 5. When these two siblings become uniquely determined remains a mystery, although a testable one.

7. CELL LINEAGE OF MIDLINE PRECURSOR 3

In the metathoracic ganglion, MP3 divides once (Fig. 4) and gives rise to two neurons which become the "H" cell and the H-cell sibling (Figs. 7, 8, and 9). Initially the two cells are bilaterally symmetrical. Later, one of the two cells differentiates into the H cell, acquiring morphological and physiological properties that are quite different from its sibling[9] (described in detail later in this chapter).

8. PROPERTIES OF THE PROGENY OF A SINGLE PRECURSOR

8.1. *Biochemistry*

Evans and O'Shea[10] had shown that DUMETi (DUM 5a, cell 3 from the MNB) contained the neurotransmitter octopamine in the adult grasshopper. We asked two questions about the progeny of the MNB.[11] First, do all of the MNB progeny contain octopamine? Second, is octopamine associated exclusively with the MNB progeny in the metathoracic ganglion? We removed large numbers of somata of individual MNB progeny from the adult metathoracic ganglion and assayed for octopamine and serotonin. Octopamine was detected in all assays in the amount of 0.14 pmol per soma. None of the somata contained ser-

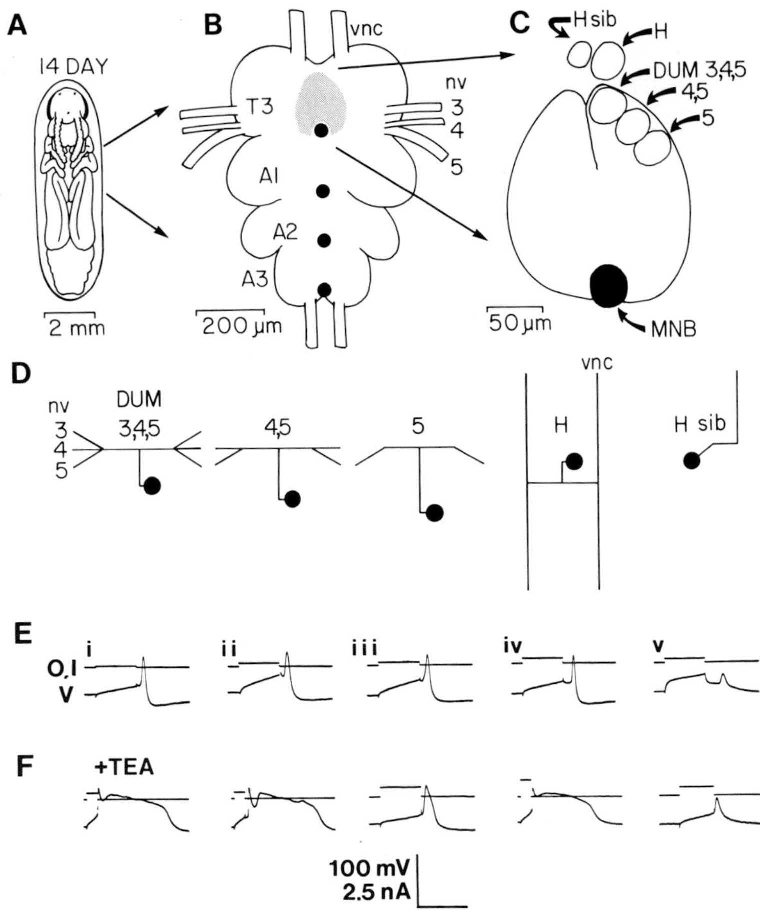

Figure 9. Grasshopper embryo (*Schistocerca nitens*) at day 14 (70%); diagrams and camera lucida drawings of living specimens viewed with Nomarski interference contrast optics (hatching occurs on day 20 at 35°C). (A) Embryo on day 14 viewed within the egg case. (B) Fused ganglion on day 14 contains the metathoracic (T3) and first three abdominal ganglia (A1–A3). Each segmental ganglion has a single MNB, shown as a filled circle. The stippled area is the packet of progeny of the MNB in the T3 ganglion. The ventral nerve cord (vnc) runs anteriorly and posteriorly; the peripheral nerves (nv) extend laterally. (C) Packet of ~100 progeny of the MNB in the T3 ganglion, showing the somata of the neurones arising from the first two cell divisions: DUM 3, 4, 5; DUM 4, 5; and DUM 5. Just anterior to the packet of progeny of the MNB are the two progeny of MP3: the H cell and the H-cell sibling. (D) Schematic diagram of the morphology of the five identified neurones: DUM 3, 4, 5; DUM 4, 5; DUM 5; the H cell; and the H-cell sib. The morphology is revealed by intracellular injection of the fluorescent dye Lucifer Yellow. (E) Action potentials of the five identified neurones in day 18 embryos, elicited by injection of current

otonin, and none showed a formaldehyde-induced fluorescence when treated with the Falck–Hillarp method, suggesting they do not contain serotonin, dopamine, adrenaline, or noradrenaline. The somata of the MNB progeny stain with neutral red, a vital dye that stains monoamine-containing neurons in the leech and lobster (see Goodman *et al.*[11] for references). To answer the second question, we removed neuronal somata along the lateral edge of the ganglion which also stain with neutral red. Octopamine is not present in significant amounts in these neurons. Thus octopamine is likely to be the transmitter of most if not all of the MNB progeny, and it appears to be exclusively associated with these cells in the metathoracic ganglion. These results led us to suggest that many if not all of the progeny of a single neuroblast have certain features in common, and one of these features may be their primary neurotransmitter,[12] a model that is clearly testable.

8.2. *Physiology*

The first three progeny of the MNB (DUM 3, 4, 5; 4, 5; and 5) are capable of generating Na^+-dependent action potentials in their axons and Na^+–Ca^{2+}-dependent action potentials in their somata[13] when mature (Figs. 9 and 10). However, there is a striking cell-specific difference among these first three progeny. Whereas tetraethylammonium (TEA) causes a 50- to 500-fold increase in the duration of the action potentials of DUM 3, 4, 5 and DUM 4, 5, it causes only a shoulder on the falling phase of the action potential of DUM 5 (Fig. 9F). We do not know whether this difference represents a difference in inward or outward current. Nevertheless, it clearly represents a biophysical difference in cells that differ by a single cell division and at most by 5 hr in birthdate.

This cell-specific difference led us to examine the range of electrical properties in the ~100 progeny of the MNB.[12] We found a broad spectrum of electrical excitability amongst these cells.

In addition to the first three cells, a few other early progeny have

---

into the somata. The three oldest progeny of the MNB all generate overshooting action potentials in their somata (i–iii). Of the two progeny of the MP3, the H cell generates an overshooting soma action potential, while the H-cell sib produces an action potential only in its axon (iv, v). (F) Action potentials of the five identified neurones in day 16 embryos, in the presence of tetraethylammonium (TEA). At the resting potential (–55 to –66 mV), the soma action potential of DUM 5 is not converted to an overshooting plateau of long duration, as observed in DUM 3, 4, 5; DUM 4, 5; and the H cell. The action potential in the H-cell sib fails to overshoot even in the presence of TEA. Calibration bar: (D, E iii, v) 25 msec; (E i, ii, iv) 100 msec. (From Goodman and Spitzer.[13])

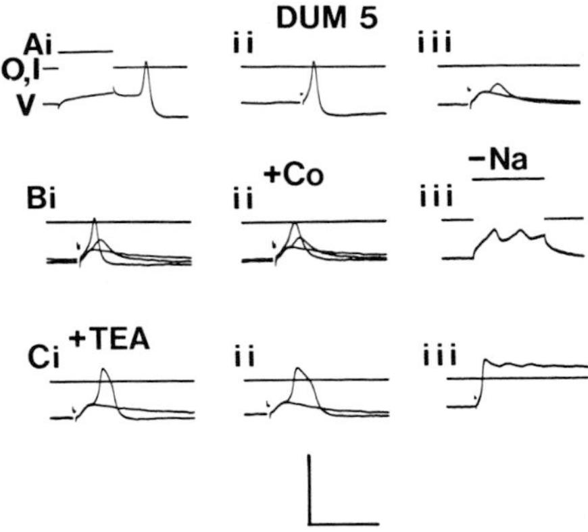

Figure 10. Action potentials in the soma and axons of DUM 5 in a day 16 embryo; all records from one cell. Somatic stimulation (A1) and antidromic invasion (A2) elicit the AP in the soma. Repetitive stimulation often fails to elicit the overshooting soma spike and reveals the double-peaked response (A3), due to separate action potentials in the two peripheral axons. (B) Ionic basis of action potentials in the soma and axons. Co^{2+} reduces the amplitude and increases the duration of the soma action potential but has little effect on the axon action potential. Removal of Na^+ abolishes the axon action potential (not shown); the remaining component of the soma action potential is elicited only by intracellular injection of current (B3). (C) Effect of TEA on soma and axon action potentials. TEA has little effect on the axon action potential at all membrane potentials tested. In contrast TEA causes the appearance of a shoulder on the soma AP at –60 mV, that broadens at –50 mV, and appears as long overshooting plateau when the soma is depolarized to –40 mV. Calibration: 100 mV, 0.5 nA, 25 msec. (Goodman and Spitzer.[13])

spiking somata and spiking axons. Several other MNB progeny generate action potentials in their neurites and axons (neurite is defined as the median process between the soma and the T-junction bifurcation leading to the two symmetrical axons), but not in their somata. Several other MNB progeny generate only axon spikes. Finally, many of the cells are incapable of producing action potentials in normal saline (Fig. 11). These nonspiking MNB progeny appear mature in all other morphological and physiological respects. By sampling many of the MNB progeny in single embryos and in many different embryos, we estimated that more than 50% of the progeny are nonspiking.

We compared the inward currents of the spiking vs. nonspiking MNB progeny (Fig. 12). The soma spikes of DUM 4, 5, for example, depend on Na^+ and Ca^{2+} inward currents. When some of the outward current is blocked by TEA, the normally nonspiking cells are capable of generating long-duration Ca^{2+} action potentials. In the presence of TEA and 10 mM Co^{2+} to block the Ca^{2+} current, we were unable to detect any evidence for Na^+ channels in these cells. Thus, we have shown a broad range of electrical properties among the progeny of the median neuroblast. Some cell-specific differences are clearly due to inward current, such as the absence of Na^+ current in the nonspiking

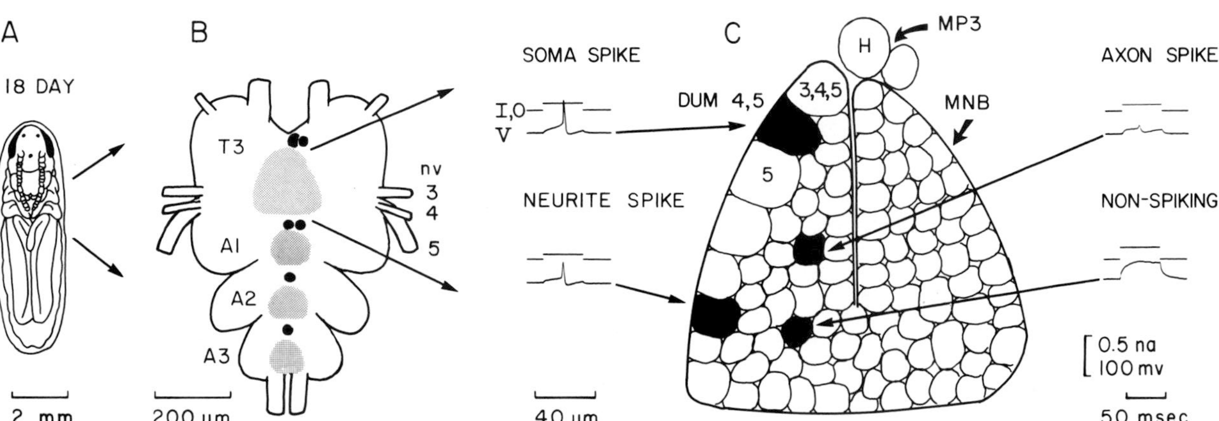

Figure 11. Grasshopper embryo at day 18 (90%); diagrams and camera lucida drawings of living specimens. (A) Embryo at day 18 viewed within the egg case. (B) Dorsal outline of metathoracic ganglion (T3) fused with first three abdominal ganglia (A1–A3), showing the location of the packets of progeny produced by the MNB in each segment (stippled areas) and the 1–2 remaining progeny of the single cell division of MP3 in each segment (black dots). (C) Camera lucida drawing of the packet of ~100 progeny of the MNB and 2 progeny of MP3. Four of the large MNB progeny are individually identified in the drawing (see text). The packet of somata of the MNB progeny appears under Nomarski optics to be encased in a glial sheath. The glial sheath has a median boundary which divides the packet into left and right portions. The progeny of the median neuroblast show the complete spectrum of electrical excitability, from soma spikes, to axon spikes, to nonspiking. This range of electrical properties is recorded in cells which appear by other criteria to have developed their mature phenotypes. (From Goodman *et al.*[12])

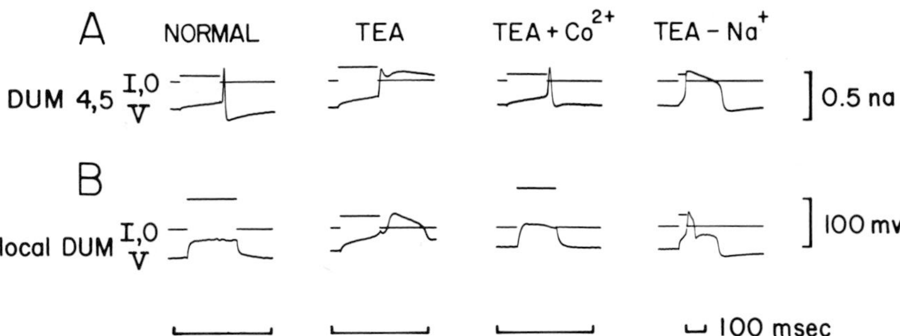

Figure 12. Comparison of electrical excitability of two progeny of the median neuroblast in the grasshopper: DUM 4, 5 and a local DUM neuron in an 18-day embryo. (A) The soma of DUM 4, 5 generates action potentials that depend on Na^+ and Ca^{2+} for their inward current. Addition of 30 mM TEA converts the brief action potential into a long and more complex response. The long plateau is abolished by the addition of 10 mM Co^{2+}, whereas the initial spike is nearly completely eliminated by removal of Na^+. (B) The local DUM neuron does not produce action potentials in normal saline. Addition of 30 mM TEA induces the cell to produce long-duration Ca^{2+} action potentials that are blocked by the addition of 10 mM Co^{2+} and are unaffected by the removal of Na^+. (From Goodman *et al.*[12])

cells; whereas other differences could be due to either inward or outward current, such as the difference between DUM 5 and DUM 3, 4, 5.

Similar differences in electrical properties have been observed between the two progeny of MP3 in the metathoracic ganglion: the H cell and H cell sib.[9,13] The H cell generates action potentials in its axons (Na^+) and soma (Na^+–Ca^{2+}), whereas its sib only generates action potentials in its axon (Fig. 9E, F). In normal saline and in TEA, the soma spike of the H cell is indistinguishable from those of DUM 3, 4, 5 and DUM 4, 5. We could find no evidence, however, for either Na^+ or Ca^{2+} inward current channels in the soma of the H-cell sib.

Thus, the progeny of two different embryonic precursor cells (MNP and MP3) show a broad spectrum of electrical properties. Electrical excitability is a mature phenotype not shared by all the progeny of a single precursor cell. In contrast, progeny from different precursor cells can share the same mature phenotype of electrical excitability (e.g., DUM 3, 4, 5 and the H cell).

8.3. *Morphology*

Earlier in this chapter I described the cell lineage for the first 12 progeny of the MNB (Fig. 7) (Goodman and Bate, in preparation). Each cell becomes a unique identified neuron in terms of its specific axonal morphology. The first 4 progeny all follow the median pathway established by the MP4 progeny, bifurcate at the anterior commissure, and extend laterally. The cell-specific morphology appears as each neuron's growth cones make their specific choices of which peripheral nerve or nerves to grow out. Similarly, the second 4 progeny follow the MP5 pathway, bifurcate, and extend laterally in the anterior commissure. They too show cell-specific morphology as they choose which peripheral nerves to grow out. The third quartet of 4 progeny follow the MP6 and bifurcate at the posterior commissure. These cells do not send axons out the peripheral nerves. Rather, their axons appear to stay within the CNS and possibly within the segment of origin (i.e., they may be intraganglionic neurons).

We penetrated the somata of many nonspiking MNB progeny (that arise from later cell divisions), in mature embryonic or adult ganglia, and filled the cells with the fluorescent dye Lucifer Yellow. These cells were all local intraganglionic neurons: each neuron had a median neurite that bifurcated at a T junction (in the posterior commissure) into bilaterally symmetrical processes, none of which left the ganglion (Fig. 13). The cells were remarkably symmetrical in their arborizations, yet quite distinct from each other. Our results led us to suggest that many of these small intraganglionic MNB progeny may also be unique and may ultimately be individually identifiable. Although all nonspiking neurons were intraganglionic, not all intraganglionic neurons were nonspiking; a few generated axon spikes.

Our results indicate that certain phenotypes are shared by the progeny of a single embryonic precursor cell in the grasshopper and may depend on the identity of that precursor cell. For example, all of the 100 MNB progeny in the T3 ganglion cluster together and are encased in a common glial sheath. All of their somata stain with neutral red, and most if not all of them make octopamine. All of them have acetylcholine (ACh) receptors with identical pharmacology.[8,12] All have certain morphological features in common (they are unpaired and bifurcate at a T junction).

Certain features, however, are unique to each individual neuron or group of neurons, and may depend on their position in the lineage. The first 12 progeny initially appear to follow the same axonal pathway in sets of four neurons or quartets. Ultimately, each of these cells becomes a unique individual based on the specific choices made by its growth cones. Some MNB progeny have axons that leave the ganglion, whereas many are intraganglionic. Some have large-diameter somata, others are medium sized, and most are small in diameter. Many of the largest MNB progeny are born first. Some MNB progeny generate both

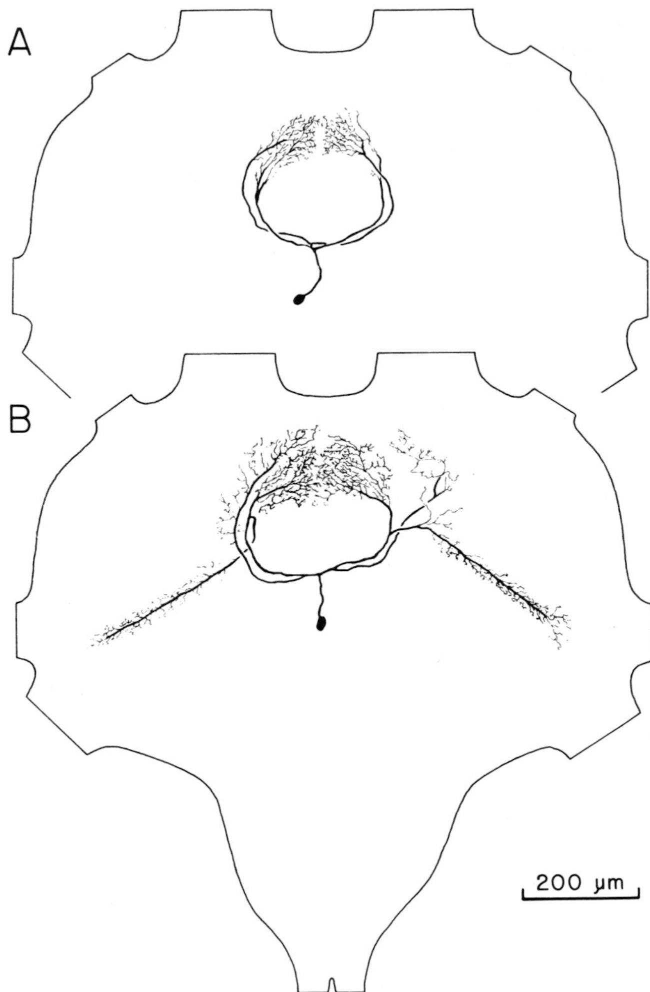

Figure 13. Morphology of two different nonspiking DUM neurons (progeny of the MNB) in the metathoracic ganglia of adult grasshoppers. Both cells are local intraganglionic neurons that were filled with Lucifer Yellow from microelectrode penetrations in their neuropil processes. (From Goodman *et al.*[12])

soma and axon action potentials, others generate neurite and axon or only axon spikes, and many are incapable of generating action potentials altogether in normal saline. The MNB appears to produce only small nonspiking progeny during its last few days of cell divisions. There appears to be a sequence of cell types generated within the MNB cell lineage from neurons with peripheral axons to those that are intraganglionic; this observation parallels descriptions of the order of birth in vertebrate nervous systems. It will be interesting to see if this pattern for grasshopper neurogenesis holds true for the other neuroblasts in this animal and for neuronal development in other animals as well.[12]

9. MORPHOLOGICAL DIFFERENTIATION

9.1. *DUM 5*

The outgrowth of processes of DUM 5a (hereafter called DUM 5) was followed as a function of developmental age by intracellular injection of Lucifer Yellow[8] (Fig. 14). DUM 5 arises from the second cell division of the MNB; the final mitosis of DUM 5 from the ganglion mother cell occurs shortly after 30% of development (after day 6). Axonal outgrowth begins at about 35%, with the extension of a growth cone along the median axonal pathway established by the MP4 progeny. DUM 5's growth cone does not make a new pathway (i.e., is not a pioneer) but rather follows preexisting pathways and continues to be confronted with choices of which pathway to take. At 38%, the growth cone approaches the anterior commissure, and at 39% the growth cone has begun to bifurcate into two separate growth cones, each of which will extend laterally on a particular commissural pathway. By 45% (day 9) the two growth cones have grown past the longitudinal axonal pathways and are extending laterally toward the edge of the CNS. By 50%, the neuron sends axons out the peripheral nerves. By 60%, the distal axon reaches the ETi muscle, the target in the femur of the limb bud. After the axon reaches its target, the central arborizations greatly increase and the cell body greatly enlarges.

The growth cone of DUM 5, just like the growth cones of other cells that we examine in these embryos, has many long, thin filopodia (which extend for at least 30–50 μm in many directions and in some cases are longer than 100 μm). At choice points, whether in the CNS or periphery, the filopodia often extend in many of the possible directions along the available pathways. The growth cone ultimately chooses which way to grow, but sometimes only after bifurcating and first growing in both the "right" and "wrong" directions (such as when it leaves the CNS). Lateral filopodia also extend from the distal axon behind the growth cone, giving the axon a "fuzzy" appearance. Whether they serve as anchors for the axon, as substrates for cell interactions, or are merely the remnants of the growth cone, we do not know. They eventually disappear and leave behind a relatively naked proximal axon (see Chapter 6).

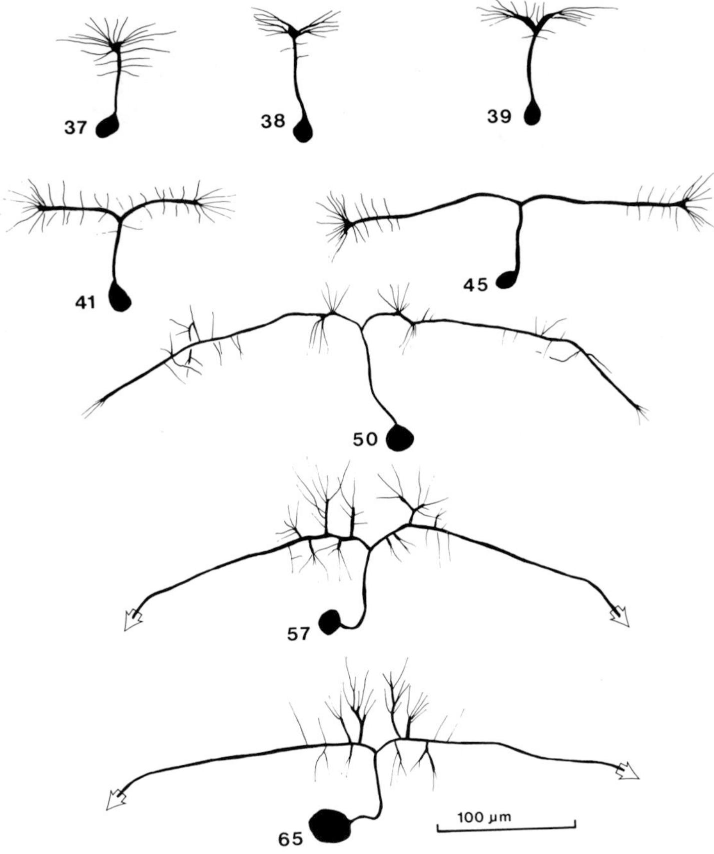

Figure 14. Morphological differentiation of DUMETi (DUM 5a) in T3, as revealed by intracellular injection of the fluorescent dye Lucifer Yellow. Development is shown only within the CNS; arrows mark where the axons extend out to the periphery. Numbers indicate percent of development.[4] The growth cones have many long, thin filopodia (0.1–0.2 μm in diameter) which extend in many directions for 30–50 μm, and sometimes for more than 100 μm.

Later, filopodia and then growth cones appear where the dendrites will form.

9.2. *The H Cell*

The H cell assumes two different roles during grasshopper embryogenesis (Fig. 15).[9] It originates in the metathoracic ganglion from the single cell division of MP3. It first appears as one of a pair of symmetrical cells with unilateral axons running anteriorly in the early fiber pathways. Later it transforms into an unpaired identified neuron.

The plane of division of the MP3 is often oblique (Fig. 4), but the two cells rapidly acquire positions on the left and right of the midline. One of the two cells usually is slightly dorsal to the other. Each of the MP3 progeny has a single contralateral axon that runs anteriorly on the MP2 pathway as one of the early processes in the developing longitudinal axonal pathways. The processes of the MP4 progeny extend in the median axonal pathway (Fig. 6) just dorsal to the somata of the MP3 progeny. The processes of the MP4 progeny here appear to contact the more dorsal of the two somata of the MP3 progeny.

One of the two progeny of MP3 in the T3 segment undergoes a transformation and it, and often its sib, survives. This secondary differentiation begins several days after its initial differentiation (Fig. 15). Either one of the two cells can undergo the transformation, but only one of them does it; the sib remains unchanged. In the cases we have ob-

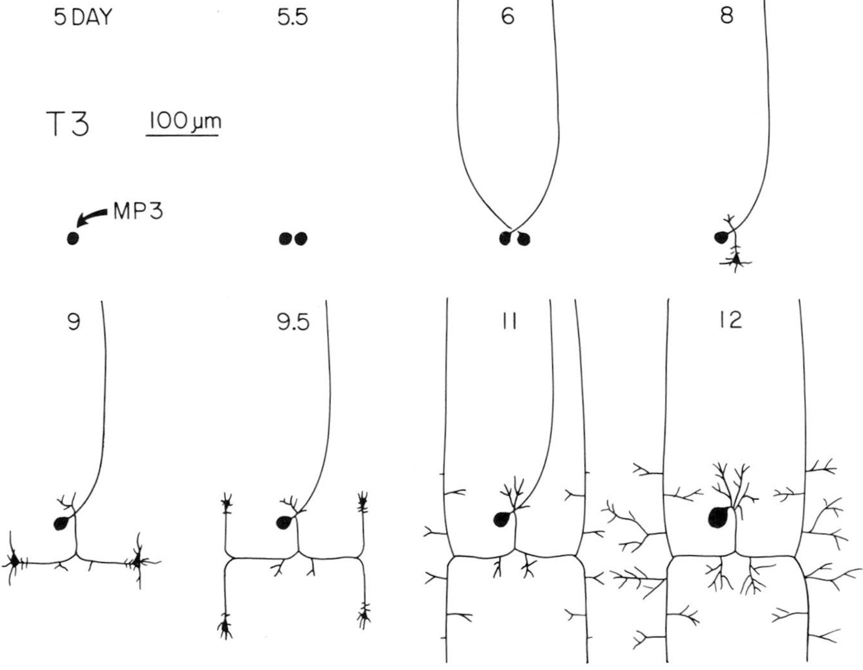

Figure 15. The transformation of the H cell in the metathoracic segment between day 5 and day 12 of embryogenesis. These are camera lucida drawings from cells injected with the fluorescent dye Lucifer Yellow. (From Goodman *et al.*[9])

served thus far, it is always the more dorsal of the two cells that transforms, regardless of its left or right position.

The transformation begins about 40% (day 8) with the appearance of a new growth cone which extends posteriorly in the median axonal pathway and then bifurcates at the posterior commissure. Each process later bifurcates in the longitudinal fiber tracts. The original unilateral process disappears between day 11 (55%) and day 12 (60%) and the transformed cell fully differentiates into the unpaired and bilaterally symmetrical identified "H" neuron. The two somata of the MP3 progeny migrate dorsally, and the soma of the H cell enlarges (Fig. 8). Thus, one of a pair of initially symmetrical cells undergoes a second phase of differentiation and transforms into an unpaired symmetrical neuron. The cell that transforms is independent of its left/right position, but is strongly correlated with its dorsal/ventral position, and this may be independent of its ancestry. The dorsal cell is contacted by the processes of the MP4 progeny and the first four progeny of the MNB. The transforming H cell then comes to acquire many of the same phenotypes as the first MNB progeny (see Section 10). These observations led us to suggest that the transformation may be an epigenetic event induced by cellular interactions with the axons of the MNB progeny, a hypothesis we plan to test by experimentally removing the MNB and MP4.

10. PHYSIOLOGICAL DIFFERENTIATION

The physiological differentiation of the three oldest progeny of the MNB (DUM 3, 4, 5; DUM 4, 5; and DUM 5) and the two progeny of MP3 (the H cell and H-cell sib) was examined in the context of their morphological development.[8,9,14,15]

10.1. Chemosensitivity

At day 7 (35%) neither the MNB nor its progeny show responses to either bath application or iontophoresis of ACh or [γ-aminobutyric acid (GABA)]. In contrast, by day 13 (65%) the oldest MNB progeny are sensitive to both bath application and iontophoresis of both of these agents (Fig. 16B). The oldest MNB progeny first become sensitive to ACh and GABA about day 8 (40%) of development, and seem to become sensitive to both transmitters at the same time. Young progeny in close proximity to the MNB show no response to iontophoretic application of ACh. In contrast, the oldest progeny at the distal end of the chain, which already possess neurites, are depolarized by iontophoretic application of ACh onto their somata.

Both the somata and processes of the oldest MNB progeny are depolarized by iontophoretic application of ACh on day 8 (Fig. 16A). Processes seem to be sensitive over their entire length out to the growth cone. It seems that chemosensitivity is distributed over the whole surface of the cell, at or soon after the time that it first appears. The reversal potential, ionic dependence, and pharmacology of the responses to ACh and to GABA appear similar at days 8, 13, and 18 of development. Furthermore, all of the MNB progeny and the MP3 progeny show similar responses to both agents. The observed reversal potential for GABA is –70 mV, and the ionic conductance appears to be Cl^-. The extrapolated reversal potential for ACh is +20 mV, and the ionic conductance appears to be Na^+. The ACh response was not fully blocked by either nicotinic or muscarinic antagonists.

10.2. *Electrical Excitability*

We have already seen the mature electrical properties of five identified neurons in the grasshopper embryo: the first three progeny of the MNB and the two progeny of MP3 (Fig. 9E and 10).[13] Midway through embryogenesis, on day 10 (50%), these five cells are highly electrically coupled (see section 10.3) and electrically inexcitable.[8] The electrical properties and cell-specific differences among the five cells develop between days 10 and 13.[14] Before day 10, the five cells have linear current–voltage (I–V) relationships and appear completely inexcitable, even in the presence of TEA. The apparent input resistance (R_{in}) of all five cells is about 100 MΩ on day 10 and greater than 200 MΩ on and after day 11. They are inexcitable even when they are electrically isolated by removing the somata from many of the cells to which they are coupled. In such cases, the measured R_{in} increases to over 300 MΩ, yet the cells still show no nonlinearities in their membrane properties and no signs of excitability.

All five cells follow the same developmental sequence. The temporal appearance of electrical excitability proceeds from no action potential, to the axon action potential, to the neurite action potential, to the soma action potential (Fig. 17 and 18), as described below. By day 10, the five neurons already have axons beginning to grow out of the metathoracic ganglion, either in peripheral nerve 5 or the ventral nerve cord. Thus, we examined the excitability of these cells by intracellular stimulation of the soma and by extracellular stimulation of the nerve bundles con-

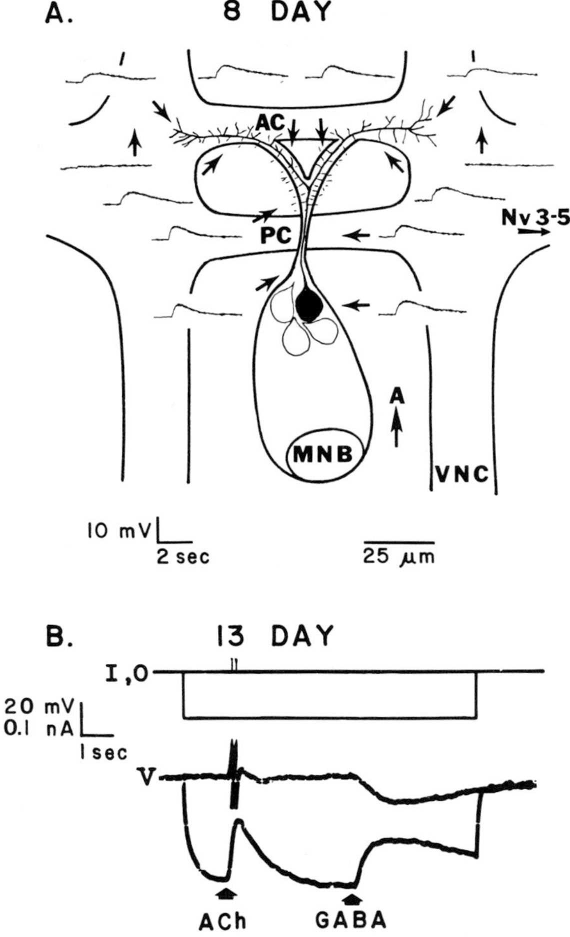

Figure 16. Chemosensitivity of identified DUM neurons (progeny of the MNB) in the grasshopper embryo (the three oldest progeny as described above). (A) Response to iontophoretic application of ACh in a day 8 embryo. The diagram shows the embryonic neuropil of a single segmental ganglion (T3), as viewed from the dorsal surface (anterior at top). The MNB is shown with its packet of progeny; those most anterior (oldest) send their axons anteriorly in a median bundle of processes which cross the posterior commissure (PC) and bifurcate near the anterior commissure (AC). The extent of branching of an individual neuron was determined by intracellular injection of Lucifer Yellow. The longitudinal connectives extend into the ventral nerve cords (VNC) and are seen on either side. The lateral neuropil extends (beyond the margin of the figure) into three fiber tracts which become peripheral nerves 3, 4 and 5. The response to application of ACh at the points indicated by the arrows were recorded by an intracellular electrode in the cell body. Processes are sensitive to ACh over their whole length. Small vertical or lateral displacements of the iontophoretic electrode abolished the response. (B) Responses to sequential

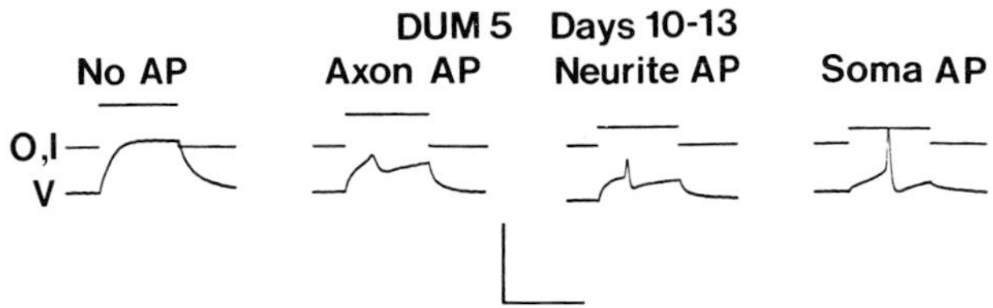

Figure 17. Onset of excitability in DUM 5 between days 10 and 13. The development of the action potential (AP) proceeds from no AP to axon AP, to neurite AP, to soma AP. Records from four cells. Calibration: 100 mV, 0.5 nA, 50 msec. (From Goodman and Spitzer.[14])

taining the axons. Between days 10 and 11, we were unable to evoke an action potential in any of these cells and the addition of TEA revealed no evidence for excitable inward current. The first nonlinear membrane property to appear was delayed rectification that is blocked by the addition of TEA. At about day 11, TEA unmasked in some cells a small, excitable Na^+-dependent response that was likely to be generated in the axon. At around this same time, some cells started to support Na^+-dependent action potentials in their axons in normal saline.

After the appearance of the axon action potential, and before the appearance of the overshooting soma action potential, we often observed an intermediate developmental stage at about day 11.5: the neurite action potential. Finally, the overshooting soma action potential appeared about day 12 (60%). The inward current is carried by both

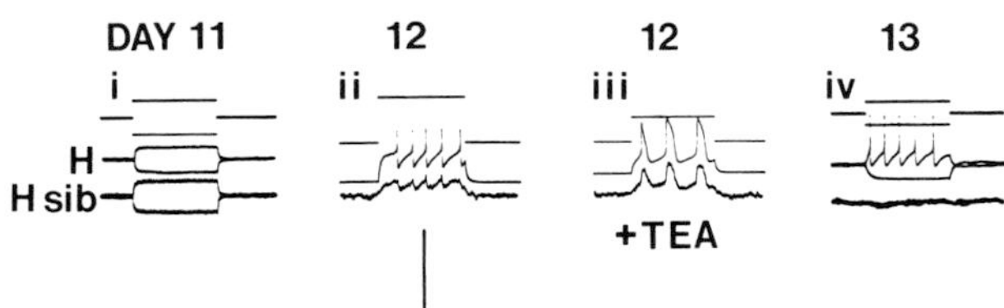

Figure 18. Electrical coupling of the two MP3 progeny: the H cell and the H-cell sib. The two cells are electrically coupled and inexcitable on day 11. They are coupled and the H cell is excitable on day 12, as shown in normal saline and in TEA. The cells are uncoupled on day 13. The records are from three pairs of cells. Calibration: 0.5 nA, 500 msec; (H cell) 100 mV; (H-cell sib) 25 mV. (From Goodman *et al.*[9])

←

iontophoretic application of ACh and GABA from a double-barreled micropipette, recorded with an intracellular electrode in a day 13 embryo. At a resting potential of −55 mV, ACh depolarizes the cell to threshold, eliciting overshooting action potentials, while GABA hyperpolarizes the cell. When the cell is hyperpolarized by injected current, the response to ACh is larger, but remains subthreshold; the cell is then depolarized by GABA. (From Goodman and Spitzer.[8])

Na^+ and Ca^{2+}. At first, the addition of TEA caused a prolonged shoulder and gradual repolarization of the action potential. Within the next day, TEA caused a long-duration soma action potential with an overshooting plateau. These two stages of the response in TEA may be the result of a developmental increase in the Ca^{2+} inward current in the soma. By day 13, all five cells showed their cell-specific electrical properties. DUM 3, 4, 5; DUM 4, 5; and the H cell generated long-duration action potentials in TEA at their resting potential. The addition of TEA only caused a shoulder in the action potential of DUM 5. The H-cell sib acquired only an axon action potential, and its soma was inexcitable.

The first three progeny of the MNB all proceed through the same temporal sequence in the development of electrical excitability. However, there is variability in the precise time of appearance of the individual stages in this sequence. For a particular neuron, the stage of excitability is not identical in every embryo of the same developmental age. The temporal sequence for the H cell appears identical to the first three progeny of the MNB, and also appears to occur in a similar length of time: 1–2 days. However, the timetable for the H cell is shifted 0.5–1 day later.

10.3. *Electrical and Dye Coupling*

All cell types examined at early embryonic stages of the grasshopper are electrically coupled to each other; development involves a process of selective uncoupling.[8,9,13,14] We also examined the movement of the fluorescent dye Lucifer Yellow (mol. wt. 450) from the interior of one cell to the interior of other cells. On day 6 (30%), neuroblasts are electrically and dye coupled to other neuroblasts and to their progeny. Interestingly, the neural epithelium is electrically coupled to the limb bud epithelium on day 6, but these two cell types do not appear to be dye coupled. At about 50% of development, the MNB becomes uncoupled from most embryonic cells other than its own progeny.

We examined in detail the development of uncoupling of the three oldest progeny of the MNB (DUM 3, 4, 5; DUM 4, 5; and DUM 5) and the two progeny of MP3 (the H cell and H-cell sib). These cells become dye uncoupled from the MNB about day 7 (35%), although they remain electrically coupled for several more days. This dye uncoupling corresponds to the timing of axonal outgrowth. The cells become secondarily dye coupled via their growth cones and axons in groups of fours, or quartets (Goodman and Bate, in preparation). The quartets of secondary dye coupling are the same quartets of MNB progeny whose axons initially follow the same axonal pathway. Within several days (by 50%) these cells have again become dye uncoupled from one another. Between days 11 and 12 (55–60%), the oldest MNB progeny become electrically uncoupled from one another. The earliest we have observed the total uncoupling among the first three progeny is on day 11.[14] In about 50% of embryos at day 12, the first three MNB progeny were totally uncoupled; by day 12.5, they were uncoupled in every embryo examined. This variability in the precise time of uncoupling is similar to the variability we observed in the precise time of appearance of different stages of electrical excitability. The onset of excitability and the cessation of coupling are not consistently correlated. We were unable, for example, to predict whether two cells on day 11.5 would be coupled or not by the particular type of action potential that each was able to generate. On day 12, pairs of cells with overshooting soma action potentials of apparently identical amplitude and shape can be coupled or uncoupled. The comparable cessation of electrical coupling between the H cell and its sib occurs 0.5–1 day later than in the MNB progeny (Fig. 18), and its timing is similarly variable with respect to their development of electrical excitability. These results led us to suggest that these two events are not causally related, but rather that they are two independent events which occur at about the same developmental stage during the differentiation of these cells.

11. BIOCHEMICAL DIFFERENTIATION

Octopamine is the neurotransmitter used by most if not all of the MNB progeny. The appearance of octopamine was studied by performing radioenzymatic assays on extracts of embryonic ganglia.[11] The detection of octopamine required pooling of chains of meso- and metathoracic ganglia dissected from embryos of known ages. The sensitivity of our assay required a minimum sample of two ganglionic chains from a 13-day (65%) embryo, and less thereafter (Fig. 19). We detected no octopamine in the ganglia before day 13, even when we pooled six ganglionic chains for a single assay. This appearance of octopamine on day 13 correlates well with the morphological differentiation of the oldest MNB progeny and with the onset of neutral red staining. Octopamine begins to appear in the MNB progeny only after the axons of DUM 5, one of the oldest progeny, have reached and extended over their peripheral target.

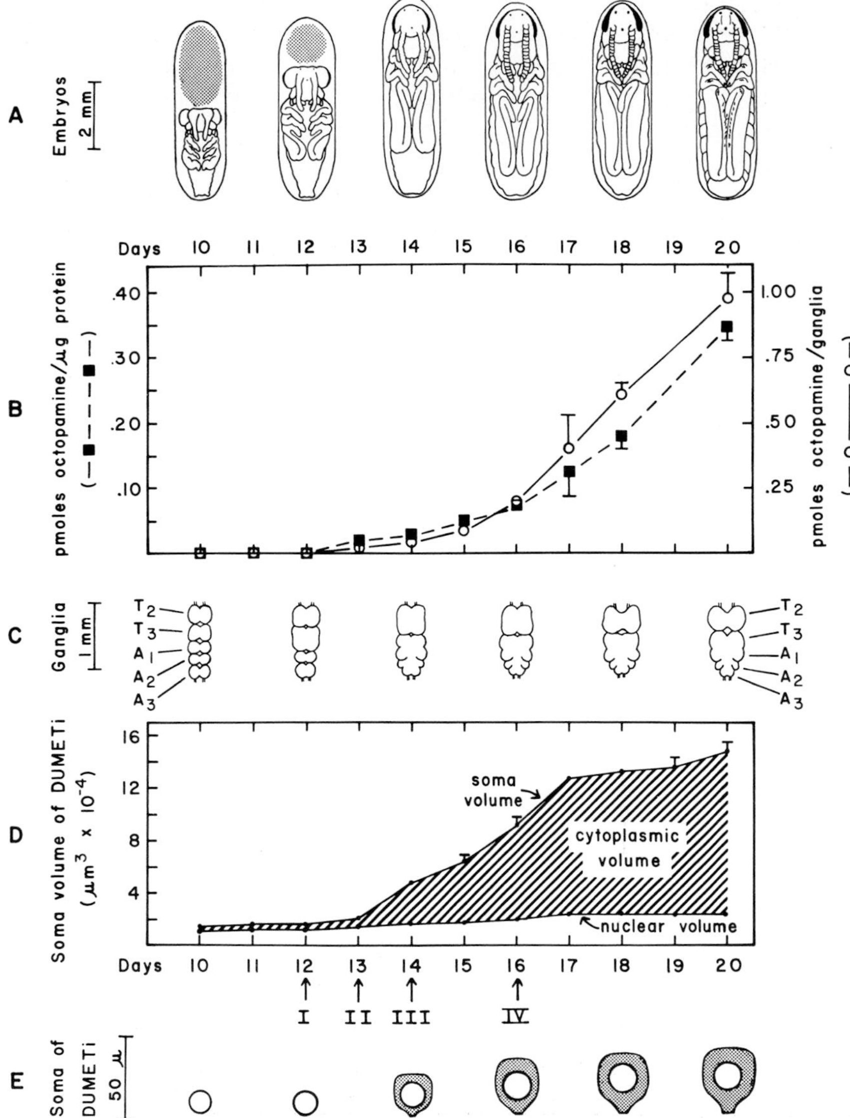

Figure 19. Temporal pattern of accumulation of octopamine and morphological development of octopaminergic DUM neurons (progeny of the MNB) during grasshopper embryogenesis. (A) Development of embryo within the egg case; major features traced from camera lucida projections. Stippling indicates yolk not yet incorporated within the embryo. Hatching occurs at day 20. (B) Time course of accumulation of octopamine in embryonic ganglia, given as picomoles of octopamine per microgram of protein (■), and as picomoles

12. TEMPORAL SEQUENCE OF DEVELOPMENT

There is a distinct order in the acquisition of particular phenotypes by the identified neurons that are the oldest progeny of the MNB. This developmental sequence occurs first in the oldest progeny; younger progeny may be as much as several days behind in their differentiation.

Day 6 (30%). The MNB has begun dividing and over the next few hours generates the two ganglion mother cells that will give rise to the first four neuronal progeny. At this stage, the MNB is highly dye and electrically coupled to its progeny, and to many other cells around it.

Day 7 (35%). The oldest MNB progeny have begun axonogenesis with the extension of growth cones along the median axonal pathway established by the MP4 progeny. These neurons with axons have become dye uncoupled from the MNB and its younger progeny (without axons). However, the neurons become secondarily dye coupled in quartets of neurons via their axons. The axons of these quartets initially follow the same axonal pathway. Chemosensitivity first appears on the oldest MNB progeny about this time, and we detect neurotransmitter receptors over the whole surface of the cells, including their growth cones.

Day 8 (40%). The growth cone has bifurcated at the anterior commissure, and the two growth cones are extending laterally.

Day 10 (50%). The axons of DUM 3, 4, 5; DUM 4, 5; and DUM 5 leave the CNS and begin growing out the peripheral nerves. The somata are still relatively small in diameter. The growth cones of DUM 5, for

---

of octopamine per set of T_2 and T_3 and A_1 to A_3 ganglia (○). Each point represents the mean of three separate determinations, each determination from four pooled chains of ganglia (T_2 and T_3 and A_1 to A_3) from animals of a given age. The standard error of the mean (S.E.M.) is indicated by error bars; where not shown, S.E.M. $\leq$ diameter of the point. (C) Development and fusion of last two thoracic (T_2 and T_3) and first three abdominal (A_1–A_3) ganglia. Outlines from camera lucida drawings of dissected ganglia are shown. (D) Developmental changes in nuclear and cytoplasmic volumes of a single identified DUM neuron (DUM 5 or DUMETi). Preparations were visualized with Nomarski optics and diameters measured with an ocular micrometer; volumes were computed by assuming the soma to be a prolate spheroid and the nucleus a sphere. Each point represents the mean of three separate determinations; the S.E.M. is indicated by error bars, and when not shown is very small. Roman numerals: I, axon of DUMETi reaches extensor tibiae muscle; II, axon of DUMETi extends over entire extensor tibiae muscle; III, soma of DUMETi stains with neutral red; and IV, DUM neuroblast stops dividing and degenerates. (E) Representative camera lucida drawings of the soma of DUMETi at different stages of development. The stippled area indicates cytoplasm. Most of the increase in volume is cytoplasmic. (From Goodman *et al.*[11])

example, often split and grow out several peripheral nerves. In time, only a single growth cone remains extending out nerve 5. By this stage, the secondary dye coupling has disappeared amongst the oldest quartet of MNB progeny.

Days 11–12 (55–60%). The axons continue to grow out the peripheral nerves. By day 12, the axon of DUM 5 has reached the proximal portion of the extensor tibiae muscle in the femur of the limb bud. This 1-day period marks the cessation of electrical coupling amongst the oldest MNB progeny and the development of electrical excitability of these cells. First the axons become excitable, and then the somata. Dendrites are already starting to appear in the CNS.

Day 13 (65%). The axon of DUM 5 has grown over its entire peripheral target. The neurotransmitter, octopamine, is appearing.

Day 14 (70%). The somata of the three oldest MNB progeny have greatly enlarged in diameter and the central arborizations of these cells have expanded. The first signs of spontaneous synaptic input are recorded about this stage.

Day 16 (80%). The MNB stops dividing and degenerates.

Day 20 (100%). Hatching.

13. SEGMENT-SPECIFIC CELL DEATH

How does the grasshopper deal with the apparent paradox of a repetitive pattern of neuronal precursor cells in the early embryo, and the subsequent specialized ganglia in each segment equipped for different functions? One difference is in cell number; the thoracic ganglia contain about 3000 neurons, the abdominal ganglia about 500 neurons. Much of this difference in the cell number between segments is due to cell death that occurs during embryogenesis[16] (Bate and Grunewald, in preparation; Goodman and Bate, in preparation). Between 45 and 60%, it is typical to see hundreds of cells simultaneously in the process of cell death in a single abdominal ganglion. Dying cells are easy to recognize because their cell bodies collapse and the condensed lipid looks like oil droplets under Nomarski optics, and the condensed lipid of the cell bodies autofluoresces in the living embryo with excitation and emission spectra similar to those of Lucifer Yellow.

The MNB produces about 100 progeny in the metathoracic segment (T3) and about 90 in A1 (it begins dividing one cell division later in A1 than in T3, and stops dividing about three cell divisions earlier). However, in A1 about 50% of the progeny die, leaving only about 45 surviving cells compared to about 100 in T3. Cells of known lineage, whose homologues survive and differentiate in the thoracic segments, predictably die in many (or sometimes all) of the abdominal segments (for example, the progeny of the MNB and MP3, as shown in Fig. 7). The first 4 progeny of the MNB (DUM 3, 4, 5; DUM 4, 5; DUM 5a; and DUM 5b) die in the abdominal segments (A1–A7). Two of the second quartet of MNB progeny often die in the abdominal segments. The cells destined to die send out axons which navigate over the axonal pathways just as their surviving homologues do in the thoracic segments. For example, DUM 5 in the abdominal segments sends out a growth cone which extends anteriorly over the median axonal pathway established by the MP4 progeny, bifurcates, and then extends laterally in a particular bundle of the anterior commissure. The growth cones of DUM 5 take the appropriate pathways to the edge of the CNS, and shortly thereafter the cell dies. DUM 5 normally innervates a muscle in the limb bud. Abdominal segments lack limb buds and also do not have the equivalent pathway to nerve 5. The cause of the death of DUM 5 in the abdominal segments is unknown, although the correlation of missing pathway and death is striking.

One consequence of segment-specific cell death is that large numbers of healthy axons and cells degenerate and disappear and in some cases whole axon bundles or pathways disappear. For example, the median axonal pathway established by the MP4 progeny disappears as all four of the first quartet of MNB progeny (which normally follow this pathway) die; the MP4 progeny may die as well. Obviously the originally identical sets of cells and axons in each segment quickly diverge as specific neurons and their axons disappear. Of the two progeny of MP3 (one of which becomes the H cell in T3), one or both often die in segments A3 to A6.[16] There is an interesting pattern of cell death of these two MP3 progeny across the thoracic and abdominal segments (Fig. 20). Although many of these cells die in segments A3–A7, there is increased survival at the posterior end in segments A8 and A9 (Loer and Goodman, in preparation). Furthermore, in any one segment, there is variability from embryo to embryo as to whether one or both MP3 progeny die, even though there is a relatively consistent pattern across the segments. For example, out of 25 embryos examined from each of two different clutches of *S. americana* eggs (a clutch comes from a single mated pair), both MP3 progeny in A2 survived in 80% of the embryos from one clutch and in only 4% of the embryos from the other clutch (Loer and Goodman, in preparation). Many of the clutches examined, however, were much more similar than these two. There are also dif-

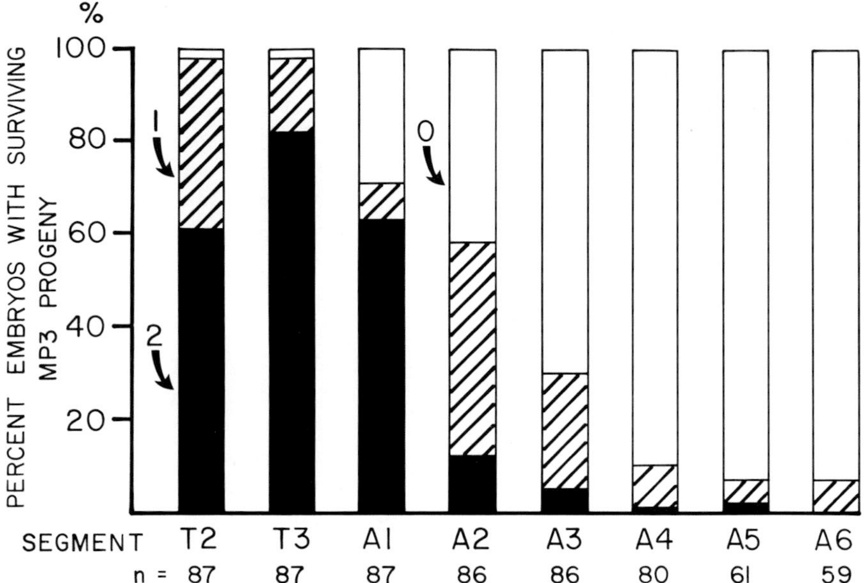

Figure 20. The survival and cell death of the two MP3 progeny in different segments of grasshopper embryos in dissected preparations examined on days 12 through 16. The percentage of embryos with two (solid bar), one (hatched bar), or no (open bar) MP3 progeny surviving per segment is scored for the mesothoracic and metathoracic (T2 and T3) and the first six abdominal ganglia (A1 to A6). The number of embryos examined is indicated (n). (From Bate *et al.*[16])

ferences between species. In *S. americana*, both of the MP3 progeny in A2 survived in 42% of the embryos (n = 151), whereas in *S. nitens* both survived in only 7% of the embryos (n = 125). Since all of the embryos from the many clutches of both species were raised in nearly constant and identical environmental conditions, these clutch-specific and species-specific differences suggest a genetic component to the probability of cell death vs. survival of the MP3 progeny (Loer and Goodman, in preparation).

14. SEGMENT-SPECIFIC DIFFERENTIATION

The differences in cell number from segment to segment are due largely to segment-specific cell death. There are also, however, segment-specific differences in the differentiation of identified neurons that survive. This segment-specific differentiation can be seen in the development of the two MP3 progeny that survive in the different thoracic and abdominal segments. The "H" cell in the metathoracic segment is one of the two progeny of MP3 (Fig. 9). The H cell has a curious developmental history (Fig. 15), but even more interesting to us is the observation that the H cell only forms an "H" shape in the thoracic segments[16] (Loer and Goodman, in preparation). In the first few abdominal segments the homologous cell (by lineage) forms other axonal arborizations (Fig. 21). In A1, for example, it forms just the posterior branches of the "H." in A2–A7, the surviving MP3 progeny rarely grow any new axons. In A8, the "H"-cell homologue forms just the posterior branches of the "H," as in A1. Thus, the H-cell homologues quite clearly undergo spe-

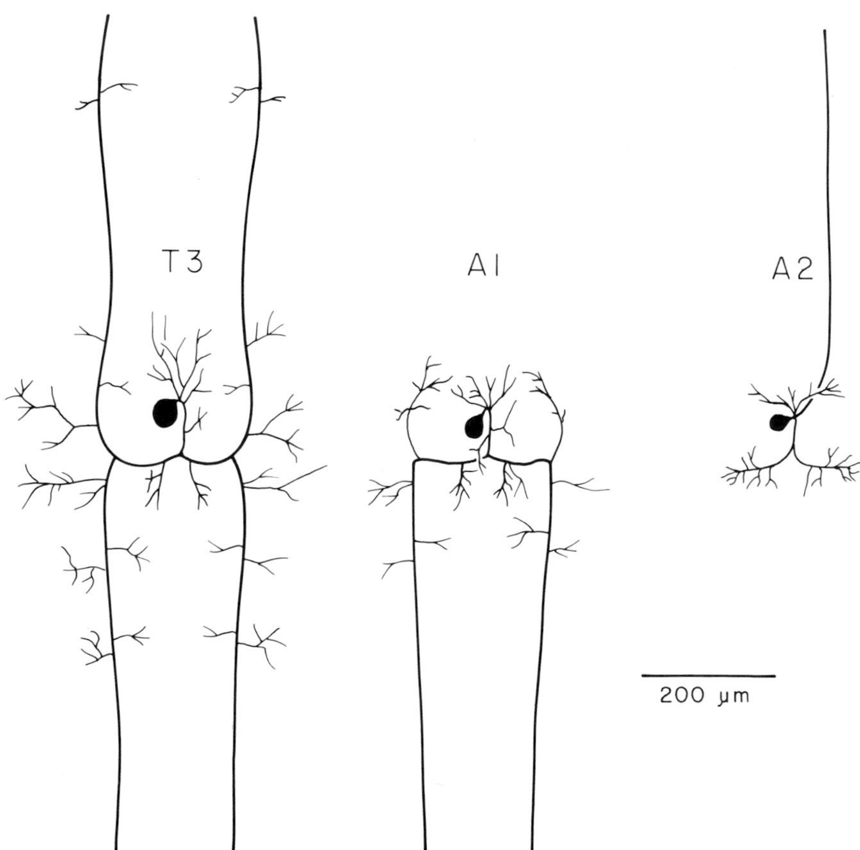

Figure 21. Segmental differences in the morphology of the MP3 progeny; camera lucida drawings from cells filled with Lucifer Yellow. (From Bate *et al.*[16])

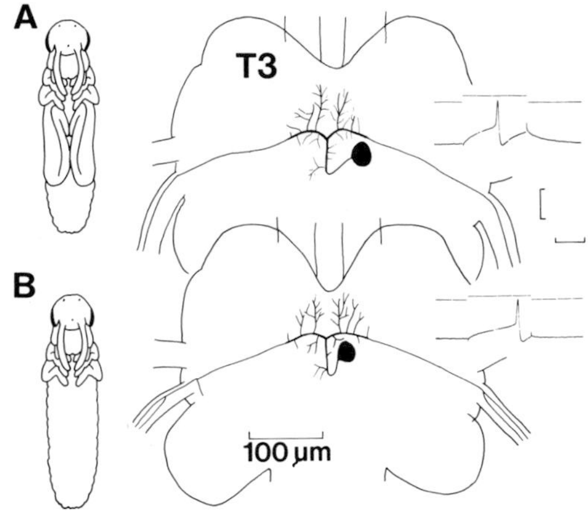

Figure 22. The differentiation of DUM 5 (DUMETi) in the metathoracic ganglion (T3) of *S. americana* embryos grown from 43 to 70% of development outside of the egg case in hanging drop cultures in (a) a control embryo and (b) an embryo in which both metathoracic legs were removed at 43%. Camera lucida drawings of cells injected with Lucifer Yellow; inserts on right show intracellular recordings of action potentials. Calibration: 40 mV, 1 nA, 20 msec. (From Whitington *et al.*[17])

cific patterns of differentiation which depend on their segment or origin. Either the cells in different segments inherit segment-specific programs of differentiation, or alternatively cells in different segments are equivalent and respond to subtle changes in their environment.

15. LIMB BUD REMOVAL EXPERIMENTS

DUM 5 survives in the metathoracic segment and dies in the abdominal segments. Similarly, the fast extensor tibiae motorneuron (FETi), which arises from a different neuroblast, survives in the metathoracic segment and dies in the abdominal segments. Both of these cells normally send an axon out nerve 5 (and into branch 5bld) to innervate the extensor tibiae muscle of the limb bud. What controls their segment-specific cell death? One clear difference between the segments is the pattern of muscles they contain. There are limbs, limb muscles, and limb-innervating neurons in the thorax but none in the abdomen. We removed the limb buds from the metathoracic (T3) segment early in embryogenesis in two ways: either by cutting them off embryos cultured outside the eggshell in hanging drops, or by using fine needles to remove limb buds from embryos inside the eggshell.[17] In both cases we found that neurons which innervate the limb muscles (in particular, DUM 5 and FETi) survived and differentiated (and even developed to adulthood) in the absence of the muscles they normally innervate (Fig. 22). This means that something other than the simple presence or absence of the target muscles is the cue for neuron survival vs. neuron death. Whether this cue is intrinsic to each prospective neuron or external to the cell remains unknown.

16. CONCLUSIONS AND QUESTIONS

We have examined the progeny of the MNB and MP3 in order to understand four topics: (1) the cell lineage of identified neurons, (2) the properties of the progeny of a single neuronal precursor, (3) the differentiation of identified neurons from birth to maturation, and (4) the development of segmental specializations. The results from these studies have confirmed our initial enthusiasm; namely, the grasshopper embryo is a particuarly attractive preparation for studying neuronal development at the cellular level.

What have we learned from these studies? First, we have described cell lineages and shown that specific identified neurons can arise from specific cell divisions (see also Chapters 1, 2, and 3). Cells arising from the same final cell division can be quite similar, yet at the same time have individually distinctive characteristics. Successive groups of four cells can have certain features in common; their growth cones follow the same pathway initially (and only later diverge), and they often become secondarily dye coupled as a quartet of cells. In the end, each cell usually becomes a unique individual, and this cell specificity unfolds during embryogenesis as the growth cones make specific choices of which axonal pathway to follow. The appropriate choice of pathway appears to be a key factor in the development of neuronal specificity. Second, all of the progeny of a single precursor can have certain features in common, such as neurotransmitter or some aspects of their morphology; other features, however, can vary widely, such as electrical properties or final axonal pathway and/or destination. Third, there is a temporal sequence in the differentiation of both morphological and physiological phenotypes, and many different cells may differentiate in the same relative order of events. Some properties, such as neurotransmitter receptors, differentiate very early; other properties, such as electrical excitability, differentiate much later. Some properties appear to be highly correlated with one another; other properties, such as the onset of electrical excitability and the cessation of electrical coupling, show some variability in their precise timing and relationship to one another. Fourth, segmental specializations can arise in two ways. Segmental differences in cell number arise largely by segment-specific cell death. Furthermore, neurons of homologous cell lineage can differentiate with segment-specific properties, giving rise to segmental specializations in cell form and function.

What are the questions for future study? Many of the basic questions raised by these studies appear solvable by further studies of grasshopper embryos. Two questions, common to all nervous systems, are particularly interesting to us. First, we would like to understand how cells know who they are (cell determination). Second, we would like to understand how their growth cones know which way to go (pathway selection). To answer the first question we will have to understand how cells acquire commitments to their cell-specific fates (see Chapter 2). One possibility is that they acquire cell specificity from their mitotic ancestry; alternatively, they may acquire this information by cell interactions. It seems likely that both mitotic ancestry and cell interactions play a role in cell determination. Since cells from a particular cell division are placed in a stereotyped temporal and spatial environment, it will be impossible to answer this question by simply observing normal development. Rather, we will have to perturb the development of these cells to uncover the different contributions to their determination (see Chapters 1 and 4). A neuron's determination need not come in one step, and may involve a series of steps as the cell becomes committed to many different phenotypes. Certain phenotypes (i.e., transmitter choice) may be determined at one time and by one mechanism, whereas another phenotype (i.e., pathway choice) may be determined at a different time and by a different mechanism.

Some of the events of differentiation may themselves play a major role in the determination of later events. One such event is pathway selection by growth cones. Growth cones contact and interact with many different cells during their sequential series of choices. Unless the entire series of specific choices is fully and independently determined from the outset, the early decisions and interactions may be of utmost importance to later decisions. The growth cones of pioneer neurons make stereotyped axonal pathways by navigating across the basement membrane in an axonless environment. Later growth cones choose specific axonal (pioneer) pathways on which to grow when confronted with a choice of several possible pathways. In both cases the key questions for the future are: what is the information marking the environment, and how are the growth cones determined to make specific responses to that information? Both questions are likely to involve discovering specific molecules that mark either basement membranes or cell surfaces in the environment, and the surfaces of the growth cones themselves (see Chapter 6). Discovering the answers to these questions of cell determination and pathway selection will require a variety of cellular and molecular techniques. Fortunately, we think it is now possible to apply these techniques to the grasshopper embryo.

ACKNOWLEDGMENTS

I wish to thank Nick Spitzer and Mike Bate for their collaboration in many of these studies. The recent studies were supported by a NSF grant and Sloan Fellowship to CSG.

17. REFERENCES

1. Wheeler, W. M., 1893, A contribution to insect embryology, *J. Morphol.* **8:**1.
2. Bate, C. M., 1976, Embryogenesis of an insect nervous system. I. A map of the thoracic and abdominal neuroblasts in *Locusta migratoria, J. Embryol. Exp. Morphol.* **35:**107.
3. Bate, C. M., and Grunewald, E. B., 1981, Embryogenesis of an insect nervous system. II. A second class of neuron precursor cells and the origin of the intersegmental connectives, *J. Embryol. Exp. Morphol.* **61:**317.
4. Bentley, D., Keshishian, H., Shankland, M., and Raymond, A., 1979, Quantitative staging of embryonic development of the grasshopper, *Schistocerca nitens, J. Embryol. Exp. Morphol.* **54:**47.
5. Bate, C. M., 1976, Pioneer neurones in an insect embryo, *Nature (London)* **260:**54.
6. Keshishian, H., 1980, The origin and morphogenesis of pioneer neurons in the grasshopper metathoracic leg, *Dev. Biol.* **80:**388.
7. Edwards, J. S., Chen, S. W., and Berns, M. W., 1981, Cercal sensory development following laser microlesions of embryonic apical cells in *Acheta domesticus, J. Neurosci.* **1:**250.
8. Goodman, C. S., and Spitzer, N. C., 1979, Embryonic development of identified neurones: Differentiation from neuroblast to neurone, *Nature (London)* **280:**208.
9. Goodman, C. S., Bate, C. M., and Spitzer, N. C., 1981, Embryonic development of identified neurons: Origin and transformation of the H cell, *J. Neurosci.* **1:**94.
10. Evans, P., and O'Shea, M., 1977, The identification of an octopaminergic neuron which modules neuromuscular transmission in the locust, *Nature (London)* **270:**275.
11. Goodman, C. S., O'Shea, M., McCaman, R., and Spitzer, N. C., 1979, Embryonic development of identified neurons: Temporal pattern of morphological and biochemical differentiation, *Science* **204:**1219.
12. Goodman, C. S., Pearson, K. G., and Spitzer, N. C., 1980, Electrical excitability: A spectrum of properties in the progeny of a single embryonic neuroblast, *Proc. Natl. Acad. Sci. U.S.A.* **77:**1676.
13. Goodman, C. S., and Spitzer, N. C., 1981, The mature electrical properties of identified neurones in grasshopper embryos, *J. Physiol.* **313:**369.
14. Goodman, C. S., and Spitzer, N. C., 1981, The development of electrical properties of identified neurons in grasshopper embryos, *J. Physiol.* **313:**385.
15. Goodman, C. S., and Spitzer, N. C., 1980, Embryonic development of neurotransmitter receptors in grasshoppers, in: *Receptors for Neurotransmitters, Hormones and*

Pheromones in Insects (D. B. Satelle, ed.), pp. 195–207, Elsevier/North-Holland Biomedical Press, Amsterdam.

16. Bate, C. M., Goodman, D. S., and Spitzer, N. C., 1981, Embryonic development of identified neurons: Segment-specific differences in the H cell homologues, *J. Neurosci.* **1**:103.
17. Whitington, P., Bate, M., Seifert, E., Ridge, K., and Goodman, C. S., 1981, Survival and differentiation of identified embryonic neurones in the absence of their target muscles, *Science*, in press.

6

Nerve Fiber Growth and Its Regulation by Extrinsic Factors

PAUL C. LETOURNEAU

1. INTRODUCTION

A remarkable feature of embryogenesis is the elaborate extension of axons by neurons to target cells in the nervous system and in other organs. This growth of nerve fibers often traces characteristic pathways to produce specific patterns of innervation. Such precise organization requires a high degree of regulation, and manipulations of embryonal and regenerating tissues have shown that axons are usually directed by cues within the environments through which they grow.[1–4] This essay discusses how axons grow and examines two factors, cell–substratum adhesion and chemotactic responses, as principal environmental regulators of axonal growth. Discussion is restricted to tissue culture studies, because growing nerve fibers are more easily observed, manipulated, and subjected to high-resolution morphological and cytochemical studies *in vitro* than *in vivo*. In addition, potential extrinsic modulators of nerve fiber growth can be tested and thoroughly evaluated *in vitro*.

The focus of this chapter is the tip of a growing nerve fiber, originally named the growth cone by Ramón y Cajal.[5] This structure has a fascinating motile behavior and a cytoskeletal ultrastructure which differentiates it from the rest of the nerve fiber. The conclusions of this chapter

PAUL C. LETOURNEAU · Department of Anatomy, University of Minnesota, Minneapolis, MN 55455.

reflect the thesis that motility of the nerve tip drives the elongation of the nerve fiber. Of course, axonal growth requires more than the nerve tip, such as the synthetic activities of the perikaryon and the anterograde axonal transport of materials. However, the nerve tip is believed to be the major site of assembly of the neurite membrane and cytoskeletal fibers, and through its motility, it constantly explores and interacts with the environment. Thus, my bias is that regulation of the directions of axonal growth happens primarily at the nerve tip.

This essay emphasizes my own efforts and outlook on axonal growth. The interested reader can refer to several recent essays[6–8] for other perspectives.

2. BEHAVIOR OF THE GROWING NERVE FIBER TIP

2.1. *Protrusion and Regression*

For nearly 80 years, since Ross Harrison invented tissue culture in order to study axonal growth, interest has centered on the movements of the nerve tip. By observing axons extending into plasma clots from explants of amphibian neural tissues, Harrison[9,10] saw that the tips of growing nerve fibers change shape continuously by the extension and movement of small protrusions (Fig. 1). These movements are largely restricted to the nerve tip and occur infrequently more proximally along the nerve fiber. With the advent of phase contrast microscopy, time lapse cinematography, and the use of optically superior planar glass and plastic substrata, these motile structures were seen to be transient cylindrical and fan-shaped expansions from the margin of the nerve tip. They undergo a series of rapid changes as a neurite grows: extending, bending, waving, resting immobile on the substratum, and usually regressing or folding back to merge with the nerve tip, often with pinocytotic uptake of the external media (Fig. 2).[11–15]

Not only are these protrusions withdrawn or retracted, but other rearward movements occur at the nerve tip. Particles are frequently picked up and transported backwards on an extended filopodium or lamellipodium to stop where the neurite expands into the growth cone.[16,17] Much smaller material, molecular complexes of added plant lectins with their polysaccharide cell surface receptors, also move back in the fluid plasma membrane of protrusions and form caps or large aggregates on the upper surface of the growth cone.[18–20] I will propose later that the forces which retract and bend protrusions and produce these other rearward movements also drive neurite growth.

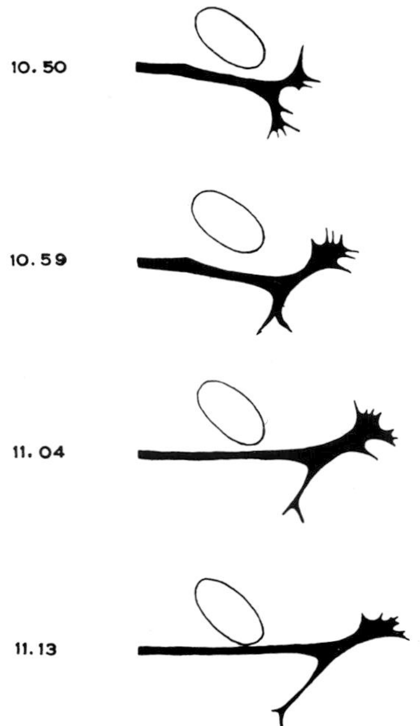

Figure 1. Drawings by Ross Harrison showing shape changes at the end of a nerve fiber growing from a neuronal explant of an amphibian embryo. The nerve fiber extended at a rate of 56 μm/hr, and its movement was accompanied by constant protrusion of fine processes from the nerve tip. (From Harrison[10] with permission of Alan R. Liss, Inc.)

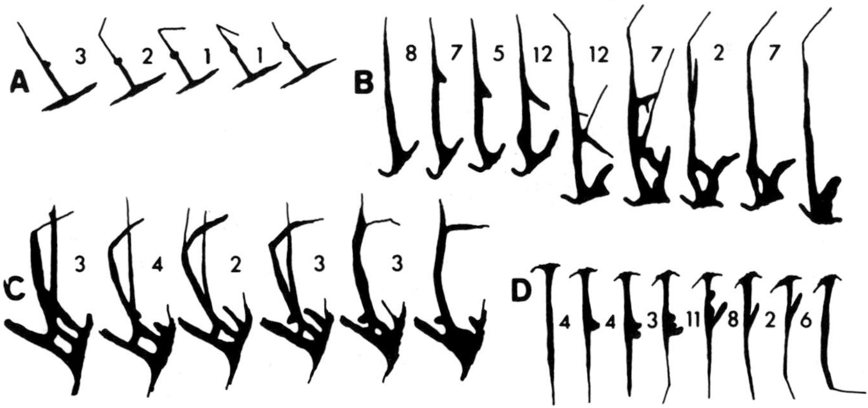

Figure 2. Tracings of frames from cinematographs, showing the rapid movements and morphological transformations of filopodia and other protrusions from the tips of growing nerve fibers. (A) Traced at ×500; (B) and (C) at ×1125; (D) at ×975. The numbers between successive frames are seconds elapsed. (From Luduena and Wessells[14] with permission of the authors and Academic Press.)

Thus, the nerve tip undergoes a constant advance and retreat of protrusions, like the ocean's lapping on a sandy shore. What do these movements have to do with neurite elongation? It has been noted that the neurite tip does not advance by an obvious forward flow of cytoplasm into a filopodium, as in the pseudopods of amoebae.[13] Furthermore, filopodial protrusion and movements can proceed for long periods without any neurite elongation. Possibly the only role of these protrusions is to imbibe fluids, nutrients, and trophic factors via endocytosis.[13,21–23] However, other studies have noted the importance to neurite growth of contacts and adhesions of these protrusions to other surfaces.

2.2. *Contacts of the Nerve Fiber Tip*

The considerable work of Weiss[24–26] emphasized cell–substratum contacts in all cell movement; their role was formalized in the concept of contact guidance by grooves and ridges in the substratum. In a general model, Weiss[26] proposed that the interplay of cell motive power with traction provided by adhesive contacts, as modulated by substratum shapes which favor adhesive contact along certain axes, can determine pathways of cell migration. Harrison[27] established that growing neurites must be in contact with a surface and will not extend into a fluid medium. The application of these ideas to neurite growth focuses attention on the nerve tip, and particularly on the exploratory palpations of other objects by filopodia. The seemingly random extension and movements of filopodia often bring them into contact with other surfaces, to which they respond alternatively by retraction, adhesion to the surface, and, occasionally, by exertion of sufficient force to distort or displace the point of attachment.[28] It was striking that filopodial traction on other neurites often preceded a nerve tip's joining to nerve fiber fascicles; in general, changes in the direction of growth cone elongation were preceded by the extension of filopodia and palpation of adjacent surfaces.[28–31]

2.3. *Cell–Substratum Adhesion and Neurite Growth*

The adhesive contacts of growth cone protrusions appeared to influence the behavior of the nerve tip as a whole. The role of cell–substratum adhesion in neurite growth was the focus of my first investigations. Studies of fibroblastic cell locomotion had revealed that anterior adhesions provide anchorage against which the cell is pulled forward,[14,32–35] and fibroblastic migration was shown to be restricted within a range of cell–substratum adhesivity; no movement was seen if adhesion was either too weak for adequate traction, or too strong, so that posterior adhesion was not released.[36] Neurite growth seemed to differ in the dynamics of adhesivity, because neurites grow in an agar matrix which does not support fibroblastic cell migration and can also extend on substrata to which fibroblasts adhere too strongly to migrate.[37,38] What is the significance of adhesion in neurite growth? Can adhesion ever be too strong, considering that the neuronal perikaryon does not move during neurite extension?

The importance of adhesion was examined by comparing neurite growth from embryonal chick sensory neurons cultured on two substrata differing only in a coating of a polycationic molecule, polyornithine (PORN). It was found that the initiation, elongation, and branching of nerve fibers were much greater on the PORN-treated substratum (Tables I and II; Fig. 3).[39] With the use of reproducible shearing forces, growth cone adhesion to PORN was found to be much greater than to untreated glass or plastic. The basis for such strong adhesion is unclear but may involve the absorption of adhesive ligands from the culture medium to the PORN-coated surface.[40–43] A strong adhesion of neurons to the PORN-treated surface was further indicated by the spreading of growth cones, flattened perikarya, and crooked neurites, which traced the routes taken by their tips (Figs. 4–6).[39,44]

Further information concerning the adhesive behavior of cultured neurons was obtained with interference reflection microscopy, a technique that displays the contours of the lower cell surface, particularly adherent areas separated from the glass substratum by only 10–30 nm.[45] When cultured on untreated glass, neurons have few of these close

Table I. Percentage of Neurons with an Axon(s) at 24 hr in Vitro

Age of embryo[a] (days)	Substratum	Neurons with axon(s) (% ± S.D.)
8	PORN or PLYS	54 ± 8.7 (n = 739)
8	Tissue culture	25 ± 2.6 (n = 642)
6	PORN or PLYS	31 (n = 165)
6	Tissue culture	7 (n = 123)
4	PORN or PLYS	21 ± 3.9 (n = 439)
4	Tissue culture	11 ± 1.6 (n = 626)

[a] Data for 8-day embryonic neurons are the combined results from five experiments; 6-day neurons from one experiment; and 4-day neurons from three experiments. Neurons were identified as spherical, refractile cells with an approximate diameter of 15 μm. Axons were identified as thin processes with a terminal growth cone, which had visible microspikes. *n*, number of neurons counted. (From Letourneau[39] with permission of Academic Press.)

Table II. Average Axon Lengths after 24 hr in Vitro

Experiment[a]	Substratum	Average lengths: μm/axon	Average lengths: μm of axon/neuron
1	PORN	291	626
	Tissue culture	68	106
2	PORN	245	524
	Tissue culture	115	189
3	PORN	285	651
	Tissue culture	105	168
Combined results	PORN	275	600
	Tissue culture	96	154

[a] The lengths of the axons of 20 randomly selected neurons were measured on each experimental substratum. In each of the three experiments the statistical significance of the differences in μm of axon/neuron between neurons on PORN and on tissue culture plastic is $p < 0.0002$, by use of the Mann–Whitney U Test. (From Letourneau[39] with permission of Academic Press.)

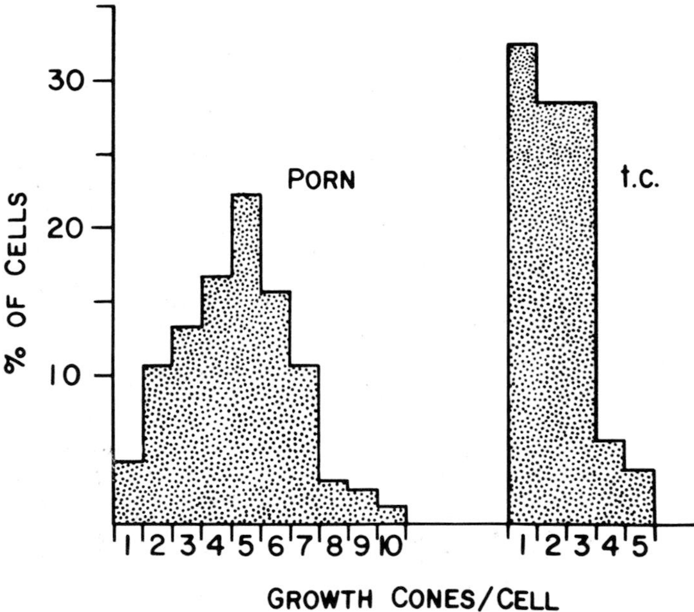

Figure 3. Frequency distribution of the number of growth cones per neuron on PORN-treated plastic and on untreated tissue culture plastic, after 24 hr *in vitro*. (From Letourneau[39] with permission of Academic Press.)

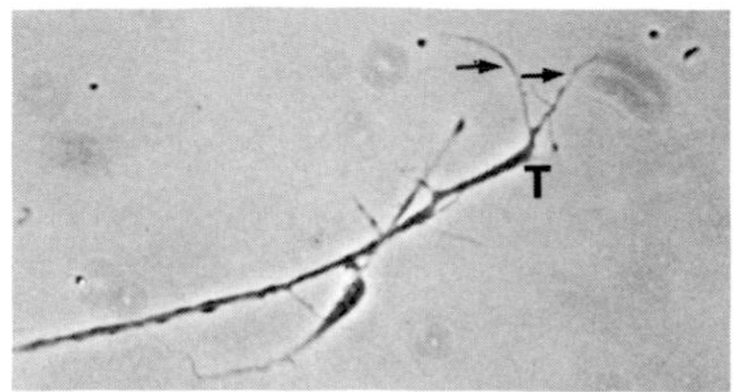

Figure 4. Neurite tip of a chick embryo sensory neuron cultured on untreated glass. Filopodia (arrows) protrude from the neurite, but the tip itself (T) is only slightly expanded. ×1050. (From Letourneau[46] with permission of Academic Press.)

adhesive contacts; typically there are just a patch beneath the cell soma and small areas beneath the growth cone.[46] Filopodia lack close contacts or adhere for only short periods, and neurites usually are not adherent to the substratum, as also seen by lightly tapping the side of the culture dish. On a PORN-treated surface, cell–substratum adhesions are much more extensive. The highly spread growth cones are underlain by broad close contacts, both centrally and at the margins, and filopodia and lamellipodia often adhere to the glass at their tips and along their edges (Figs. 7 and 8).[46] Frequently, a linear adhesive contact runs the length of a protrusion and continues inward beneath the growth cone margin. These linear adhesions are associated only with areas where filopodia and lamellipodia protrude. Extensive adhesive contacts run beneath the crooked neurites and flattened somata on a PORN-treated surface, but again discrete linear adhesions are absent unless protrusion is evident. Although the stabilizing action of these extensive adhesive contacts of cultured neurons to the substratum might be a factor in enhancing neuronal morphogenesis on PORN, it is my view that these linear adhesions of the protrusions are more generally important to neurite growth and its regulation at the nerve tip.

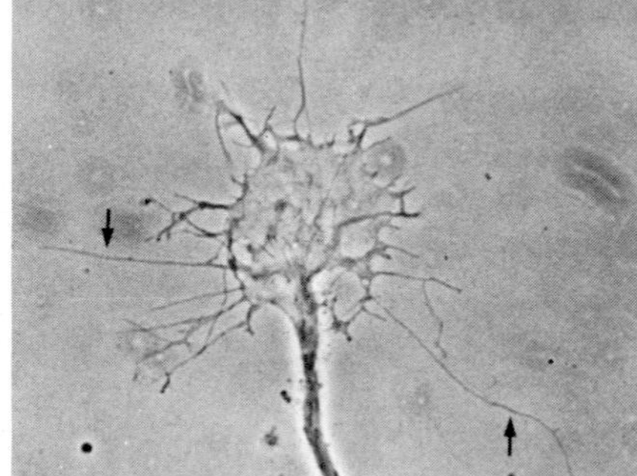

Figure 5. Neurite tip of a sensory neuron cultured on polyornithine-treated glass. Spreading of the neurite tip is clearly evident, as is the extreme length of some filopodia (arrows). ×1125. (From Letourneau[46] with permission of Academic Press.)

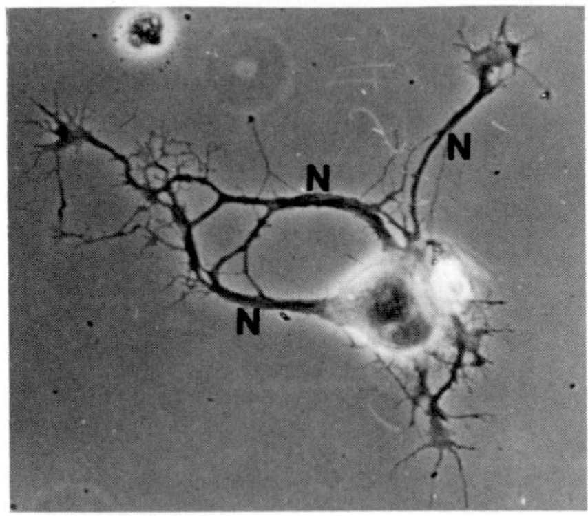

Figure 6. A sensory neuron cultured 20 hr on polyornithine-treated glass. The curved neurites (N) indicate high adhesion to the substratum. ×550. (From Letourneau[39] with permission of Academic Press.)

3. STRUCTURE OF THE GROWING NERVE FIBER

Before considering a mechanism of neurite growth, the structure of growth cones and neurites will be described. The motile and adhesive properties of growth cones reflect a cytoskeletal organization different from that of the neurite.

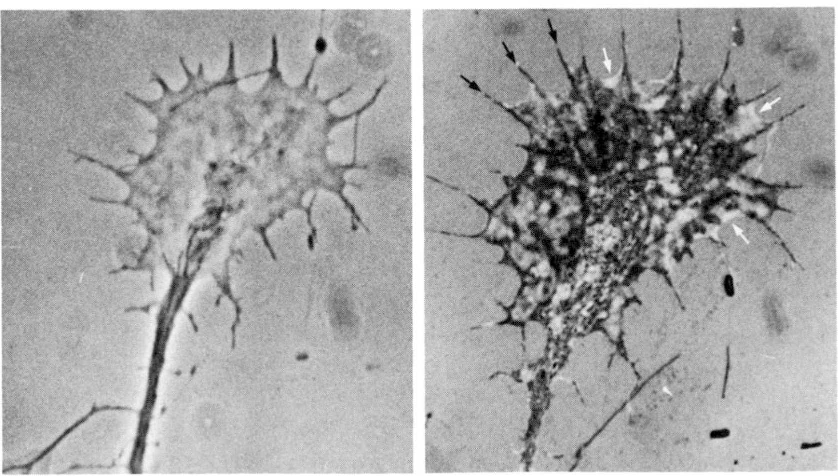

Figure 7. Phase contrast photomicrograph of a well-spread growth cone on polyornithine-treated glass. ×1500. (From Letourneau[46] with permission of Academic Press.)
Figure 8. Interference reflection micrograph revealing the adhesive contacts of this growth cone. Black-appearing adhesive contacts underlie filopodia and continue inward beneath the growth cone margin (black arrows). White arrows indicate concave portions of cell margin widely separated from substratum. ×1800. (From Letourneau[46] with permission of Academic Press.)

3.1. *The Neurite*

The neurite has a cytoskeletal core of 10 nm neurofilaments and microtubules, oriented longitudinally from the soma to the growth cone (Fig. 9).[47–49] These fibers are long, maybe over 100 μm long,[50] and they seem well suited for structural support of the neurite and for a role in axoplasmic transport.[51–53] Pharmacological studies implicate microtubules in these functions,[51,54] but no experimental evidence supports the morphological implication of neurofilaments in these activities. A third cytoskeletal component, microfilaments, do not run as long, parallel fibers down the neurite. Rather, microfilaments form a three-dimensional network consisting of either crisscrossed, short segments intersecting at many points, or articulated, sharply bent filaments.[49,55,56] This network fills the cell cortex without any particular orientation, contacts

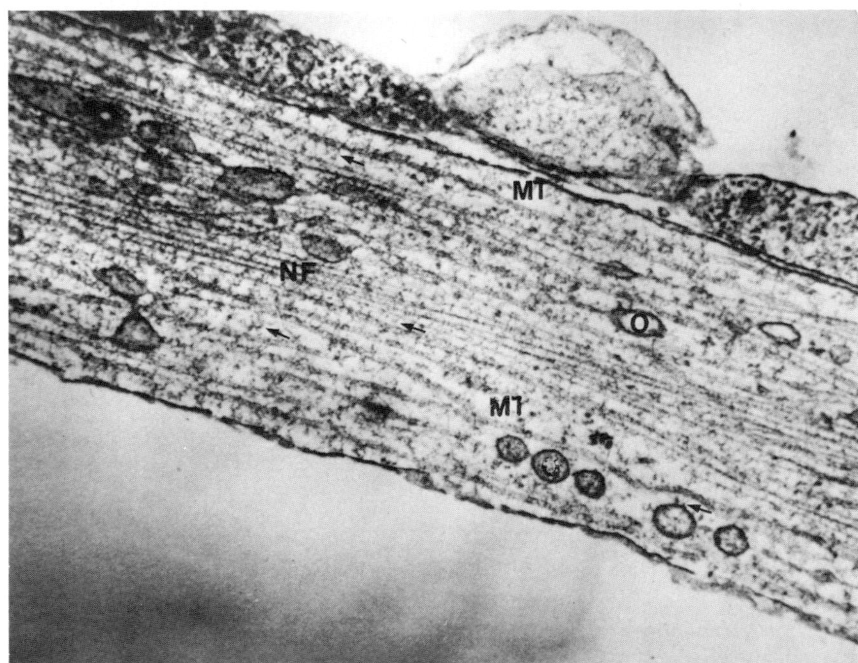

Figure 9. Longitudinal section along a neurite of a sensory neuron. Neurofilaments (NF) and microtubules (MT) are conspicuously long and straight. Microfilaments form an indistinct network beneath the plasmalemma and centrally among the other cytoskeletal fibers. Short microfilament segments (arrows) seem to contact neurofilaments and microtubules, as well as membranous organelles (O) that may be in transit within the neurite. ×31000. (From Yamada *et al.*[49] with permission of the authors and Rockefeller University Press.

the plasmalemma at many points, and penetrates inward among the more centrally located neurofilaments and microtubules (Fig. 9).[14,48,49] In this region, segments of microfilaments appear to interlink the longer cytoskeletal fibers and form bridges with other neuritic organelles.[49,57] In many cells microfilaments are made of actin,[58,59] thus suggesting that this filamentous network may act in axoplasmic transport and accounting for the infrequent protrusion of filopodia along a neurite.[49,60–62] This pervasive network of microfilaments may also contribute to the structural support of the neurite by cross-linking the longitudinally oriented neurofilaments and microtubules into a dense fibrous matrix.[52]

Lysosomes, mitochondria, and sacs of agranular reticulum are also seen in growing neurites.[63–66] Presumably many of these organelles are in transit between the perikaryon and nerve tip in both directions, and they are linked to neurofilaments and microtubules by short microfilaments which may shuttle them along the longitudinal cytoskeletal fibers.[49,57] Many of the agranular sacs rapidly incorporate exogenous tracers, indicating an endocytic origin, but other sacs may be outbound and include precursors of the neurite and growth cone plasmalemma or secretory products.[63,66,67]

3.2. *The Nerve Fiber Tip*

The orderly arrangement of organelles and fibers in the neurite is disrupted at the nerve tip. Neurofilaments and microtubules diverge and splay out into the broadened growth cone, with mitochondria and other membranous components entangled among the cytoskeletal fibers (Fig. 10).[14,17,49,63] The motile growth cone margin and its protrusions consists largely of a network of microfilaments attached to the plasma membrane at many points (Figs. 11–13).[48,49,63] As in neurites, most of this network is not polarized, but in filopodia and portions of lamellipodia, one often sees denser, more linear arrays of microfilaments, which extend centrally within the growth cone margin as small bundles (Figs. 12 and 13).[14,46,68] Whether these filament bundles are formed by reorganization of the filament network is unclear, though the filament bundles connect with the network at many points. Few other organelles are present in the growth cone margin, except that microtubules and sacs are seen extending out from the mass of organelles in the base of the growth cone in association with the proximal ends of microfilament bundles (Fig. 13).[46,69] This association is a clue to the link between growth cone motility and neurite elongation.

Immunocytochemical probing of growth cone structure reveals that actin and myosin are concentrated in these linear arrays of microfila-

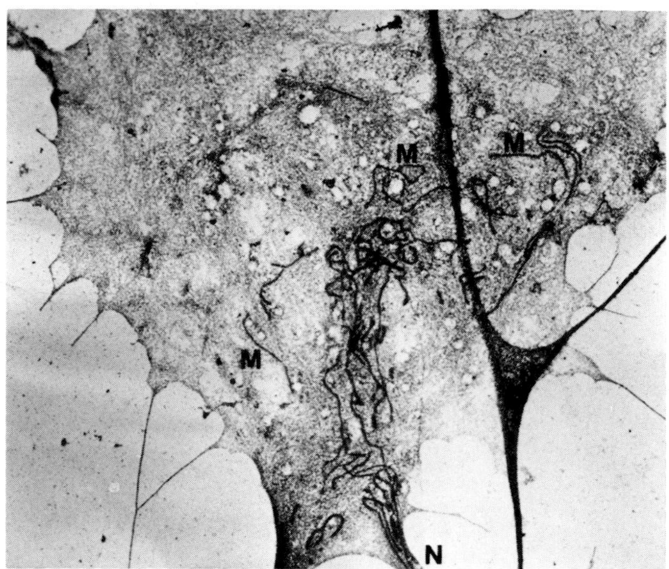

Figure 10. A whole growth cone cultured on a formvar-coated gold grid. Mitochondria (M) swirl around within the base of the growth cone. The neurite (N) extends from below the photograph. ×3300.

ments (Figs. 14 and 15).[70] An added significance of these filament bundles is that they are frequently seen at the sites where the growth cone has made linear adhesions to the substratum (Figs. 16 and 17). Thus, the motile margin of a growth cone resembles the locomotory portions of other cells, because it contains actomyosin complexes anchored within the cell to sites of cell–substratum adhesion.[32,34,35] As in a muscle cell, these complexes may interact to exert tension on other surfaces or on intracellar structures.

4. MECHANISM OF NERVE FIBER GROWTH

This section presents a model for nerve fiber growth, which lacks direct evidence for several features, but will be useful in examining how axons are directed to their targets. First I will consider how the major neurite structures, the plasmalemma and cytoskeleton, grow in the neurite, and then discuss how basic motile activities of protrusion, adhesion, and the generation of mechanical energy, drive the elongation of a neurite.

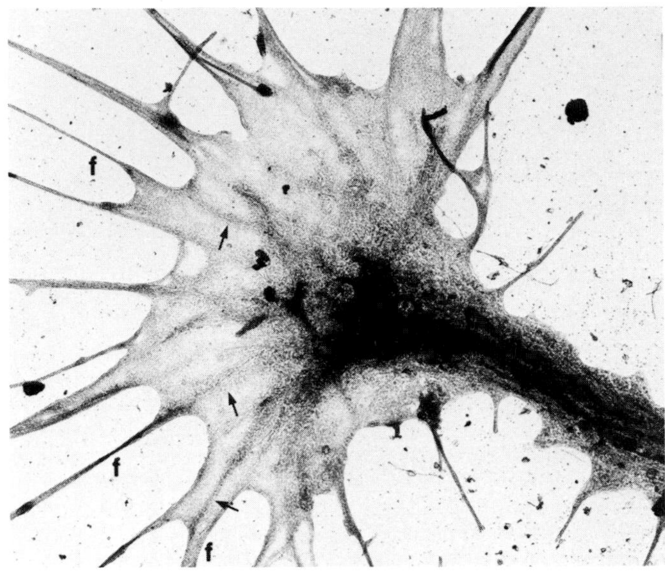

Figure 11. A whole growth cone cultured on a formvar-coated gold grid. Note the linear cytoplasmic densities (arrows) aligned on the same axes as filopodia (f) extended from the cell margins. The distribution of these denser cytoplasmic areas resembles the linear adhesive contacts seen with interference reflection microscopy. ×3700. (From Letourneau[46] with permission of Academic Press.)

4.1. *Expansion of the Neurite Membrane*

The formation of a neurite requires the synthesis and assembly of large areas of neuritic plasma membrane. One might imagine that the membrane expands by addition to the neurite near the cell soma, at the distal tip, or by intercalation all along its length. Although direct evidence for any mode of membrane expansion in the neurite is lacking, the indirect evidence suggests that membrane expansion occurs primarily at the nerve tip.[17,20,67] When a neurite is severed into proximal and distal segments by microsurgery, the distal segment can continue to elongate with a normally active growth cone for several hours.[13,71,72] Thus, the proximal neurite is not where membrane is added. Intercalation at many points does not seem to occur, because markers placed on the neurite plasmalemma neither move apart nor become farther from the soma as a neurite grows.[16,73] In addition, the lower neurite membrane can be immobilized by extensive adhesion to a PORN-treated surface without slowing neurite growth.[39,46] It seems as though membrane is spun out at the nerve tip to become stably incorporated into the neurite plasmalemma.

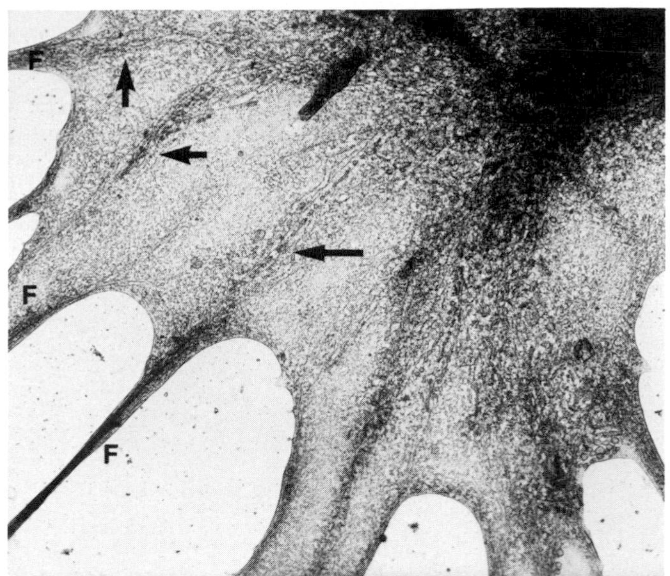

Figure 12. Higher magnification of same growth cone seen in Fig. 11, showing that microtubules and small agranular vesicles (arrows) are aligned on the axis of several filopodia (F). ×10500. (From Letourneau[46] with permission of Academic Press.)

How the membrane expands at the nerve tip is controversial. Preformed membrane vesicles, derived from the golgi apparatus, may be transported in the neurite and fuse with the cell surface at the nerve tip as during exocytosis.[63,65,74] Certainly many glycoproteins, including possible membrane components, travel to the ends of axons by fast axoplasmic transport. Tracer studies reveal that some agranular sacs in the growth cone are endocytic, but there are thousands, and others may be precursors of the plasmalemma.[64,66,75] Alternative to a vesicular mode of assembly, single molecules or small molecular aggregates may insert into the plasma membrane from the cytoplasm.[76] These two modes of membrane addition are not mutually exclusive; rather the timing of addition and nature of particular membrane molecules may dictate their route of incorporation into the plasma membrane.

4.2. *Growth of the Cytoskeleton*

Microtubules and neurofilaments are present all along a neurite, in all branches, and in the bases of growth cones. Where are these fibers assembled and how do they reach the growth cone? Individual fibers may be assembled in the cell soma, transfered intact into the neurite

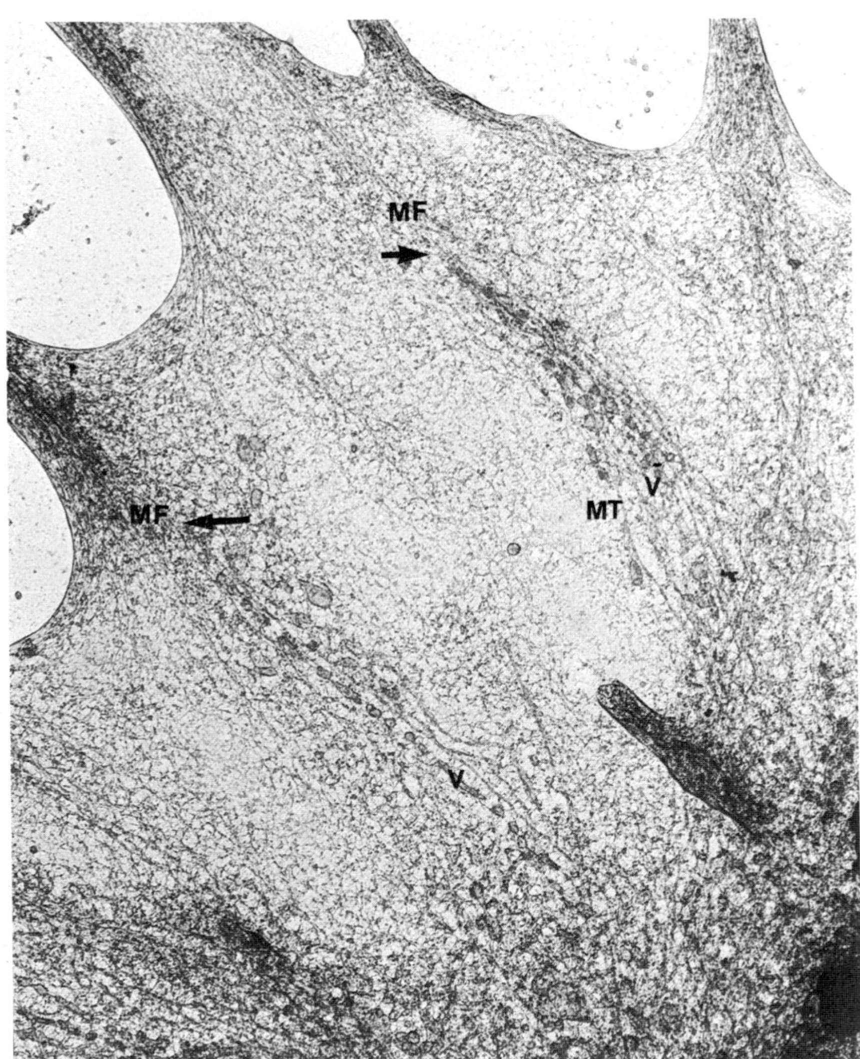

Figure 13. Same growth cone as Figs. 11 and 12. Contacts of the aligned vesicles (V) and microtubules (MT) with bundles of microfilaments (MF) can be seen (arrows). This interaction may be responsible for the positions of these vesicles and microtubules in the growth cone margin. ×24,500. (From Letourneau[46] with permission of Academic Press.)

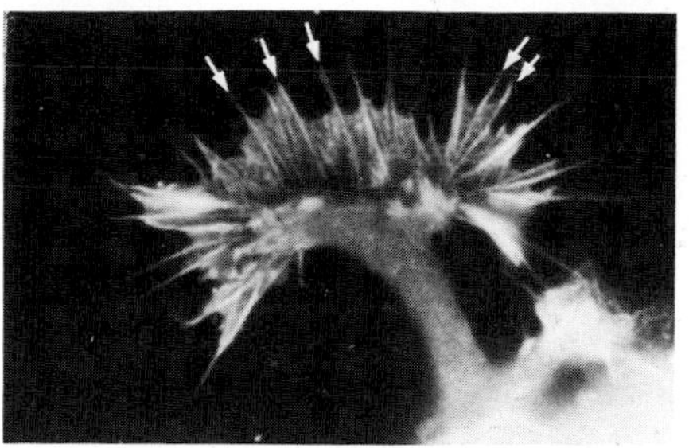

Figure 14. Immunocytochemical localization of actin in a growth cone of a sensory neuron. Fluorescent antibodies are concentrated into linear arrays (arrows) in the growth cone margin, which often are aligned with filopodia. These may coincide with microfilament bundles. ×1075. (From Letourneau[70] with permission of Academic Press.)

and transported forward as the growth cone advances. Alternatively, assembled fibers do not move great distances, but free subunits of these fibers are transported into the neurite where they polymerize onto the ends of intact fibers or participate in the initiation and assembly of new fibers. In either case, these cytoskeletal fibers grow only by addition of subunits to an end, not by intercalation within a fiber,[77,78] so that if the concentration of subunits is not limiting in a neurite, the location of ends of microtubules and neurofilaments determines where these fibers grow. Far more ends of these fibers are seen in the growth cone than elsewhere in a neurite, indicating that the nerve tip may be a major site of cytoskeletal growth (Letourneau, submitted for publication).

The microfilaments of a neurite are functionally and structurally separate from the microtubules and neurofilaments, and their assembly must be considered independently. In adult axons, actin and associated proteins are transported separately and more rapidly than these other cytoskeletal components.[79–81] Microfilaments of the cell cortex are rapidly disrupted by cytochalasin B,[49] and the microfilament network of the growth cone and neurite is quickly extracted by detergents, leaving intact the microtubules and neurofilaments of the neurite core (Letourneau, submitted for publication). The rapid protrusion and movements of the growth cone margin further indicate that the microfilaments are a labile, dynamic structural component of the neurite. Interactions of actin monomers with other regulatory proteins and ionic conditions

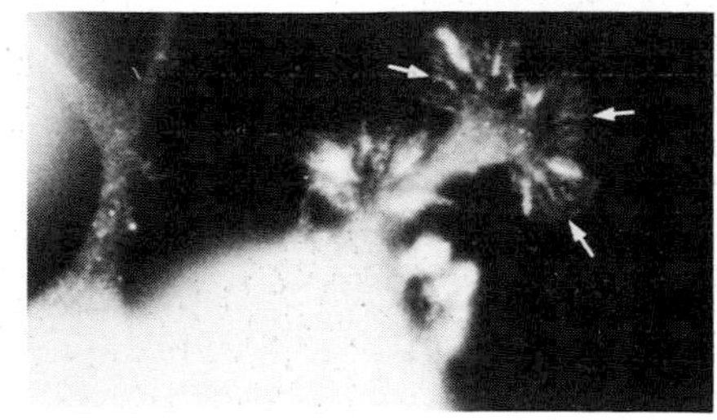

Figure 15. Immunocytochemical localization of myosin in a growth cone of an NGF-treated PC12 cell. Linear arrays of fluorescence (arrows) are seen with the same type of distribution as actin, indicating that actomyosin complexes may exist in the growth cone margin. ×1075. (From Letourneau[70] with permission of Academic Press.)

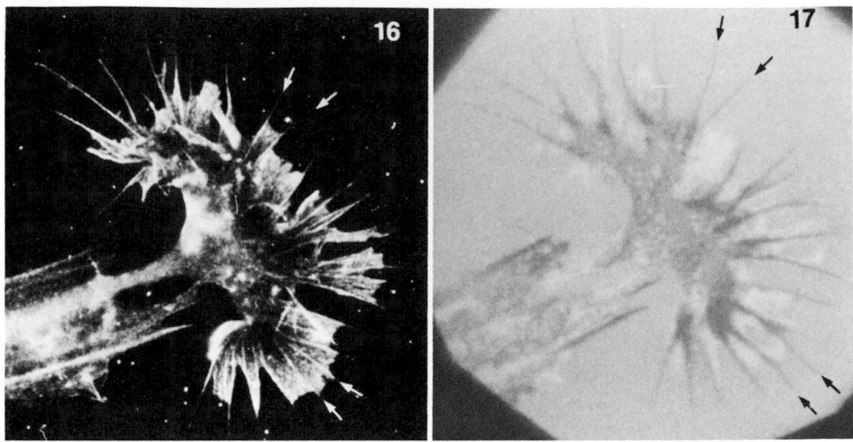

Figure 16 and 17. (Fig. 16) Immunocytochemical localization of actin in a growth cone and (Fig. 17) interference reflection image of growth cone–substratum adhesion of a sensory neuron. Many linear actin arrays (white arrows) coincide with linear adhesions (black arrows) of the growth cone margin to the substratum. ×1075. (From Letourneau[70] with permission of Academic Press.)

throughout the neurite may determine the state of assembly and activity of the microfilamentous network.

4.3. *Protrusion, Adhesion, and Actomyosin Action*

Unlike the seeming stability of the neurite membrane, the membrane of the nerve tip is dynamic, expanding locally as filopodia and lamellipodia protrude, and regressing with endocytotic uptake of membrane where these protrusions are withdrawn.[64,66,67] If these activities are equal, the net membrane area will not change. However, adhesion of protrusions to a surface may counteract their retraction so that membrane addition by protrusion exceeds membrane withdrawal during retraction. The highly spread growth cones on PORN (Fig. 5), and the rapid expansion of growth cone surface area when cell-substratum adhesion is increased, indicate that membrane expansion at the growth cone is favored by adhesion of protrusions.[39,46] Since protrusion occurs mainly at the nerve tip, this form of membrane expansion occurs primarily at the nerve tip. When protrusion is stabilized by adhesion, no other form of membrane addition is needed to provide a plasmalemmal sheath for the growing neurite. At later times, specific individual molecules may be added to the membrane by other means.[82]

By anchoring protrusions, adhesive contacts have an important role in membrane growth. I will now propose that adhesive contacts are equally important for their role in force exertion in the growth cone. I have already noted that actin and myosin are colocalized in linear arrays of microfilaments in the growth cone margin (Figs. 14–17). During the contraction of striated muscle, actin filaments slide past immobile myosin filaments and exert force on their attachments to the Z lines at the boundary of the sarcomeres. In nonmuscle cells, these contractile filaments must also be associated with other structures to transmit mechanical energy; but unlike striated muscle, whether the actin filaments or the myosin filaments slide may depend on the relative masses of structures linked to the filaments and on other forces impinging on these structures. Actin filaments in nonmuscle cells are linked to the plasma membrane with the same polarity as actin filaments are connected to the Z lines of a sarcomere.[68,83–85] The structural associations of myosin in nonmuscle cells are less clear, but may include the plasma membrane, membranous organelles, and elements of the cytoskeleton.[79,80,86,87] With these associations, actin and myosin can interact to exert force on the plasmalemmal attachments of the actin filaments (Figs. 18–21) or may slide the myosin filaments toward the membrane insertions of actin filaments.

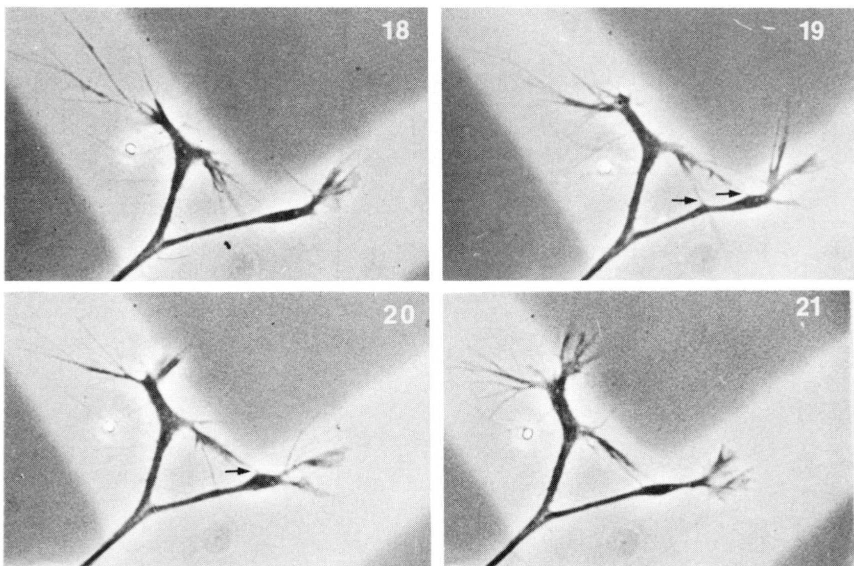

Figures 18–21. Frames from a time lapse movie, showing the exertion of force by filopodia upon contact points with an adjacent neurite branch. The neurite branch is transiently distorted (arrows) at the point of attachment with a filopodium. Elapsed time between successive frames: 18–19, 230 sec; 19–20, 113 sec; 20–21, 524 sec. ×650.

4.4. *Force Exertion in the Growth Cone Margin; How the Neurite Grows*

The growth cone margin exhibits cycles of protrusion and retraction. The underlying basis of protrusion is not presently known, though the polarity of actin filaments in contact with the plasma membrane indicates that this actin cannot push the membrane out in an actomyosin interaction.[83,88] Retraction may occur when actomyosin complexes pull on the plasma membrane of protrusions that are weakly adherent or not adherent to a surface. If, however, a protrusion has strong adhesive contacts, the actin filaments may not slide backwards, but instead the membrane remains anchored at the adhesive point, and force is exerted to draw the myosin filaments forward. Those structures that are linked to myosin, such as sacs of membrane precursor, neurofilaments, or microtubules, will be pulled toward the adhesive contacts. This forward movement promotes neurite growth by drawing new membrane to the front of the nerve tip, as well as by pulling cytoskeletal fibers forward from the base of the growth cone to positions where they may be further lengthened by terminal additions of monomers.

This proposal is supported by electron-microscopic observations that microtubules, neurofilaments, and vesicles extend into the growth cone margin only where they are associated with the small bundles of microfilaments protruding inward from filopodia and lamellipodia (Figs. 11–13). It seems as though these organelles are drawn out from the base of the growth cone by virtue of their linkage to microfilament bundles.

Thus, common locomotory activities, protrusion, adhesions, and force generation, are expressed in neurons to build a unique structure, the axon. The genetic program for development of neuronal morphology is not known, but it must also provide for the sustained motile activity at the nerve tip, the structural transformation of the spread growth cone base to the cylindrical shaft of a neurite, and the continuous synthesis and transport of components for the growing neurite. These, too, may be based upon common cellular activities, but their coordinate regulation is unique to neurons.

5. REGULATION OF NERVE FIBER GROWTH BY ENVIRONMENTAL FACTORS

Axons normally grow to their targets along characteristic routes, yet axons can also reach their targets when forced to cross foreign environments.[89–92] In other cases axons respond to manipulation of their environment with new, but repeatable growth patterns.[1,2,93,94] These observations suggest that both intrinsic cellular properties and extrinsic environmental features can determine axonal pathways. I will focus on the nerve tip as the site where axonal growth is regulated by extrinsic factors. Cell–substratum or cell–cell adhesion and soluble chemotactic factors will be examined as modulators of neurite growth, with attention directed to the ways in which they affect growth cone motility.

5.1. *Regulation by Cell–Substratum Adhesion*

When growth cone–substratum adhesion is strong, neurons sprout many neurites; the neurites grow fast and branch frequently (Tables I and II; Fig. 3).[39] These data can be explained by the influence of adhesive contacts on force exertion in the growth cone. On an adhesive surface, forces applied by actomyosin complexes on membrane insertion points are likely to result in forward movement of the nerve tip and its contents; on a poorly adhesive surface retraction is more common. Thus growth cone motility more effectively advances the neurite on adhesive substrata, leading to faster neurite growth.

The role of adhesion in neurite initiation is nicely illusrated by Collins's[95] findings that embryonal chick ciliary neurons sprout neurites within minutes of adding heart conditioned medium (HCM) to the dish. Before neurites emerge, however, the first response is that filopodia which protruded but did not adhere in the absence of HCM, now attach firmly to the substratum, which has absorbed components of the conditioned medium. Perhaps actin filaments, attached to the plasmalemma of firmly anchored protrusions, now no longer withdraw the cell margin during actomyosin interactions. Instead force can now be exerted by myosin filaments in the cell margin to pull out microtubules and neurofilaments, organizing a neurite from organelles available within the perikaryon.

A critical feature of the role of cell–substratum adhesions is their action on local actomyosin movements to promote the advance of organelles in the vicinity of firmly adherent protrusions. Consequently, if protrusions make stronger or more frequent adhesions at one side of a growth cone, neurite organelles will be transported predominantly to the more adherent side, and the neurite will grow in that direction. Such directed growth has been demonstrated *in vitro* on substrata containing patterned variation in adhesivity (Fig. 22).[96,97] Besides moving organelles, mechanical forces in the growth cone margin may be transmitted via cytoskeletal linkages from regions of strong cell–substratum adhesion to detach weakly adherent areas.[98] This will also direct neurites towards regions of stronger adhesivity.

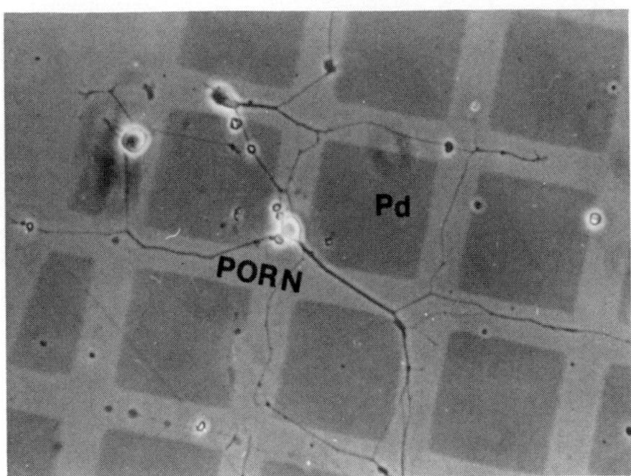

Figure 22. Preferential extension of neurites on the more adhesive portions of a patterned substratum. Growth cones branch, turn, or continue straight upon the PORN-treated plastic (PORN) and rarely cross onto the palladium (Pd)-coated squares, which is a less adhesive surface. ×140. (From Letourneau[97] with permission of Academic Press.)

Local effects of adhesion in the growth cone margin may also explain increased neurite branching on PORN. Branches most often occur by the division of a growth cone into several nerve tips.[73] On a PORN-treated surface, branching can be induced rapidly through micromanipulation by lifting and detaching from the substratum the middle of a widely spread growth cone.[99] This manipulation may isolate and thus accentuate the outwardly directed tensions being exerted in the sides of the growth cone that remain attached, inducing a division of the growth cone and its contents. On PORN, the neurite organelles projecting into the growth cone may often be divided into several streams by the actomyosin forces exerted at several points around an adherent, widely spread growth cone (Fig. 23).

5.2. *Regulation by Spatial Variations in Adhesivity*

These *in vitro* studies lead to the proposal that spatial and temporal variations in neuron–substratum and growth cone–substratum adhesion determine the time and place of neurite initiation, neurite branching patterns and pathways of neurite growth. These variations may stem from the distribution of environmental adhesion-mediating molecules into gradients and other spatial patterns or may arise from intrinsic asymmetries in the distribution of adhesion-mediating molecules on the surfaces of neurons and their extensions.

Asymmetries in cell surface components could be established by prior asymmetric interactions of a neuron with other cells or environmental features. One potential cue may be the early contact of the neuroblasts with the basal lamina of the ventricular layer.[100] The organelles and cytoskeletal filaments of epithelial cells are often polarized relative to the basal lamina. Perhaps the transmembrane linkage of adhesive ligands to cytoskeletal fibers[101–103] organizes asymmetry in the distribution of these cell surface components. In addition, the orderly movements of glial and neuronal precursors as they traverse the cell cycle during early proliferative periods may preserve a cellular orientation which defines the apical-basal axis of mature neuronal shapes.[100]

Certainly neuronal specificity is an intriguing property, which involves the specification of a particular topographic locus for each cell in a field of innervation.[100,104] This property is probably determined by positional information acquired from extrinsic sources at an early stage prior to initial neurite outgrowth.[105–107] This information becomes fixed within neurons and cannot be changed.[105–107] How it is stored and interpreted remains a mystery, although studies have suggested that positional information is expressed in the adhesive interactions of axons and target cells.[108,109]

5.2.1. Evidence for Spatial Variations in Adhesivity. Besides the response of neurites to artificially patterned substrata, there is evidence that spatial variations in the adhesive ligands of cells and cell products

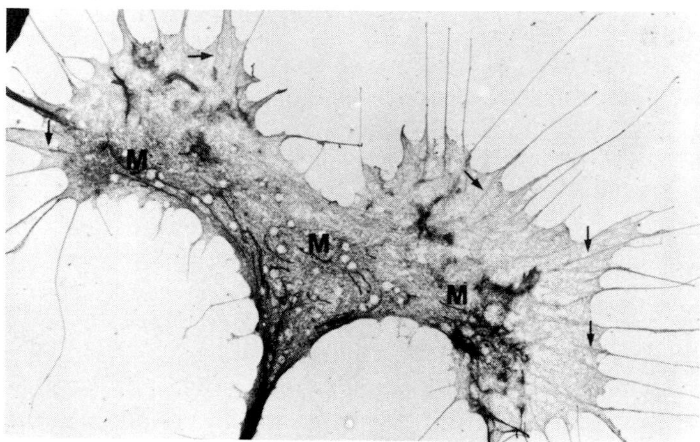

Figure 23. A growth cone in the process of dividing into two neurite branches. Mitochondria (M) have moved into the two diverging sides of the growth cone, and bundles of microfilaments (arrows) are present in the growth cone margin at the two sides. Compare distribution of these bundles to the actin fibers seen in Fig. 16. ×4000.

direct axonal growth. The adhesive affinities of dissociated embryonal retinal cells for explanted optic tecta comprise a spatial gradient which mimics the distribution of retinotectal synapses.[108,109] Thus, neuronal locus specificity may be expressed in the topographic distribution of cellular adhesive ligands across the interacting fields of retinal axons and tectal surfaces. Recent work indicates that these regional adhesive affinities are based on regional differences in protein and carbohydrate determinants of the retinal cell surface.[110] However, it has not yet been demonstrated that retinal axons and the tectal surfaces they contact in the embryo actually contain the adhesive asymmetries measured by these *in vitro* assays.

The *in vitro* growth of neurites from chick autonomic neurons is strikingly enhanced on substrata coated either with molecules released by fibroblasts and muscle cells into conditioned media or with microexudates deposited by these cells onto the substratum.[40,111,112] These materials may form tracks for axonal growth, because they are produced by cells that growing axons encounter *in vivo.* The significance of these substances seems to be that they are adhesive ligands for neurites and growth cones, for their distribution on the substratum rigidly defines the extent of axonal growth.[41,113] The location of these substances *in vivo* may resemble that of fibronectin, an adhesive molecule for fibroblastic cells that is located on cell surfaces, in basement membranes, and in extracellular matrices.[114–116] Although these molecules may mark pathways for axonal growth through nontarget areas, they have not been shown to contain heterogeneity sufficient to sort out the organization of synaptic fields.

5.2.2. Regulation by Contact Guidance. The shape of the substratum, alone, may influence the pathways of axonal growth in the absence of regional differences in adhesive ligands. In recent examination of the principle of contact guidance, fibroblastic cell movement was shown to be restricted along ridges, in grooves, and by highly curved substrata.[117] It was proposed that microfilament bundles cannot assemble and operate in association with adhesive sites in the highly bent states necessary to protrude and spread the cell margin over ridges, into steep grooves, or around sharp curves. As a corollary, protrusion and movement are favored on a surface whose shape allows the assembly of more or larger adhesions linked to filament bundles within the cell margin.

The asymmetric growth of neurites within oriented collagen matrices may reflect the ability of filopodia to form longer and more numerous adhesions by extending along the axes of collagen fibrils rather than by contacting fibrils from the side.[118,119] In addition, less force is dissipated and lost for use in neurite extension when filopodia pull along the longitudinal axis of collagen fibrils rather than pulling from the side and displacing fibrils.

Contact guidance has often been cited as a determinant of axonal growth *in vivo*. Instead of the homogeneous planar surface of tissue culture dishes, axons *in vivo* encounter fibrous mats or layers, more open matrices of connective tissue, or the variously rounded and elongated shapes of other cells. As expected, the restricted opportunities for adhesive contacts *in vivo* dictate that growth cones tend to be bulbous with thin filopodial protrusions, rather than having highly spread margins, as on PORN.[120–126] Contact guidance may explain axonal growth along other axons and glial processes, in channels or along tissue interfaces, but it cannot explain why a particular pathway is chosen among several or why axons grow in a certain direction along the pathway.[2,127–129] In the following section I discuss how neurites become associated with guidance pathways such as pioneering axons or glial fibers, and will suggest that intrinsic adhesive affinities are important in the interactions of neurites with other cells.

5.2.3. *Interactions of Neurites with Other Cells; Entering and Leaving Nerve Bundles.* Protrusions from nerve tips have been observed to contact and pull on nearby neurites with enough force to distort the neurites (Figs. 18–20). If this adhesion is weak, the protrusion withdraws, but if the contact persists, the nerve tip may expand its contacts with the encountered neurite and grow along it.[28–31,130] Whether a growth cone follows a pioneer fiber may be determined by the resistance of this initial filopodial–neurite contact to tensions applied within the filopodium. Thus, adhesive affinities between neurites and nerve tips might regulate which fascicle a nerve tip joins and hence the target area to which the neurite grows[25,131] (see Chapters 4, 5, 7, and 8). Even within a bundle, neurite–neurite relationships may shift as growth cones maximize their adhesive contacts as they advance. If nerve tips prefer adhesion to neurites from neighboring cells over neurites of distant origin, these interactions may establish topographic order within a nerve trunk even before a target is reached.[132,133]

On entering a target area, individual axons or small groups leave nerve bundles for specific zones of innervation. *In vitro* studies indicate that this exit may be prompted by decreases in neurite–neurite adhesion or by the availability of new, more adhesive substrata. When sensory ganglia are cultured on regular substrata, neurites leave the explants grouped into large fascicles. However, in the presence of antiserum to the nerve cell adhesion molecules, CAM, neurite–neurite adhesion is inhibited while neurite–substratum adhesion is not; in this case fascicles do not form, and neurites leave the explant as individual fibers.[134,135]

The same results occur without adding anti-CAM when ganglia are cultured on substrata of high adhesivity. Again, fascicles are rare, and single crooked, adherent nerve fibers extend from explants, as growth cones prefer the PORN-treated substratum to the surfaces of other fibers (Letourneau, unpublished data).

These observations indicate that the total adhesive environment must be considered in predicting the outcome of a particular interaction of a nerve tip with other neurites or cells. A recent model proposes that a hierarchical sequence of adhesive interactions among optic fiber growth cones, other optic fibers, and tectal cells determines the pattern of retinotectal connectivity.[136] Optic fiber growth cones interact with other fibers and surfaces within the optic stalk until they reach the tectum, where the fibers spread out across surfaces of greater adhesivity. This model is supported by the recent finding that optic fiber growth cones extend more readily on a layer of tectal cells than on retinal cells.[137]

6. REGULATION OF NERVE FIBER GROWTH BY CHEMOTAXIS

The orientation of morphogenetic cell movements by concentration gradients of soluble chemicals, i.e., chemotaxis, is an old idea, though only recently has the chemotactic potential of vertebrate cells been examined in detail.[138–140] Ramón y Cajal[141] proposed that axons are drawn forward by alluring substances, and since then positive and negative evidence[142] for chemotactic growth of axons has been reported. Explants of neural tissues extend neurites preferentially toward a piece of tissue which is assumed to release a chemoattractant.[143–145] These results are open to other interpretations, such as preferential survival or adhesion of neurites situated closest to the tissue source. In addition, differences in neurite interactions with each other and with nonneuronal cells may produce the observed growth. These possibilities are interesting and relevant to understanding how target tissues direct axonal growth, but they are *not* chemotaxis. To prove chemotaxis one must demonstrate that the *motility of the nerve tip* is oriented by a chemical gradient.

6.1. *NGF as a Chemoattractant*

The powerful hormonal action of nerve growth factor (NGF) on the metabolism and differentiation of sympathetic and sensory neurons is well known,[22] but the possibility that NGF is also a chemoattractant is a relatively new and inadequately tested idea. *In vitro* studies show that neurites appear to extend preferentially from explants toward a source of NGF,[146] and a dramatic *in vivo* finding is that NGF, when injected into the brains of young rats, induces abnormal growth of axons from peripheral sympathetic neurons into the spinal cord and up to the site of injection.[147] Because NGF is well characterized and can be applied in its pure form at known concentrations, it is the focus of this discussion. Similar conclusions should hold for other potential chemoattractants (see Chapter 9).

6.2. *Behavorial Responses of Growth Cones That Indicate a Chemotactic Response to NGF*

When dispersed sensory neurons were cultured in agar matrices containing an NGF gradient, the nerve tips displayed a partial, yet repeatable orientation up the gradient.[148] In addition, neurites tended to be extended further up the gradient than down, indicating a long-term directional response to the NGF gradient. However, to really understand chemotactic behavior, one must define the short-term responses of growth cones to an attractant. When NFG is released from a micropipette placed near the tips of sensory neurites, the tips turn and extend toward the pipette within 20 min.[149,150] This growth toward the pipette was not measurably faster than normal, but was a reorientation to the assumed gradient.[150] Whether this response persists for long periods of neurite growth must be investigated further.

The sensory responses of bacteria and leukocytes to chemoattractants have been probed by rapidly changing the concentration of the attractant.[151,152] This approach was used to further define the neurite response to NGF, and we found, surprisingly, that sensory neurites retracted within 5 min when NGF concentrations were elevated to a level corresponding to a large increase in occupancy of a high-affinity cell surface NGF receptor.[153] Parasympathetic ciliary neurons, which do not respond trophically to NGF, do not retract their neurites when NGF levels are raised. Because retraction can be elicited from sensory neurites severed from their perikarya by microsurgery, local NGF receptors on the neurites must be involved. We also found that cytochalasin B, a microfilament-disrupting drug, inhibits this retraction. Though paradoxical, retraction demonstrates a rapid effect of changes in NGF levels on growth cone motility. Retraction is obviously not a positive chemotactic event, but may be a supernormal response of the motile apparatus to large increases in occupancy of NGF receptors.

6.3. *Mechanisms of Chemotactic Response to NGF*

The elements of a chemotactic response are (1) sensation of the attractant, (2) determination of the gradient, and (3) modulation of locomotion.[154] NGF receptors are present on neurites, and gradients may be sensed because of spatial differences in occupancy of NGF receptors along a neurite or growth cone. As in chemotaxis of the best-studied vertebrate cell, the leukocyte, changes in NGF levels may rapidly alter such neuronal membrane properties as ion fluxes, calcium binding, or adhesivity.[140,155] These responses may mediate the attractant's influence on growth cone motility by stimulating protrusive activity, increasing actomyosin contractility, or increasing adhesivity of the cell surface at the point of greatest NGF binding. Changes in intracellular concentrations of ions or other small molecules might also influence the assembly of cytoskeletal fibers. Any of these responses is capable of regulating the direction of axonal growth, but as previously proposed for regulation by cell–substratum adhesion (Section 5.1), the requirement for a chemotactic response to NGF is a *local* change in growth cone motility.

The chemotactic role of NGF *in vivo* appears to be unsubstantiated except for the study mentioned above.[147] The degree of connection specificity that might be determined by chemotactic responses to NGF is unclear because NGF is synthesized by many organs, and NGF-responsive neurons are located throughout the body. Perhaps a chemotactic response to NGF acts in concert with directive interactions of growth cones with substratal features, to determine the vector of movement along particular pathways. There is question whether chemical gradients could be established or maintained in an organism as large as an embryo.[156] In many cases, however, the distance between neuronal somata and targets is short at early times of axonal extension, and chemotaxis may operate most effectively in early stages or may operate only in the vicinity of target cells.

6.4. *NGF Receptors and Electrical Currents*

A regulatory action of NGF–receptor complexes on growth cone motility has been suggested in recent investigations of the influence of electrical potential differences on neurite growth. Studies in the laboratory of Jaffe and co-workers have indicated that neurite growth from explants is asymmetric in a steady electrical field.[157] Ganglia placed in fields of 70 mV/mm or more showed significantly greater neurite growth toward the cathode than the anode. In spite of this oriented general response, many single neurites were not directed toward the cathode.

As he found for other surface receptors on other cells, Jaffe proposes that the steady electrical current electrophoreses plasmalemmal NGF receptors toward the cathodal side of neurons and neurites.[157,158] Presumably, interactions of NGF with unequally distributed receptors on the neurites facilitates neurite growth toward the cathode, but not in the direction of the anode. How this occurs is unclear, but just as in a chemotactic response, asymmetric influences on protrusion, adhesion, or force exertion may enhance neurite growth toward the cathode. In chemotaxis, asymmetry in environmental concentrations of NGF is the crucial feature in producing local differences in receptor occupancy, while electrical fields may produce an asymmetry of occupied NGF receptors by inducing mass movements of molecules in the membrane. Electrophoresis of other membrane components, such as adhesive ligands, could also influence the directions of neurite growth, but it is intriguing that a single cellular mechanism may account for the effects of both chemotaxis and electrical fields on neurite growth. Further investigation is needed to corroborate Jaffe's proposal. It will be helpful to study the responses of dissociated single neurons and demonstrate that the electrical currents act directly on the neurons rather than on components of the culture medium or substratum. Yet the idea that electrical fields influence cellular migrations is a compelling alternative to prevalent proposals based on mechanical factors.

7. FUTURE PROSPECTS

Exciting and substantial increases in our understanding of how neuronal connections are established are likely to come in the next few years. Biochemical and immunological approaches are on the track of unraveling the molecular basis of neuronal cell identity, possibly the ultimate determinant of synaptic specificity.[159–163] In addition, monoclonal antibodies directed to neuronal surface components may be used to follow determinative interactions and subsequent events comprising the developmental history of neuronal phenotypes (see Chapter 3). This section highlights areas of inquiry that are particularly related to my own interests in future work.

7.1. *Regulation of Actin Structure and Function*

Neurite growth is based on the motility of the growth cone margin, itself the product of dynamic activities and structural transformations of the microfilamentous network within the nerve tip. How are filopodial and lamellipodial protrusions formed? How are the linear bundles of microfilaments assembled, and what is their relationship to the linear adhesions? What are the ultrastructural associations of myosin, and what triggers contractile tensions in the growth cone margin? These crucial questions for neurite growth are related to all cell motility and are more easily investigated in other cellular systems.

The rapid protrusion and other surface movements of locomotory cells require that actin be labile in its position and state of assembly, unlike the stable organization of sarcomeres. There are proteins and enzymes in a variety of nonmuscle cells that regulate the organization of actin: interactions with monomeric and F-actin cross-link polymerized filaments into bundles, inhibit or promote polymerization of actin filaments, and mediate the attachment of filaments to membranes.[164–168] In addition, ionic conditions and pH may modify actin organization and function either by direct effects on actin or by influencing the accessory proteins.[169,170] These endogenous regulators allow actin assembly and function to be modulated by numerous stimuli, such as the adhesive contacts and chemotactic gradients that may regulate axonal growth.

Because growth cones cannot be harvested in sufficient quantities for biochemical analyses of actin regulation, these endogenous regulators must be investigated by other means. Growth cones are severely disrupted by many of the fixatives used for immunological staining of fibroblastic cells; subsequently, little more than the presence of a particular molecule in neurites can be indicated.[68,171,172] Only careful attention to the preservation of structure and detailed observations of cellular behavior will provide the most useful information about the activities of growth cones. As an example, stress fibers, the dense bundles of actin filaments in fibroblastic cells, do not occur in cultured neurons.[14] Thus, conclusions about the associations and roles of myosin, tropomyosin, or other cytoskeletal proteins in stress fibers do not necessarily hold for the growth cone.[58,173–176]

On the other hand, the growing nerve fiber offers a unique opportunity for study of eukaryotic cell locomotion. The nerve tip acts solely as a locomotory apparatus and is well separated from the diverse synthetic and other activities of the cell soma. Thus, examination of its cytoskeleton and behavior may reveal more clearly the structural basis and regulation of cell locomotion than the study of fibroblasts, macrophages, etc.

7.2. *Intrinsic Regulation of Neuronal Morphogenesis*

Environmental factors are a major influence on the directions of axonal growth, yet the formation of neurites by isolated neurons *in vitro* reveals that intrinsic activities are responsible for neurite formation. Do intrinsic factors determine the distinctive shapes of vertebrate pyramidal and Purkinje neurons or the regular morphologies of identified invertebrate nerve cells? Can an *in vitro* approach identify intrinsic features of axonal or dendritic growth, and reveal the cellular basis for internal regulation of cell shape?

Vertebrate neurons do not attain a single generalized shape *in vitro*. Morphological types seen *in vivo* can frequently be correlated with those seen in culture, although rigorous comparisons of *in vivo* and *in vitro* shapes have rarely been done.[7,73,177] Should characteristic morphologies emerge from a study, they might merely reflect the retention and regeneration in culture of the dendritic and axonal stumps of differentiated neurons. Cultures of appropriately immature neurons, plated at low cell density to isolate neurons from cell contact, may indicate that undifferentiated neurons generate characteristic morphological features free of environmental cues.

Advances in the culture of inverterate neurons offer an additional opportunity to examine the intrinsic regulation of neuronal shape. In these smaller systems many neurons are characteristically located and possess individual, characteristic axonal and dendritic patterns.[178–182] Identified neurons can be plucked from their ganglia and grown in culture, where they extend neurites and form synapses with other neurons.[183,184] *In vitro* morphologies and connectivity can be compared to those *in vivo*, providing hints about the roles of intrinsic and extrinsic factors in the elaboration of these two important neuronal properties, cell shape, and connectivity. It would be very exciting if young neurons or neuroblasts from invertebrate embryos could be cultured to look for rudimentary versions of their normal axonal and dendritic patterns[185] (see also Chapter 5). Neurons of known lineage and ontogenetic relationships might be cultured and their *in vitro* shapes compared for indication of inherited characteristics.

A direct influence on neuronal shape could be exerted by regulating the positions within perikarya of the golgi apparatus or cytoskeletal components, organelles that contribute to neurite structure. Asymmetrical cell shapes are commonly associated with asymmetric localizations of microtubules, and similar correlations may be involved in the generation of neuronlike shapes by neuroblastoma cells. After recovery from colcemid, a microtubule disruptor, small microtubule initiation sites form and then coalesce into a single large initiation site.[186] The position of this structure seems to determine the position of the first neurite formed, possibly by focusing the polymerization of microtubules from this site toward the plasma membrane. Another interesting finding is that daughter neuroblastoma cells frequently generate mirror image neuritic forms in the first hours after their mitotic separation.[187] Eventually, the mirror image resemblance of the sister cells is destroyed by disparate growth of the neurite tips, yet these data suggest that cytoplasmic asymmetries, perhaps based on cytoskeletal and adhesive organization, act as heritable epigenetic determinants of neuronal morphology.

These studies suggest that intracellular polarity determines the initiation points of axons, and the number and orientation of dendritic shapes.[188,189] As an axon or dendrite extends further from the perikaryon, environmental factors may exert their influence on neuronal morphogenesis. Yet the intrinsic organization of organelles, and microtubules in particular, may continue to influence neuronal shape at distal locations in a neurite. Each segment of nerve fiber has a cytoskelton of microtubules and neurofilaments; whenever a growth cone divides or a collateral branch is formed along a neurite, the existing cytoskeletal fibers must be subdivided or new fibers must be assembled. This requirement limits the potential for branching of neurites. For example, a neurite with only one microtubule cannot branch without assembly or provision of additional fibers. Because microtubules grow at their ends, the location of microtubular ends along a neurite may determine where collaterals sprout. In view of findings that axonal microtubules average 100 μm in length[50] and that many microtubules may be continuous from the perikaryon to the nerve tip (Letourneau, submitted for publication), it seems likely that microtubular termini are uncommon along young neurites. Thus collateral sprouts may be rare in early neurite growth, and branching will be restricted to the division of growth cones,[73] where the highest density of microtubular ends is found.

7.3. *Interactions of Neurites with Other Cells and in Vivo Surfaces*

What are the adhesive interactions that support neurite growth *in vivo* and how do these contacts regulate axonal pathways? My bias is that more can be learned from the observation of living cells than from fixed preparations. Unfortunately, the opacity of many tissues prohibits observation of living growth cones (there are a few exceptions[125]). However, tissue culture can be used to approximate substratal features of the environment *in vivo* and probe the affinities and interactions of growing neurites with other cells (see Chapter 9).

The stimulation of neurite growth on collagen-coated surfaces is well known,[119,190] though cultures of hydrated matrices of collagen may be a closer rendition of the connective tissues *in vivo*.[191] Within these optically clear matrices nerve tips do not flatten as on a PORN-treated surface; rather they resemble growth cones within tissues, being bulbous with filopodial protrusions. The matrices may be modified by incorporation of other extracellular materials, glycosaminoglycans, and fibronectin.[192,193] Of particular interest are molecules like the neurite-promoting component in chick HCM. Since this component acts when bound to PORN-treated plastic or cellular microexudates,[40,111,112] its effects on nerve fibers in a collagen matrix should be examined. For example, these materials may bind to collagen and modify the interaction of nerve tips with the matrix fibrils. One might find differences in growth cone morphology or protrusive activity that indicate differences in the interaction of nerve tips with the collagen fibrils and added components of the matrix. In addition, collagen matrices can be used to examine the responses of nerve tips to contacts with other neurites and nonneuronal cells in an environment which may resemble *in vivo* situations.[28,130]

The neurons and supportive cells of sensory and autonomic ganglia probably differentiate in the periphery where the neural crest cells aggregate into ganglionic masses.[194,195] Neurites are extended in distinct fascicles or along pathways of supportive cells.[131,196,197] Are there ganglion-specific adhesive affinities that guide cells of shared developmental history? Would a sympathetic fiber prefer to grow along another sympathetic fiber, or is a sensory neurite as good? Does a Schwann cell from a sensory nerve trunk follow a sympathetic axon as avidly as a sensory axon?

Data argue for and against any type of surface specificity in the interaction of peripheral neurons with nonneuronal cells. Sensory neurons initiate neurites just as frequently when sitting on heart fibroblasts as on sensory ganglionic nonneuronal cells.[190] Chick HCM stimulates neurite outgrowth by all chick peripheral neurons,[90,190,198] but on the other hand, mouse HCM stimulates outgrowth by mouse autonomic neurons but not sensory neurons.[199] In addition, ganglionic supportive cells associate with neurites and migrate along them, while fibroblastic cells in the same dishes do not recognize neurites.[130,200] Nonneuronal cells of sensory and sympathetic ganglia may have surface receptors for NGF.[201] Do the neurons and supportive cells of parasympathetic ganglia, which are unresponsive to NGF, have NGF receptors?

Neurons, supportive cells, and fibroblastic cells from peripheral ganglia can be separated into fairly homogeneous populations with plating techniques and use of mitotic poisons.[201–204] However, the ganglionic identity of these cells cannot be established by mere inspection. Specific markers, such as monoclonal antibodies, could allow ganglionic origin to be determined in mixed cultures. A simple answer may be to label the cells with a nontoxic, long-lasting dye, such as the fluorochromes recently used.[137] With these dyes cell suspensions or adherent cultures could be labeled and mixed with neurons or nonneuronal cells of different origin. Intercellular adhesion, cell migration and association, neurite elongation, and cell proliferation are phenomena that might be investigated in these cultures, where ganglionic identity can be determined by the color of cell label.

8. CONCLUSIONS

Axonal growth is driven by the motile activity of the nerve fiber tip or growth cone. This structure exhibits a constant extension and retraction of cytoplasmic processes which move about to sample soluble and surface features of the local environment. Some of these exploratory movements will result in the adhesion of a protrusion to another surface. Mechanical force is exerted on these contacts by actomyosin within the microfilaments of the protrusions, and if the adhesive bonds withstand the applied tension, then force is effectively transmitted intracellularly via cytoskeletal associations to pull on microtubules, neurofilaments, and membranous organelles that project into the growth cone. This action promotes neurite growth by sustaining the forward movement of neurite structures and by determining the positions of microtubular and neurofilament ends, which may be lengthened by terminal addition of subunits.

A key concept is that actomyosin acts locally to move neurite organelles within the growth cone; hence growth of the neurite is a local event. This is the foundation of extrinsic regulation of the morphogenesis of neurite pathways. Spatial variation in the adhesion of protrusions from the growth cone margin will produce asymmetry in the advance of neurite organelles. This may prompt division of one growth cone into several, each following adhesive pathways, or a growth cone may turn and elongate toward the more adhesive side.

Growth cones are also sensitive to concentration gradients of chemicals that may be chemoattractants. Sensory neurons extend neurites further up NGF gradients than down gradients over long periods, and within minutes growth cones turn toward an introduced NGF source. Cell surface receptors for NGF on growth cones and neurites are involved in the modulation of growth cone motility. As proposed for the regulation of neurite growth by adhesive interactions, local influences on growth cone motility, whether protrusion, adhesion, or force generation, underlie the chemotactic responses of nerve tips.

In an embryo, growth cones encounter axons, other growth cones, nonneuronal cells, and extracellular materials. Each of these interactions is a potential influence on the path of axonal growth, depending on the responses of growth cones to the shapes of available surfaces and the adhesive bonds which form. Positional information to direct axonal growth may be expressed as topographic differences in the adhesive affinities between growth cones and their substrata within a field of cells. Target tissues may release chemicals which attract appropriately sensitive axons. These chemotactic responses may act in concert with the influences of surface features to direct axons toward their target tissues. At the time of axon and dendrite formation, asymmetries established in the intracellular organization of neuritic structures may determine initial neuronal shape, but as neurites extend further from the perikaryon, environmental features determine the paths taken.

ACKNOWLEDGMENTS

The author thanks Dr. Stanley Kater for helpful comments on the manuscript. The technical assistance of Alice Ressler, photographic work of Walter Gutzmer, and secretarial skills of Roberta Andrich were valuable contributions. This work was supported by the National Science Foundation, Minnesota Medical Foundation, the Graduate School of the University of Minnesota, and an Institutional Grant from the American Cancer Society to the University of Minnesota.

9. REFERENCES

1. Constantine-Paton, M., 1979. Axonal navigation, *Biosci.* **29**:526.
2. Katz, M. J., and Lasek, R. J., 1980, Guidance cue patterns and cell migration in multicellular organisms, *Cell Motil.* **1**:141.
3. Landmesser, L. T., 1980, The generation of neuromuscular specificity, *Ann. Rev. Neurosci.* **3**:279.
4. Sidman, R. L., and Wessells, N. K., 1975, Control of direction of growth during the elongation of neurites, *Exp. Neurol.* **48**:237.
5. Ramón y Cajal, S., 1980, Sur l'origine et les ramifications des fibres nerveuses de la moelle embryonaire, *Anat. Anz.* **5**:609, 631.
6. Bray, D., 1982, Filopodial contraction and growth cone guidance, in: *Cell Behaviors* (G. Dunn, Contis, and Bellairs, eds.), Cambridge University Press, Cambridge.
7. Johnston, R., and Wessells, N. K., 1980, Regulation of the elongating nerve fiber, *Curr. Top. Dev. Biol.* **16**:165.
8. Wessells, N. K., 1982, in: *Cell Behaviors* (G. Dunn, Contis, and Bellairs, eds.), Cambridge University Press, Cambridge.
9. Harrison, R. G., 1907, Observations on the living developing nerve fiber, *Anat. Rec.* **1**:116.

10. Harrison, R. G., 1910, The growth of the nerve fiber as a mode of protoplasmic movement, *J. Exp. Zool.* **9:**787.
11. Costero, I., and Pomerat, C. M., 1951, Cultivation of neurons from adult cerebral and cerebellar cortex, *Am. J. Anat.* **89:**405.
12. Godina, G., 1963, The morphological and structural features of neurons *in vitro* studied by phase contrast and time-lapse movies, in *Cinemicrography in Cell Biology* (G. G. Rose, ed.), pp. 313–338, Academic Press, New York.
13. Hughes, A., 1953, The growth of embryonic neurites, *J. Anat.* **87:**150.
14. Luduena, M. A., and Wessells, N. K., 1973, Cell locomotion, nerve elongation, and microfilaments, *Dev. Biol.* **30:**427.
15. Pomerat, C. M., Hendelman, W. J., Raiborn, C. W. and Massey, J. F., 1967, Dynamic activities of nervous tissue *in vitro,* in: *The Neuron* (H. Hyden, ed.), pp. 119–178, Elsevier, Amsterdam.
16. Bray, D., 1970, Surface movements during the growth of single explanted neurons, *Proc. Natl. Acad. Sci. U.S.A.* **65:**905.
17. Bray, D., and Bunge, M. B., 1973, The growth cone in neurite extension, in *Locomotion of Tissue Cells,* Ciba Foundation Symposium 14 (new series), pp. 195–209, Associated Scientific Publishers, Amsterdam.
18. Carbonetto, S., and Argon, Y., 1980, Lectins induce the redistribution and internalization of receptors on the surface of cultured neurons, *Dev. Biol.* **80:**364.
19. Letourneau, P. C., 1979, Inhibition of intercellular adhesion by canavalin A in association with conA-induced redistribution of surface receptors, *J. Cell Biol.* **80:**128.
20. Pfenninger, K. H., and Maylie-Pfenninger, M. F., 1978, Characterization, distribution, and appearance of surface carbohydrates on growing neurites, in: *Neuronal Information Transfer* (A. Karlin, V. M. Tennyson, and H. J. Vogel, eds.), pp. 373–386, Academic Press, New York.
21. Campenot, R. B., 1977, Local control of neurite development by nerve growth factor, *Proc. Natl. Acad. Sci. U.S.A.* **74:**4516.
22. Harper, G. P. and Thoenen, H., 1980, Nerve growth factor: Biological significance, measurement, and distribution, *J. Neurochem.* **34:**5.
23. Stoeckel, K., Schwab, M., and Thoenen, H., 1975, Specificity of retrograde transport of nerve growth factor (NGF) in sensory neurons: A biochemical and morphological study, *Brain Res.* **89:**1.
24. Weiss, P., 1934, *In vitro* experiments on the factors determining the course of the outgrowing nerve fiber, *J. Exp. Zool.* **68:**393.
25. Weiss, P., 1941, Nerve patterns: The mechanics of nerve growth, *Growth* (*Third Growth Symp. Suppl.*) **5:**163.
26. Weiss, P., 1961, Guiding principles in cell locomotion and cell aggregation, *Exp. Cell Res. Suppl.* **8:**260.
27. Harrison, R. G., 1914, The reaction of embryonic cells to solid structure, *J. Exp. Zool.* **7:**521.
28. Nakai, J., 1960, Studies on the mechanism determining the course of nerve fibers in tissue culture. II. The mechanism of fasciculation. *Z. Zellforsch. Mikrosk. Anat.* **52:**427.
29. Dunn, G. A., 1971, Mutual contact inhibition of extension of chick sensory nerve fibers *in vitro, J. Comp. Neurol.* **143:**491.
30. Nakai, J., and Kawasaki, Y., 1959, Studies on the mechanism determining the course of nerve fibers in tissue culture. I. The reactions of the growth cone to various obstructions. *Z. Zellforsch. Mikrosk. Anat.* **51:**108.

31. Nakajima, S., 1965, Selectivity in fasciculation of nerve fibers *in vitro*, *J. Comp. Neurol.* **125:**193.
32. Abercrombie, M., Dunn, G. A., and Heath, J. P., 1977, The shape and movement of fibroblasts in culture, in: *Cell and Tissue Interactions* (J. W. Lash and M. M. Burger, eds.), pp. 57–70, Raven Press, New York.
33. Harris, A., 1973, Location of cellular adhesions to solid substrata, *Dev. Biol.* **35:**83.
34. Huxley, H. E., 1973, Muscular contraction and cell motility, *Nature* (*London*) **243:**445.
35. Hynes, R. O., and Destree, A. T., 1978, Relationships between fibronectin (LETS protein) and actin, *Cell* **15:**875.
36. Gail, M. H., and Boone, C. W., 1972, Cell-substrate adhesivity, *Exp. Cell. Res.* **70:**33.
37. Letourneau, P. C., and Wessells, N. K., 1974, Migratory cell locomotion versus nerve axon elongation. Differences based on the effects of Lanthanum ion, *J. Cell Biol.* **61:**56.
38. Strassman, R. J., Letourneau, P. C., and Wessells, N. K., 1973, Elongation of axons in an agar matrix that does not support cell locomotion, *Exp. Cell Res.* **81:**482.
39. Letourneau, P. C., 1975, Possible roles for cell-to-substratum adhesion in neuronal morphogenesis, *Dev. Biol.* **44:**77.
40. Collins, F., 1978, Induction of neurite outgrowth by a conditioned-medium factor bound to the culture substratum, *Proc. Natl. Acad. Sci. U.S.A.* **75:**5210.
41. Collins, F., and Garrett, J. E., 1980, Elongating nerve fibers are guided by a pathway material released by embryonic non-neuronal cells, *Proc. Natl. Acad. Sci. U.S.A.* **77:**6226.
42. Grinnell, F., 1978, Cellular adhesiveness and extracellular substrata, *Int. Rev. Cytol.* **29:**65.
43. Grinnell, F., and Minter, D., 1978, Attachment and spreading of baby hamster kidney cells to collagen substrata. Effects on cold-insoluble globulin, *Proc. Natl. Acad. Sci. U.S.A.* **75:**4408.
44. Luduena, M. A., 1973, The growth of spinal ganglion neurons in serum-free medium, *Dev. Biol.* **33:**470.
45. Izzard, C. S., and Lochner, L. R., 1976, Cell-to-substrate contacts in living fibroblasts: An interference reflexion study with an evaluation of the technique, *J. Cell. Sci.* **21:**129.
46. Letourneau, P., 1979, Cell-substratum adhesion of neurite growth cones and its role in neurite elongation, *Exp. Cell. Res.* **124:**127.
47. Palay, S. L., and Chan-Palay, V., 1977, General morphology of neurons and neuroglia, in: *Handbook of Physiology I: The Nervous System* (E. R., Kandel, ed.), pp. 5–37, Waverly Press, Baltimore, MD.
48. Tennyson, V. M., 1970, The fine structure of the axon and growth cone of the dorsal root neuroblast of the rabbit embryo, *J. Cell Biol.* **44:**62.
49. Yamada, K. M., Spooner, B. S., and Wessells, N. K., 1971, Ultrastructure and function of growth cones and axons of cultured nerve cells, *J. Cell. Biol.* **49:**614.
50. Bray, D., and Bunge, M. B., 1981, Serial analysis of microtubules in cultured rat sensory axons, *J. Neurocytol.* (in press).
51. Daniels, M., 1975, Role of microtubules in growth and stabilization of nerve fibers, *Ann. N.Y. Acad. Sci.* **253:**535.
52. Lasek, R. J., and Hoffman, P. N., 1976, The neuronal cytoskeleton, axonal transport and axonal growth, in: *Cell Motility* (R. Goldman, T. Pollard, and J. Rosenbaum, eds.), pp. 1021–1049, Cold Spring Harbor Laboratory, Cold Spring Harbor, NY.
53. Lazarides, E., 1980, Intermediate filaments as mechanical integrators of cellular space, *Nature* (*London*) **283:**249.

54. Daniels, M. P., 1973, Fine structural changes in neurons and nerve fibers associated with colchicine inhibition of nerve fiber formation *in vitro*, *J. Cell Biol.* **58:**463.
55. Heuser, J. E., and Kirschner, M. W., 1980, Filament organization revealed in platinum replicas of freeze-dried cytoskeletons, *J. Cell Biol.* **86:**212.
56. Spooner, B. S., Yamada, K. M., and Wessells, N. K., 1971, Microfilaments and cell locomotion, *J. Cell Biol.* **49:**593.
57. Ellisman, M. H., and Porter, K. R., 1980, Microtrabecular structure of the axoplasmic matrix; visualization of cross-linking structures and their distribution, *J. Cell Biol.* **87:**464.
58. Bray, D., and Gilbert, D., 1980, Cytoskeletal elements in neurons, *Ann. Rev. Neurosci.* **4:**505.
59. Chang, C.-M., and Goldman, R. D., 1973, The localization of actin-like fibers in cultured neuroblastoma cells as revealed by heavy meromyosin binding, *J. Cell Biol.* **57:**867.
60. Bray, D., Thomas, C., and Shaw, G., 1978, Growth cone formation in cultures of sensory neurons, *Proc. Natl. Acad. Sci. U.S.A.* **75:**5226.
61. Fernandez, H. L., and Samson, F. E., 1973, Axoplasmic transport: Differential inhibition by cytochalasin-B, *J. Neurobiol.* **4:**201.
62. Ochs, S., and Worth, R. M., 1978, Axoplasmic transport in normal and pathological systems, in: *Physiology and Pathobiology of Axons* (S. G. Waxman, ed.), pp. 251–264, Raven Press, New York.
63. Bunge, M. B., 1973, Fine structure of nerve fibers and growth cones of isolated sympathetic neurons in culure, *J. Cell Biol.* **56:**713.
64. Bunge, M. B., 1977, Initial endocytosis of peroxidase or ferritin by growth cones of cultured nerve cells, *J. Neurocytol.* **6:**407.
65. Droz, B., Rambourg, A., and Koenig, H. L., 1975, The smooth endoplasmic reticulum: Structure and role in the renewal of axonal membrane and synaptic vesicles by fast axonal transport, *Brain Res.* **93:**1.
66. Wessells, N. K., Luduena, M. A., Letourneau, P. C., Wrenn, J. T., and Spooner, B. S., 1974, Thorotrast uptake and transit in embryonic glia, heart fibroblasts and neurons *in vitro*, *Tissue Cell* **6:**757.
67. Bray, D., 1973, Model for membrane movements in the neural growth cone, *Nature* (*London*) **244:**93.
68. Kuczmarski, E. R., and Rosenbaum, J. L., 1979, Studies on the organization and localization of actin and myosin in neurons, *J. Cell Biol.* **80:**356.
69. Nuttall, R. P., and Wessells, N. K., 1979, Veils, mounds, and vesicle aggregates in neurons elongating *in vitro*. *Exp. Cell Res.* **119:**163.
70. Letourneau, P. C., 1981, Immunocytochemical evidence for colocalization in neurite growth cones of actin and myosin and their relationship to cell-substratum adhesions, *Dev. Biol.* **85:**113.
71. Shaw, G., and Bray, D., 1977, Movement and extension of isolated growth cones, *Exp. Cell Res.* **104:**55.
72. Wessells, N. K., Johnson, S. R., and Nuttall, R. P., 1978, Axon initiation and growth cone regeneration in cultured motor neurons, *Exp. Cell Res.* **117:**335.
73. Bray, D., 1973, Branching patterns of individual sympathetic neurons in culture, *J. Cell Biol.* **56:**702.
74. Teichberg, S., and Holtzman, E., 1973, Axonal agranular reticulum and synaptic vesicles in cultured embryonic chick sympathetic neurons, *J. Cell Biol.* **57:**88.
75. Birks, R. I., Mackey, M. C. and Weldon, P. R. 1972, Organelle formation from

pinocytotic elements in neurites of cultured sympathetic ganglion. *J. Neurocytol.* **1:**311.
76. Rothman, J. E., and Lenard, J., 1977, Membrane asymmetry, *Science* **195:**743.
77. Kirschner, M., 1980, Implications of treadmilling for the stability and polarity of actin and tubulin polymers *in vivo, J. Cell Biol.* **86:**330.
78. Margolis, R. L., and Wilson, L., 1978, Opposite end assembly and disassembly of microtubules at steady state *in vitro, Cell* **13:**1.
79. Black, M. M., and Lasek, R. J., 1980, Slow components of axonal transport: Two cytoskeletal networks, *J. Cell Biol.* **86:**616.
80. Hoffman, P. N., and Lasek, R. J., 1975, The slow component of axonal transport. Identification of major structural polypeptides of the axon and their generality among mammalian neurons, *J. Cell Biol.* **66:**351.
81. Willard, M., Wiseman, M., Levine, J., and Skene, P., 1979, Axonal transport of actin in rabbit retinal ganglion cells, *J. Cell Biol.* **81:**581.
82. Carbonetto, S., and Fambrough, D. M., 1979, Synthesis, insertion into the plasma membrane and turnover of α-bungarotoxin receptors in chick sympathetic neurons, *J. Cell Biol.* **81:**555.
83. Begg, D. A., Rodewald, R., and Rebhum, L. I., 1979, The visualization of actin filament polarity in thin sections, *J. Cell Biol.* **79:**846.
84. Mooseker, M. S., 1976, Actin filament-membrane attachment in the microvilli of intestinal epithelial cell, in: *Cell Motility,* (R. Goldman, T. Pollard, and J. Rosenbaum, eds.), pp. 631–650, Cold Spring Harbor Laboratory, Cold Spring Harbor, NY.
85. Small, J. V., Isenberg, G., and Celis, J. E., 1978, Polarity of actin at the leading edge of cultured cells, *Nature (London)* **272:**638.
86. Herman, I. M., and Pollard, T. D., 1981, Electron microscopic localization of cytoplasmic myosin with ferritin-labelled antibodies, *J. Cell Biol.* **88:**346.
87. Shizuta, Y., Davies, P., Olden, K., and Pastan, I., 1976, Diminished content of plasma membrane-associated myosin in transformed cells, *Nature (London)* **261:**414.
88. Mooseker, M. S., Pollard, T. D., and Fujiwara, K., 1978, Characterization and localization of myosin in the brush border of intestinal epithelial cells, *J. Cell Biol.* **79:**444.
89. Arora, H. L. and Sperry, R. W., 1962, Optic nerve fiber regeneration after surgical cross-union of medial and lateral optic tracts, *Am. Zool.* **2:**61.
90. Attardi, D. G., and Sperry, R. W., 1963, Preferential selection of central pathways by regenerating optic fibers, *Exp. Neurol.* **7:**46.
91. Lance-Jones, C., and Landmesser, L. T., 1978, Effect of spinal cord deletions and reversals on motorneuron projection patterns in the embryonic chick hindlimb, *Soc. Neurosci.* **4:**118.
92. Lance-Jones, C., and Landmesser, L. T., 1979, Pathway selection by embryonic chick lumbrosacral motorneurons, *Soc. Neurosci.* **5:**Abst.
93. Constantine-Paton, M., and Capranica, R. P., 1975, Central projection of optic tract from translocated eyes in the leopard frog (*Rana pipiens*), *Science* **189:**480.
94. Katz, M. J., and Lasek, R. J., 1979, Substrate pathways which guide growing axons in *Xenopus* embryos, *J. Comp. Neurol.* **183:**817.
95. Collins, F., 1978, Axon initiation by ciliary neurons in culture, *Dev. Biol.* **65:**50.
96. Helfand, S. L., Smith, G. A., and Wessells, N. K., 1976, Survival and development in culture of dissociated parasympathetic neurons from ciliary ganglia, *Dev. Biol.* **50:**541.
97. Letourneau, P. C., 1975, Cell-to-substratum adhesion and guidance of axonal elongation, *Dev. Biol.* **44:**92.

98. Bray, D., 1979, Mechanical tension produced by nerve cells in tissue culture, *J. Cell Sci.* **37**:391.
99. Wessells, N. K., and Nuttall, R. P., 1978, Normal branching, induced branching, and steering of cultured parasympathetic motor neurons, *Exp. Cell Res.* **115**:111.
100. Jacobson, M., 1978, *Developmental Neurobiology,* Plenum Press, New York.
101. Ash, J. F., Louvard, D., and Singer, S. J., 1977, Antibody-induced linkages of plasma membrane proteins to intracellular actomyosin-containing filaments in cultured fibroblasts, *Proc. Natl. Acad. U.S.A.* **74**:5584.
102. Condeelis, J., 1979, Isolation of Concanavalin A caps during various stages of formation and their association with actin and myosin, *J. Cell Biol.* **80**:751.
103. Toh, B. H. and Hard, G. C., 1977, Actin co-caps with concanavalin A receptors, *Nature (London)* **269**:695.
104. Sperry, R. W., 1963, Chemoaffinity in the orderly growth of nerve fiber patterns and connections, *Proc. Natl. Acad. Sci. U.S.A.* **50**:703.
105. Fraser, S. E., and Hunt, R. K., 1980, Retinotectal specificity, *Ann. Rev. Neurosci.* **3**:319.
106. Gaze, R. M., and Keating, M. J., 1972, The visual system and neuronal specificity, *Nature (London)* **237**:375.
107. Hunt, R. K., and Jacobson, M., 1972, Development and stability of positional information in *Xenopus* retinal ganglion cells, *Proc. Natl. Acad. Sci. U.S.A.* **69**:780.
108. Barbera, A., 1975, Adhesive recognition between developing retinal cells and the optic tecta of the chick embryo, *Dev. Biol.* **46**:167.
109. Gottlieb, D. I., Rock, K., and Glaser, L., 1976, A gradient of adhesive specificity in developing avian retina, *Proc. Natl. Acad. Sci. U.S.A.* **73**:410.
110. Marchase, R. B., 1977, Biochemical investigations of retino-tectal adhesive specificity, *J. Cell Biol.* **75**:237.
111. Collins, F., 1980, Neurite outgrowth induced by substrate-associated material from nonneuronal cells, *Dev. Biol.* **79**:247.
112. Hawrot, E., 1980, Cultured sympathetic neurons: Effects of cell-derived and synthetic substrata on survival and development, *Dev. Biol.* **74**:136.
113. Adler, R., and Varon, S., 1981, Neurite guidance by polyornithine-attached materials of ganglionic origin, *Dev. Biol.* **81**:1.
114. Chen, L. B., Murray, A., Segal, R. A., Bushnell, A., and Walsh, M. L., 1978, Studies on intercellular LETS glycoprotein matrices, *Cell* **14**:377.
115. Linder, E., Vaheri, A., Ruoslahti, E., and Wartiovaara, J., 1975, Distribution of fibroblasts surface antigen in the developing chick embryo, *J. Exp. Med.* **142**:41.
116. Yamada, K. M., Olden, K., and Hahn, L. H. E., 1980, Cell surface protein and cell interactions, *Soc. Dev. Biol. Symp.* **38**:43.
117. Dunn, G. A., and Heath, J. P., 1976, A new hypothesis of contact guidance in tissue cells, *Exp. Cell Res.* **101**:1.
118. Dunn, G. A. and Ebendal, T., 1978, Some aspects of contact guidance, *Zoon Suppl.* **6**:65.
119. Ebendal, T., 1976, The relative roles of contact inhibition and contact guidance in orientation of axons extending on aligned collagen fibrils *in vitro, Exp. Cell Res.* **98**:159.
120. Hinds, J. W., and Hinds, P. L., 1972, Reconstruction of dendritic growth cones in neonatal mouse olfactory bulb, *J. Neurocytol.* **1**:169.
121. Meinertzhagen, I. A., 1973, Development of the compound eye and optic lobe of insects in *Developmental Neurobiology of Arthropods* (D. Young, ed.), pp. 51–104, Cambridge, University Press, Cambridge.

122. Muller, K. J., and Scott, S. A., 1980, Removal of the synaptic target permits terminal sprouting of a mature intact axon, *Nature* (*London*) **283:**89.
123. Murphy, A. D., and Kater, S. B., 1980, Sprouting and functional regeneration of an identified neuron in *Helisoma*, *Brain Res.* **186:**251.
124. Skoff, R. P., and Hamburger, V., 1974, Fine structure of dendritic and axonal growth cones in embryonic chick spinal cord, *J. Comp. Neurol.* **153:**107.
125. Speidel, C. C., 1933, Studies of living nerves. II. Activities of ameboid growth cones, sheath cells, and myelin segments, as revealed by prolonged observation of individual nerve fibers in frog tadpoles, *J. Anat.* **52:**1.
126. Vaughn, J. E., Hendrikson, C. K., and Grieshaber, J. A., 1974, A quantitative study of synapses on motor neuron dendritic growth cones in developing mouse spinal cord, *J. Cell Biol.* **60:**664.
127. Anderson, H., Edwards, J. S., and Palka, J., 1980, Developmental neurobiology of invertebrates, *Ann. Rev. Neurosci.* **3:**97.
128. Nordlander, R. H., and Singer, M., 1978, The role of ependyma in regeneration of the spinal cord in the urodele amphibian tail, *J. Comp. Neuronal.* **180:**349.
129. Suburo, A., Carri, N., and Adler, R., 1979, Environment of axonal migration in the developing chick retina—A scanning electron-microscopic study, *J. Comp. Neurol.* **184:**519.
130. Wessells, N. K., Letourneau, P. C., Nuttall, R. P., Luduena-Anderson, M., and Geiduschek, J. M., 1980, Responses to cell contacts between growth cones, neurites and ganglionic non-neuronal cells, *J. Neurocytol.* **9:**647.
131. Bray, D., Wood, P., and Bunge, R. P., 1980, Selective fasciculation of nerve fibers in culture, *Exp. Cell Res.* **130:**241.
132. Rusoff, A. C., and Easter, S. S., 1979, Order in the optic nerve, *Science* **208:**31.
133. Letourneau, J. G., 1976, Somatotopic organization of afferent axons in peripheral nerves, *J. Comp. Physiol.* **110:**25.
134. Rutishauser, U., and Edelman, G. M., 1980, Effect of fasciculation on the outgrowth of neurites from spinal ganglia in culture, *J. Cell Biol.* **87:**370.
135. Rutishauser, U., Gall, W. E., and Edelman, G. M., 1978, Adhesion among neural cells of the chick embryo. IV. Role of the cell surface molecule CAM in the formation of neurite bundles in cultures of spinal ganglia, *J. Cell Biol.* **79:**382.
136. Fraser, S. E., 1980, A differential adhesion approach to the patterning of nerve connections, *Dev. Biol.* **79:**453.
137. Bonhoeffer, F., and Huf, J., 1980, Recognition of cell types by axonal growth cones *in vitro, Nature* (*London*) **288:**162.
138. Postlethwaite, A. E., Seyer, J. M., and Kang, A. H., 1978, Chemotactic attraction of human fibroblasts of type I, II, and III collagens and collagen-derived peptides, *Proc. Natl. Acad. Sci. U.S.A.* **75:**871.
139. Ramsey, W. S., 1972, Analysis of individual leukocyte behavior during chemotaxis, *Exp. Cell Res.* **70:**129.
140. Zigmond, S. H., 1978, Chemotaxis by polymorphonuclear leukocytes, *J. Cell Biol.* **77:**269.
141. Ramón y Cajal, S., 1928, *Degeneration and Regeneration of the Nervous System*, (R. M. May, trans.), Hafner, New York, 1959.
142. Weiss, P., and Taylor, A. C., 1944, Further experimental evidence against "neurotropism" in nerve regeneration, *J. Exp. Zool.* **95:**233.
143. Chamley, J. H., Goller, I., and Burnstock, G., 1973, Selective growth of sympathetic nerve fibers to explants of normally densely innervated autonomic effector organs in tissue culture, *Dev. Biol.* **31:**362.

144. Coughlin, M. D., 1975, Target organ stimulation of parasympathetic nerve growth in the developing mouse submandibular gland, *Dev. Biol.* **43:**140.
145. Ebendal, T., and Jacobson, D. O., 1977, Tissue explants affecting extension and orientation of axons in cultured chick embryo ganglia, *Exp. Cell Res.* **105:**379.
146. Charlwood, K. A., Lamont, D. M. and Banks, B. E. C., 1972, Apparent orienting effects produced by nerve growth factor, in: *Nerve Growth Factor and Its Antiserum* (E. Zaimis and J. Knight), pp. 102–107, Athlone Press, University of London, London.
147. Levi-Montalcini, R., 1976, The nerve growth factor: Its role in growth, differentiation and function of the sympathetic axon, in: *Perspectives in Brain Research, Progress in Brain Research,* vol. 45 (M. A. Corner and D. F. Swaab, eds.), pp. 235–258. Elsevier/North Holland Biomedical Press, Amsterdam.
148. Letourneau, P., 1978, Chemotactic response of nerve fiber elongation to nerve growth factor, *Dev. Biol.* **66:**183.
149. Gunderson, R. W., and Barrett, J. N., 1979, Neuronal chemotaxis: Chick dorsal root axons turn forward high concentration of nerve growth factor, *Science* **206:**1079.
150. Gunderson, R. W., and Barrett, J. N. 1980, Characterization of the turning response of dorsal root neurites toward nerve growth factor, *J. Cell Biol.* **87:**546.
151. McNab, R. M., and Koshland, D. E., 1972, Gradient-sensing mechanism in bacterial chemotaxis, *Proc. Natl. Acad. Sci. U.S.A.* **69:**2509.
152. Zigmond, S. H., and Sullivan, S. J., 1979, Sensory adaptation of leukocytes to chemotactic peptides, *J. Cell Biol.* **82:**517.
153. Griffin, C. G., and Letourneau, P. C., 1980, Rapid retraction of neurites by sensory neurons in response to increased concentrations of nerve growth factor, *J. Cell Biol.* **86:**156.
154. Adler, J., 1976, Chemotaxis in bacteria, *J. Supramol. Struct.* **4:**305.
155. Schubert, D., LaCorbiere, M., Whitlock, C., and Stallcup, W., 1978, Alterations in the surface properties of cells responsive to nerve growth factor, *Nature* (*London*) **273:**718.
156. Crick, F., 1970, Diffusion in embryogenesis, *Nature* (*London*) **225:**420.
157. Jaffe, L. F., and Poo, M. M., 1979, Neurites grow faster towards the cathode than the anode in a steady field, *J. Exp. Zool.* **209:**115.
158. Jaffe, L., 1977, Electrophoresis along cell membranes, *Nature* (*London*) **265:**600.
159. Fields, K. L., 1979, Cell type-specific antigens of cells of the central and peripheral nervous system, *Curr. Top. Devel. Biol.* **13:**237.
160. Fields, K. L., Brockes, J. P., Mirsky, R., and Wendon, L. M. B., 1978, Cell surface markers for distinguishing different types of rat dorsal root ganglion cells in culture, *Cell* **14:**43.
161. Gottlieb, D. I., and Glaser, L., 1980, Cellular recognition during neural development, *Ann. Rev. Neurosci.* **3:**303.
162. Schachner, M., 1979, Cell surface antigens of the nervous system, *Curr. Top. Dev. Biol.* **13:**259.
163. Soltor, D., and Schachner, M., 1976, Brain and sperm cell surface antigen (NS-4) on preimplantation mouse embryos, *Dev. Biol.* **52:**98.
164. Geiger, B., 1979, A 130K protein from chicken gizzards. Its localization at the termini of microfilament bundles in cultured chicken cells, *Cell* **18:**193.
165. Geiger, B., Tokuyasu, K. T., and Singer, S. J., 1979, Immunocytochemical localization of α-actinin in intestinal epithelial cells, *Proc. Natl. Acad. Sci. U.S.A.* **76:**2833.
166. Stossel, T. P., and Hartwig, J. H., 1976, Interaction of actin, myosin, and a new actin-binding protein of rabbit pulmonary macrophages, *J. Cell Biol.* **68:**602.

167. Uyemura, D. G. and Spudich, J. A., 1980, Biochemistry and regulation of nonmuscle actins, in: *Biological Regulation and Development,* vol. 2, (R. Goldberger, ed.), pp. 315–338, Plenum Press, New York.
168. Wang, K., and Singer, S. J., 1977, Interaction of filamin with F-actin in solution, *Proc. Natl. Acad. Sci., U.S.A.* **74:**2021.
169. Begg, D. A. and Rehbun, L. I., 1979, pH regulates the polymerization of actin in the sea-urchin egg cortex, *J. Cell Biol.* **83:**241.
170. Pardee, J. D., and Spudich, J. A., 1980, Mechanism of K^+-induced actin assembly, *J. Cell Biol.* **87:**226*a*.
171. Marchisio, P. C., Osborn, M., and Weber, K., 1978, Changes in intracellular organization of tubulin and actin in N-18 neuroblastoma cells during the process of axon extension induced by serum deprivation, *Brain Res.* **155:**229.
172. Roisen, F., Inczedy-Marcsek, M., Hsu, L. and Yorke, W., 1978, Myosin: Immunofluorescent localization in neuronal and glial cultures, *Science* **199:**1445.
173. Heggeness, M. H., Wang, K., and Singer, S. J., 1977, Intracellular distributions of mechanochemical proteins in cultured fibroblasts, *Proc. Natl. Acad. Sci. U.S.A.* **74:**3883.
174. Lazarides, E., 1975, Tropomyosin antibody: The specific localization of tropomyosin in nonmuscle cells, *J. Cell Biol.* **65:**549.
175. Lazarides, E., 1971, Two general classes of cytoplasmic actin filaments in tissue culture cells: The role of tropomyosin, *J. Supramol. Struct.* **5:**531.
176. Zigmond, S. H., Otto, J. J., and Bryan, J., 1979, Organization of myosin in a submembranous sheath in well-spread human fibroblasts, Exp. Cell Res. **119:**205.
177. Banker, G. A., and Cowan, W. M., 1978, Further observations on hippocampal neurons in dispersed cell culture, *J. Comp. Neurol.* **187:**469.
178. Goodman, C. S., 1974, Anatomy of locust ocellar interneurons: Constancy and variability, *J. Comp. Physiol.* **95:**185.
179. Goodman, C. S., 1978, Isogenic grasshoppers: Genetic variability in the morphology of identified neurons, *J. Comp. Neurol.* **182:**681.
180. Macagno, E. R., 1980, Genetic approaches to invertebrate neurogenesis, *Curr. Top. Dev. Biol.* **15:**319.
181. Pitman, R. M., Tweedle, C. D., and Cohen, M. J., 1973, The form of nerve cells: Determination by cobalt impregnation, in: *Intracellular Staining in Neurobiology* (S. B. Kater and C. Nicholson, eds.), pp. 83–98, Springer-Verlag, New York.
182. Stretton, A. O. W., and Kravitz, E. A., 1973 Intracellular dye injection: The selection of procion yellow and its application in preliminary studies of neuronal geometry in the lobster nervous system, in: *Intracellular Staining in Neurobiology* (S. B. Kater and C. Nicholson, eds.), pp. 21–40, Springer-Verlag, New York.
183. Ready, D. F., and Nicholls, J., 1979, Identified neurons isolated from leech CNS make selective connections in culture, *Nature (London)* **281:**67.
184. Wong, R. G., Hadley, R. D., Kater, S. B., and Hauser, G. C., 1981, Neurite outgrowth in molluscan organ and cell cultures: The role of conditioning factor(s), *J. Neurosci.*, in press.
185. Goodman, C. S., Pearson, K. G., and Spitzer, N. C., 1980, Electrical excitability: A spectrum of properties in the progeny of a single embryonic neuroblast, *Proc. Natl. Acad. Sci. U.S.A.* **77:**1676.
186. Spiegelman, B. M., Lopata, M. A., and Kirschner, M. W., 1979, Aggregation of microtubule initiation sites preceding neurite outgrowth in mouse neuroblastoma cells, *Cell* **16:**253.

187. Solomon, F., 1979, Detailed neurite morphologies of sister neuroblastoma cells are related, *Cell* **15:**165.
188. Hibbard, E., 1965, Orientation and directed growth of Mauthner's cell axons from duplicated vestibular nerve roots, *Exp. Neurol.* **13:**289.
189. Van der Loos, H., 1965, The "improperly" oriented pyramidal cell in the cerebral cortex and its possible bearing on problems of growth and cell orientation, *Bull. Johns Hopkins Hosp.* **117:**228.
190. Luduena, M. A., 1973, Nerve cell differentiation *in vitro, Dev. Biol.* **33:**268.
191. Elsdale, T., and Bard, J., 1972, Collagen substrata for studies in cell behavior, *J. Cell Biol.* **54:**626.
192. Derby, M. A., 1978, Analysis of glycosaminoglycans within the extracellular environments encountered by migrating neural crest cells, *Dev. Biol.* **66:**321.
193. Polansky, J. R., Toole, B. P., and Gross, J., 1974, Brain hyaluronidase: Changes in activity during chick development, *Science* **193:**862.
194. LeDouarin, N., 1980, The ontogeny of the neural crest in avian embryo chimaeras, *Nature (London)* **286:**663.
195. Nichols, D. H., Kaplan, R. A., and Weston, J. A., 1977, Melanogenesis in cultures of peripheral nerve tissue. II. Environmental factors determining the fate of pigment-forming cells, *Dev. Biol.* **60:**226.
196. Hill, C. E., Chamley, J. H., and Burnstock, G., 1974, Cell surfaces and fiber relationships in sympathetic ganglion cultures: A scanning electron-microscopic study, *J. Cell Sci.* **14:**657.
197. Kalderon, N., 1979, Migration of Schwann cells and wrapping of neurites *in vitro*: A function of protease activity (plasmin) in the growth medium, *Proc. Natl. Acad. Sci. U.S.A.* **76:**5992.
198. Helfand, S. L., Riopelle, R. J., and Wessells, N. K., 1978, Non-equivalence of conditioned medium and nerve growth factor for sympathetic, parasympathetic, and sensory neurons, *Exp. Cell Res.* **113:**39.
199. Couglin, M. D., Bloom, E. M., and Black, I. B., 1981, Characterization of a neuronal growth factor from mouse heart-cell conditioned medium, *Dev. Biol.* **82:**56.
200. Wood, P. M., 1976, Separation of functional Schwann cells and neurons from normal peripheral nerve tissue, *Brain Res.* **115:**361.
201. Sutter, A., Riopelle, R. J., Harris-Warrick, R. M., and Shooter, E. M., 1979, Nerve growth factor receptors, *J. Biol. Chem.* **254:**5972.
202. Dvorak, D. J., Gipps, E., and Kidson, C., 1978, Isolation of specific neurons by affinity methods, *Nature (London)* **271:**564.
203. Okun, L. M., Ontkean, F. K., and Thomas, C. A., 1972, Removal of non-neuronal cells from suspensions of dissociated embryonic dorsal root ganglia, *Exp. Cell Res.* **73:**226.
204. Sotelo, S., Gibbs, C. J., Gajdusek, D. G., Toh, B. H., and Wurth, M., 1980, Method for preparing cultures of central neurons: Cytochemical and immunochemical studies, *Proc. Natl. Acad. Sci. U.S.A.* **77:**653.

7

Pioneer Fibers

The Case for Guidance in the Embryonic Nervous System of the Cricket

JOHN S. EDWARDS

1. INTRODUCTION

The vocabulary and the *dramatis personae* may have changed somewhat, but most current concepts and mechanisms proposed for the development of the nervous system are about as old as the subject itself. The idea that the neurons must be guided or led or must find their way to targets during development was implicit as early as 1887 when His[1] proposed that all nerves originate as outgrowths from single cells. The hypothesis arising from his observations opened up a new view of neurogenesis. His[2] described the first events in prophetic words that have a contemporary ring: *"the way which Nature follows in forming the nervous system is very simple. There is nothing more simple than the formation of the process of the cell, nothing more simple than the straight outgrowing of these processes until they find an obstacle, or until they come to a terminal station."* This surely summarizes nearly all that can be said today about the pathways of insect peripheral pioneer fibers, as will become apparent in what follows. But first some other relevant properties of growing neurons deserve attention in a historical perspective.

JOHN S. EDWARDS · Max-Planck-Institut für Verhaltensphysiologie, Abteilung Huber, D-8131 Seewiesen, West Germany, on leave from Department of Zoology, University of Washington, Seattle, WA.

The embryonic axons of the vertebrate central nervous system grow out from the cell bodies, as Ramón y Cajal also abundantly proved. They do so in an organized, seemingly directed way, so that structural patterns emerge, even though some axons do go astray.[3] And they do their growing on a solid substrate: they cannot invade a fluid medium, but they do not need whole cells; fibrin, or even spider's web as Ross Harrison showed,[4,5] will do. Impressed with the sensitive directional responses of growing axons to substrate microstructure, Weiss[6] coined the term *contact guidance* to describe that behavior and emphasized the significance of *pioneering fibers,* recognizing with his predecessors the crucial morphogenetic role of the first neuronal outgrowths. So, together with the *growth cone,* whose role was appreciated by Ramón y Cajal long before it was seen in action, and with his hypothesis of chemical attraction (*chemotaxis*), some principal elements of modern developmental neuroembryology were established. Subsequent theory has built upon these pioneer ideas like neurons upon pioneer fibers.

The developing neurons with which all the fundamentals of neurogenesis were realized came from vertebrates, but when the development of insect sensory systems received serious attention many years later, it was clear that similar principles applied. In due course it was found that arthropod sensory neurons, unlike those of vertebrates, originate in the epidermis, sending their axons to the center,[7–9] and it became evident that in the periodic addition of sensory axons during postembryonic development, new axons found and followed preexisting nerves to the central nervous system. The behavior of the centripetally growing sensory axon is consistent with the concept of contact guidance. By following existing nerves the tip of a growing axon may thus travel several tortuous centimeters in a large insect on its way to a central termination. Of course, this explanation of the pattern of postembryonic development leads inevitably back to the different question of how the *initial* connections are made between center and periphery.

New axons from regenerating sensilla can also find their central targets and establish functional connections even after they have been subjected to a variety of spatial, temporal, and genetic manipulations in insects[10] (see Chapter 4). The almost unerring capacity to locate appropriate central neurons even when approaching from abnormal directions implies a capacity for pathfinding and cell recognition that must be based on a rather flexible set of rules and certainly argues against a unitary isolable mechanism. Rather such observations suggest a sequence of interactions between the neuron and its milieu. A first requisite is the location by the newly elongating afferent axon of a pathway to the center. It need not be a particular pathway, and it seems that any available pathway across the hemocoelic body cavity to the central ganglia can serve. Once within the ganglia new interactions may come into play, but our concern here is with the path from the periphery.

It should be emphasized at this point that the topological challenge to the growing insect afferent axon appears different in principle from that to the vertebrate, where from the outset of development neurons are growing over surfaces more or less within contiguous tissues. The insect on the other hand consists of an outer epidermal layer from which sensory axons originate, and a central nervous system "floating" in a hemocoel or blood space. This "surface within a surface" organization implies that the peripheral nerve must desert one surface and find another by traversing the body cavity. However, the axons are never in fact faced with the impossible challenge of bridging a fluid medium, for the two surfaces are at first connected, and separate only in the later embryo. In metamorphosis, as in regeneration, passage of centripetal fibers occurs along preexisting pathways, using peripheral nerves of the obsolete larva, and neural connections that were established with the imaginal disks soon after their segregation as islands of suspended embryogeny. Once again we are brought back to the question of the *initial* contacts, the first pathways that will serve as the fasciculation foci for all subsequent peripheral sensory nerve development.

2. FIRST CONNECTIONS BETWEEN PERIPHERY AND CENTER: HOW AND WHEN?

It has been shown in orthopteroid insects[11–16] and it is plausibly so in all insects, that the earliest embryonic neural connections between periphery and center are made when distances are short and pathways simple (see Chapter 5). Such connections appear to be invariably the pathway for all afferent axons during later embryonic and postembryonic development. This chronology is paralleled in the central nervous system.[17]

2.1. *Sensory Embryogenesis in the House Cricket Acheta domesticus*

The embryogenesis of the abdominal cerci of a cricket[13] will serve as an example of the pattern now known for several appendages. The abdominal cerci are elongate sensory appendages, rather like posterior antennae that arise from the terminal segment of the abdomen (Fig. 1, top right). Their anatomy and mechanosensory input to the terminal ganglion of the ventral nerve cord are known in some detail. The basic

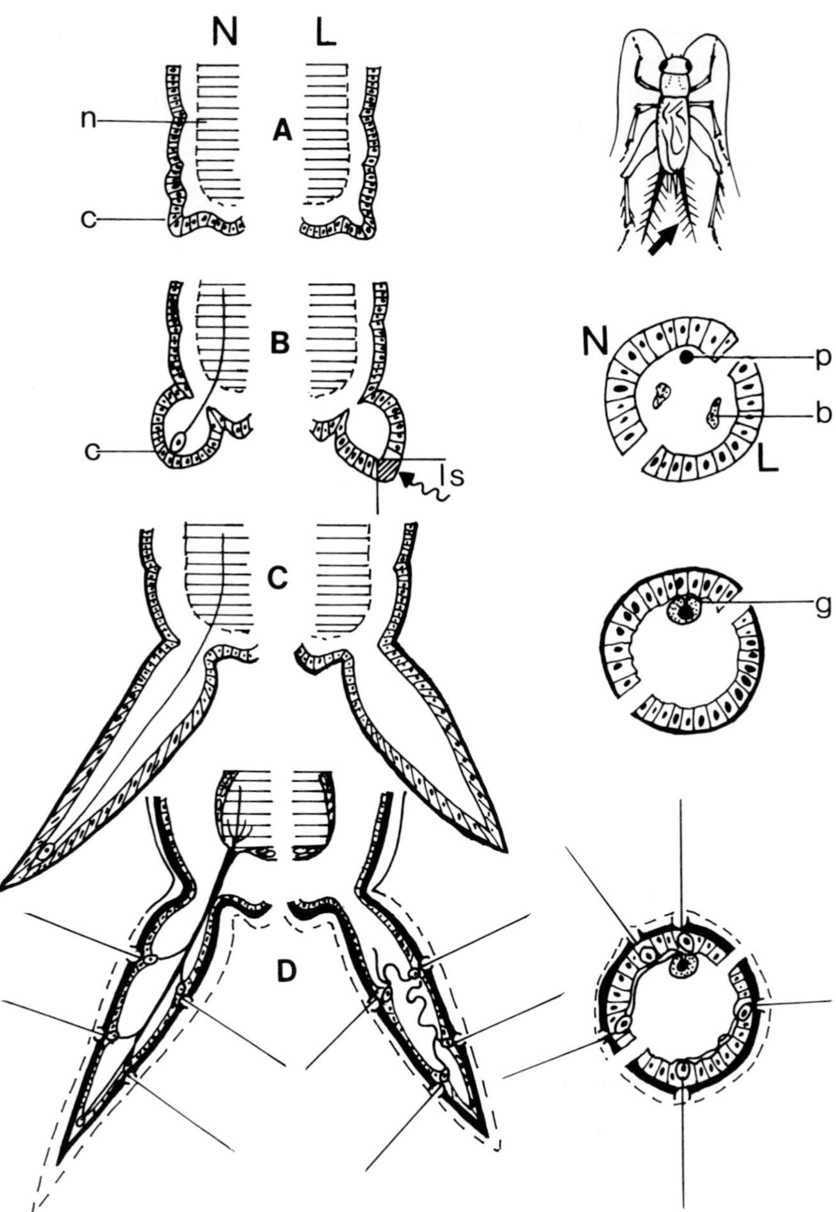

Figure 1. Schematic summary of cercal sensory development in *A. domesticus*. The abdominal cerci are posterior sensory appendages (arrow top right, adult cricket). Normal (N) and lesioned (L) cerci are shown at successive stages, in longitudinal sections on the left, and in transverse basal sections on the right. (A) Early embryo showing the epidermis

structure of the system is described by Edwards and Palka[18]; more recent aspects of structure, function, and development are covered in reviews.[10,19]

Cercal embryogenesis may be divided into three phases. The first phase covers the generation of the cercal rudiment at the posterior angles of the abdomen (Fig. 1A), during a phase of ebullient mitosis that terminates after about 30–40% of development has elapsed, with the embryo enclosed in a delicate sheath. The second phase begins with a dramatic migration of the embryo out of the yolk to take up its definitive position within the egg, a process termed katatrepsis. In the course of these embryonic movements, the abdomen unfolds until the cerci reach the posterior pole of the egg (Fig. 1B). At this point there is a brief pause in development; then the cerci enter a phase of rapid elongation that terminates with the secretion of a chitinous cuticle, the second sheath to be formed over the embryo (Fig. 1C). In the third phase, certain epidermal cells at specific points on the surface of the embryo generate sensilla whose cuticular components are incorporated into the continuous cuticle that will be the functional integument of the hatchling cricket (Fig. 1D). For present purposes the key event occurs at about 50% through the course of development, when cells emerge through the epidermis at the tip of the cercal rudiment and take up positions on the basal lamina. These cells, which have been observed *in vivo* in the legs of the grasshopper *Schistocerca nitens*[14] produce centripetal processes that move over the basal lamina of the cercal epidermis immediately before the cercus undergoes rapid elongation, and they enter the rudimentary terminal ganglion. When the cercus elongates, these cell pro-

---

with cercal rudiments at the posterior lateral angles (c); the presumptive neuropil region (n) is hatched in all figures. (B) Immediately before elongation of the cercus, a pioneer fiber normally grows to a region of the terminal ganglion. A laser lesion (site ls) removes the presumptive pioneer fiber cell body. In transverse section the mid-dorsal pioneer fiber strand (p) lies against the basal lamina of the normal cercus, but is absent from the lesioned structure. Embryonic "blood cells" (b) circulate in the lumen. (C) The cercus has elongated, carrying the pioneer fiber cell bodies along with the apex of the cercus, thus creating mid-dorsal and mid-ventral pioneer fiber tracts with glial sheaths. The mid-dorsal fiber tract is shown in the normal cercus, but fails to form in the lesioned cercus. This pioneer tract is shown surrounded by glial cells (g) in the transverse section of the normal embryo. The epidermis has secreted a cuticle devoid of sensilla (thick line over epidermis). (D) Hatchling cricket. To simplify the diagram, the sensilla of the first-instar integument are shown in their erect functional position. (The overlying embryonic cuticle shown in dashed line is normally shed shortly after hatching, but is retained in the diagram to signify the contrast between it and the first instar cuticle.) In the normal animal the axons of the dorsal sensilla follow the mid-dorsal pioneer tract to the terminal ganglion, where they terminate in specific regions, while in the lesioned cercus these sensillar axons fail to form a single organized bundle. They are not shown reaching the ganglion, but it is not implied that such axons never reach the ganglion.

cesses are stretched out between the apex of the cercus and the ganglion. Within a short period they acquire enveloping cells similar in form and ultrastructural texture to the glia. By the time the cercus has fully elongated and formed the second cuticular sheath, a small population of axonlike profiles accompanies the original processes from the apical cells. This pattern of events, first described from the antennae of a locust[11] and the cerci of a cricket,[12] demonstrated that the first cell processes were in effect pioneer fibers, establishing connections between periphery and center.

The similarity of developmental sequence in grasshoppers and crickets, despite differences in detailed chronology, establishes the likelihood that the pioneer fibers serve to organize the peripheral nerves, but are they essential? In order to test the hypothesis that the pioneer fibers are indeed necessary for the normal organization of the peripheral nerves, it was necesessary to show that in the absence of pioneer tracts subsequent neural development is disrupted.

2.2. *Technical Approaches to the Ablation of Pioneer Cell Bodies*

Ablation of the presumptive pioneer fiber cell bodies requires that the tip of the cercal rudiment be treated after it has become visible in the katatrepsis migration, but before the cells have formed their centripetal processes just prior to cercal elongation. Microsurgical manipulation with needles inserted through the egg membranes caused excessive damage and adhesion of damaged cells to the inner egg membrane so that subsequent development was massively affected. A second approach using ultraviolet cautery with the cooperation of Drs. Klaus Sander and Klaus Kaltoff at the University of Freiburg gave partial success, in that some treated embryos developed without adhesion to egg membranes at the lesion site, but damage to the cercus was not sufficiently localized. In a third approach using laser radiation, initial attempts, made possible by Dr. David Auth at the University of Washington, led to successful, localized lesions made with the microlaser facility at the University of California at Irvine, in collaboration with Dr. M. Berns.[20]

2.3. *Results of Laser Ablation of Embyonic Cerci*

The capacity to make controlled localized lesions led us to compare the morphogenesis of the cercal nerve when the apical cell bodies of pioneer fibers were ablated before (Fig. 1B), or after, the passage of their centripetal processes to the terminal ganglion.[20] The effect of lesions was assessed in terms of the normality of the dorsal and ventral sensory axon bundles within the cercus at a stage near the completion of embryogenesis (Fig. 1D). In essence we found that the bundle was disorganized if lesions were made *before* the time at which pioneer centripetal processes should be formed, but that seemingly normal bundles could be organized if the apical region of the cercal rudiment was ablated *after* formation of the pioneer tracts. It seems then that once the pathway is established, and glial cells have multiplied and wrapped themselves around the original pioneer cell processes, the empty glial sleeve that remains following degeneration of the pioneer fibers can function as a focus for the later developing afferent axons of the functional sensilla. In contrast, if the pioneer processes never travel their appointed route along the surface of the basal lamina, a signal is lost, and the glial cells do not sit down. After the cercus has elongated, it is too late: the glial sleeve is absent and the trace followed by the pioneers has evidently gone; either the sensory axons do not recognize it or it has disappeared from the basal lamina.

3. THE EVENTS OF SENSORY EMBRYOGENESIS: A HYPOTHETICAL PROGRAM

Our results are consistent with the following hypothesis for the role of pioneer fibers as organizing tracts for sensory nerves in an insect.

1. Cells at specific loci in the embryonic epidermis, notably at the apices of appendage rudiments, and probably at other sites as well, are committed during the course of early pattern formation to differentiate from their fellow epidermal cells and to form processes that grow toward the central nervous system. Because the embryonic epidermis and presumptive neuroblasts are at first close neighbors (Fig. 1A), it is plausible that the cells destined to make the first contacts from the appendage are closely related to their central targets.

2. The cell processes so formed—the pioneer fibers—make their way to the center over the basal lamina of the epidermis. They perhaps do so by following a specific pathway that can be read on the surface of the basal lamina: it may be a differential adhesivity as envisaged in Steinberg's models of cell aggregation,[21] due to marker substances laid down on the basal lamina by the mid-dorsal and mid-ventral epidermal cells (see Chapter 6). Alternatively, intramembranous particle arrays in the form of straight ridges[22] may provide guidance cues. The pioneer cell processes start to grow centripetally because the outgrowth is so oriented from the outset: it is determined by the position of the cells—

a mechanism proposed by Harrison[5] for orientation of growth in peripheral nerve development. Specific cellular differentiation as a consequence of cellular orientation is a common occurrence in morphogenetic events within the insect epidermis,[22] although the mechanism is still unknown.

The pathmarkers upon epithelia or their basal laminae seem impermanent, but it is likely that they are related to the radial polarity of the cercal epidermis. Dorsal and ventral cells know their place, at least in postembryonic animals, as grafting experiments show,[23] and the cells of the dorsal and ventral midline make sensilla of very specific orientation, different from the remainder of the cercus. It is not unreasonable to suppose that they can specifically mark their underlying basal lamina during an early stage of differentiation[24] and that embryonic gradients of extracellular materials[25–29] might guide the growth cones of the pioneer cells.

3. Glial cells aggregate along the pathway of the dorsal and ventral pioneer fibers. They may respond to the basal lamina or to signals from the epidermal cells, but it seems more probable that they respond to the presence of the pioneer fibers for they do not appear to settle in their absence. They wrap the pioneers to form a sleeve that separates them from the epidermis. Later the entire structure will separate from the epidermis and come to lie in the lumen of the cercus.

The embryonic source of the peripheral glia is unknown. They are perhaps derived from epidermal cells, but more likely they arise from circulating cells in the embryonic hemocoel—blood cells for want of a better term—which are similar in texture to the early glia. The source of these embryonic blood cells is not known. Central glia probably derive from neuroblasts.[30] While blood cells should have a mesodermal origin, by analogy with vertebrates, these distinctions may be spurious in the insect embryo, and the matter of glial origin must be considered an open and urgent question.

4. The dorsal and ventral tracts serve as fasciculation foci for axons of the functional sensilla when they differentiate much later in embryogenesis. The first sensillar axons need only grow toward the nearer (dorsal or ventral) pole to find pioneer tracts. Their axons can in turn serve as tributary pathways to the main dorsal and ventral nerves for later recruited axons.

5. Removal of the pioneer cell bodies prevents the formation of the tracts, and in consequence the subsequently developing sensory axons do not aggregate in dorsal and ventral bundles. They seem instead to fasciculate randomly and wander blindly. Whether such fibers can none-

theless find their way to appropriate central terminations is, as yet, unknown.

The guiding role of the substratum, in this case the basal lamina of the cercal epithelium, emerges as a continuous theme in the analysis of neural development. Our results and interpretation fit well with the combined mechanical and chemically based guidance mechanisms proposed by Hamburger[31] and with the specific formulation of these ideas proposed by Singer *et al.*[32] Guidance channels in vertebrates[33] seem to have their counterparts in the developing Urochordate (tunicate) larvae described by Cloney.[34] The basal lamina of developing insect epithelia may carry instructions to the growing axons placed upon them.[27] If that were the case, the question arises: Why could not later differentiating functional axons use the same cue as a route to the ganglion in the absence of the pioneer fibers? The answer may be that the pathway is an evanescent spoor, lasting only until the elongation of the cercus, by which time it will have served its purpose, and dissipating when major changes in cell position and conformation supervene.

4. A MATTER OF SCALE

All the events outlined in the descriptions given above occur within domains measuring at most a few hundred micrometers, and often a few tens of micrometers. Completed insect embryos are tiny by comparison with those of vertebrates, but it seems clear that in all embryos the distance traversed by the *first* connecting processes within the nascent nervous system are at most a few hundred microns. Of course, long migrations and distant projections occur in the later embryogenesis of vertebrates, but only after patent pathways are established through the structured embryo.

First contacts over short distances would require relatively simple directional cues. The capacity of insect epidermal cells to respond at a distance was dramatically demonstrated by Wigglesworth,[35,36] who found that cells deprived of their tracheal supply, and thus of their source of oxygen, thrust out processes toward the nearest intact trachea, attach to it, and pull it toward the deprived cells. The epidermal cells behave as if responding to a gradient of oxygen availability, but whatever the effective cue, the generation of axonlike strands up to 200 μm in length provides a parallel to the outgrowths of pioneer cell bodies which are themselves products of the epidermal layer. Bearing in mind the "grappling hook" response of oxygen-starved epidermal cells, it is tempting to propose that a growth-directing substance is released from the embryonic terminal ganglion and that this substance develops a diffusion gradient along dorsal and ventral basal lamina pathways, guiding the already centripetally oriented growth cone of the pioneer fibers to the center (see Chapter 6). The distance involved, from the cell body at the apex of the cercus to the terminal ganglion, is less than 100 μm, and is thus well within the dimensions at which diffusion phenomena or membrane particle arrays[22] could provide morphogenetic signals.[37]

5. PERIPHERY AND CENTER

The organization of pathways in the insect central nervous system seems also to depend on the establishment of a fundamental framework of pioneer cell processes[17] whose pattern of longitudinal trunks and transverse commissures reflects the ordered pattern of the cells of the original neuroectodermal cell sheet (see also Chapters 5 and 8).

The guidance of neurons from the periphery to the center must await the organization of the central patterning. It is clear from the detailed studies of Shankland[15,16] that the pioneer cells from the embryonic cerci in the grasshopper *S. nitens* do indeed pick up axons of the primary longitudinal tracts as they turn sharply to enter the ganglion; they grow directly along these tracts for several hundred microns within the ganglion without forming secondary growth cones or side branches. With that connection established, the pathways are forged for subsequent projection of the functional sensilla in successive batches throughout postembryonic development. The geometry of the final product is complex, but it had simple origins.

Acknowledgments

My work discussed in this study was supported by N.I.H. grant NB07778, and the study was written during the tenure of an Alexander von Humboldt Award as a guest of Professor Franz Huber M.P.I.V., Seewiesen. I wish to thank Drs. C. Elliot and O. Edwards and Ms. G. Stuart for help in preparing the manuscript.

6. REFERENCES

1. His, W., 1887, Die Entwicklung der ersten Nervenbahnen beim menschlichen Embryo: Uebersichtliche Darstellung, *Arch. Anat. Physiol. Leipzig Anat. Abt.* [illegible]2:368.

2. His, W., 1887, On the development of the nerves and on their propagation to the central organs and to the periphery, *Br. Assoc. Adv. Sci. Rep. Trans. Sect. D* **1887**:773.
3. Ramón y Cajal, S., 1908, Nouvelles observationes sur l'evolution des neuroblasts avec quelques remarques sur l'hypothése neurogenetique de Hensen-Held, *Anat. Anz.* **23**:1.
4. Harrison, R., 1910, The outgrowth of the nerve fiber as a mode of protoplasmic movement, *J. Exp. Zool.* **9**:787.
5. Harrison, R., 1914, The reaction of embryonic cells to solid structures, *J. Exp. Zool.* **17**:521.
6. Weiss, P., 1941, Nerve patterns: The mechanics of nerve growth, *Third Growth Symp.* **5**:163.
7. Henke, K., and Rönsch, G., 1951, Über Bildungsgleichheiten in der Entwicklung epidermaler Organe und die Entstehung des Nervensystems im Flügel der Insekten, *Naturwissenschaften* **14**:335.
8. Krumins, R., 1952, Die Borstenentwicklung bei der Wachsmotte *Galleria mellonella* L. *Biol. Zentralbl.* **71**:183.
9. Wigglesworth, V. B., 1953, The orgin of sensory neurones in an insect *Rhodnius prolixus* (Hemiptera), *Q. J. Microsc. Sci.* **94**:93.
10. Anderson, H., Edwards, J. S., and Palka, J., 1981, Developmental neurobiology of invertebrates, *Ann. Rev. Neurosci.* **3**:97.
11. Bate, C. M., 1976, Pioneer neurones in an insect embryo, *Nature* (*London*) **260**:54.
12. Edwards, J. S., 1977, Pathfinding by insect sensory neurons, in: *Identified Neurons and Behavior of Arthropods* (G. Hoyle, ed.) pp. 483–493, Plenum Press, New York.
13. Edwards, J. S., and Chen, S. W., 1979, Embryonic development of an insect sensory system, the abdominal cerci of *Acheta domesticus, Wilhelm Roux Arch. Entwicklungsmech. Org.* **186**:151.
14. Keshishian, H., 1980, The origin and morphogenesis of pioneer neurons in the grasshopper metathoracic leg, *Dev. Biol.* **80**:388.
15. Shankland, M. 1981, Development of a sensory afferent projection in the grasshopper embryo. I. Growth of peripheral pioneer axons within the central nervous system, *J. Embryol. Exp. Morphol.*, **64**:169.
16. Shankland, M., 1981, Development of a sensory afferent projection in the grasshopper embryo. II. Growth and branching of peripheral sensory axons within the central nervous system, *J. Embryol. Exp. Morphol.*, **64**:187.
17. Bate, C. M., and Grunewald, E. B., 1981. Embryogenesis of an insect nervous system II. A second class of neuron precursor cells and the origin of the intersegmental connectives, *J. Embryol. Exp. Morphol.* **61**:317.
18. Edwards, J. S., and Palka, J., 1974, The cerci and abdominal giant fibers of the house cricket *Acheta domesticus.* I. Anatomy and physiology of normal adults, *Proc. R. Soc. London Ser. B* **185**:59.
19. Edwards, J. S., and Palka, J., 1976, Neural generation and regeneration in insects, in: *Simpler Networks and Behavior* (J. C. Fentress, ed.), pp. 167–185, Sinauer, Sunderland, MA.
20. Edwards, J. S., Chen, S. W., and Berns, M. W., 1981, Cercal sensory development following laser microlesions of embryonic apical cells in *Acheta domesticus, J. Neurosci.* **1**:250.
21. Steinberg, M. S., 1970, Does differential adhesion govern self assembly processes in histogenesis? Equilibrium configurations and the emergence of a hierarchy among populations of embryonic cells, *J. Exp. Zool.* **73**:395.

22. Lane, N. J., 1979, Intramembranous particles in the form of ridges, bracelets, or assemblies in arthropod tissues. *Tissue Cell* **11**:1.
23. Lees, A. D., and Waddington, C. H., 1942, The development of the bristles in normal and some mutant types of *Drosophila melanogaster*. *Proc. R. Soc. London Ser. B* **131**:87.
24. Palka, J., and Schubiger, M., 1975, Central connections of receptors on rotated and exchanged cerci of crickets, *Proc. Natl. Acad. Sci. U.S.A.* **72**:966.
25. Sperry, R., 1963, Chemoaffinity in the orderly growth of nerve fiber patterns and connections. *Proc. Natl. Acad. Sci. U.S.A.* **50**:703.
26. Sidman, R. L., and Wessells, N. K., 1975, Control of direction of growth during the elongation of neurites, *Exp. Neurol.* **48**:237.
27. Revel, J.-P., 1974, Some aspects of cellular interactions in development, in: *The Cell Surface in Development* (A. Moscona, ed.), pp. 51–56, Wiley, New York.
28. Letourneau, P., 1975, Cell to substratum adhesion and guidance of axonal elongation. *Dev. Biol.* **44**:92.
29. Toole, B., 1976, Morphogenetic role of glycosamine glycans (acid mucopolysaccharides) in brain and other tissues, in: *Neuronal Recognition* (S. Barondes, ed.), pp. 275–329, Plenum Press, New York.
30. Edwards, J. S., 1969, Postembryonic development and regeneration of the insect nervous system, *Adv. Insect Physiol.* **6**:97.
31. Hamburger, V., 1962, Specificity in Neurogenesis, *J. Cell Comp. Physiol. Suppl.* **60**:81.
32. Singer, M., Nordlander, R. H., and Egar, M., 1979, Axonal guidance during embryogenesis and regeneration in the spinal cord of the newt: The blueprint hypothesis of neural pathway patterning. *J. Comp. Neurol.* **185**:1.
33. Katz, M. J., Lasek, R. J., and Nauta, H. J. W., 1980, Ontogeny of substrate pathways and the origin of the neural circuit pattern, *Neuroscience* **5**:821.
34. Cloney, R. A., 1978, Ascidian metamorphosis: Review and analysis, in: *Settlement and Metamorphosis of Marine Invertebrate Larvae* (F. S. Chia, ed.), pp. 255–282, Elsevier/North Holland, Amsterdam.
35. Wigglesworth, V. B., 1958, The role of the epidermal cells in the migration of tracheoles in *Rhodnius prolixus* (Hemiptera), *J. Exp. Biol.* **36**:632.
36. Wigglesworth, V. B., 1977, Structural changes in the epidermal cells of *Rhodnius* during tracheole capture, *J. Cell Sci.* **26**:161.
37. Crick, F. H. C., 1971, The scale of pattern formation, *Symp. Soc. Exp. Biol.* **25**:429.

8

Mechanisms for the Formation of Synaptic Connections in the Isogenic Nervous System of *Daphnia Magna*

MURRAY S. FLASTER, EDUARDO R. MACAGNO, and ROBERT S. SCHEHR

1. INTRODUCTION

Most neurobiologists think that a nervous system, in order to function properly, must be wired together in a very accurate manner. Even in a relatively simple system containing a few hundred neurons, only a small fraction of the possible synaptic connections are made, in a pattern which is repeated from individual to individual within a species. Explaining this phenomenon is one of the most important tasks faced by developmental neurobiologists.

A number of explanations have been suggested. At one extreme is the idea that cells have a unique set of labels on their surfaces which match those of a restricted number of other cells, allowing each neuron as it grows to recognize, among all the neurons it touches, the appropriate synaptic targets. Sperry[1] proposed such a theory to explain the

MURRAY S. FLASTER, EDUARDO R. MACAGNO, and ROBERT S. SCHEHR · Department of Biological Sciences, Columbia University, New York, NY 10027.

fact that optic nerve regeneration in lower vertebrates restores normal function and apparently normal synaptic connectivity. At another extreme is the idea that it is the accurate timing and spatial ordering of developmental events that yield the end result, without any requirement for individual cell labels. For example, the temporal order of arrival of two populations of fibers which compete for the same target neurons can explain connectivity in the mammalian dentate gyrus.[2] In our work on *Daphnia* we find that some aspects of the formation of eye–optic ganglion projections can be explained in terms of the spatiotemporal organization of optic axon growth. A number of arguments can be made on theoretical grounds against the validity of either of these proposed mechanisms in their pure form, particularly as they would apply to more complex systems. It is likely, however, that elements of both will appear in any ultimate explanation.

The goal of the studies reviewed in this article is to explain the mechanisms by which topographically ordered synaptic connections are established between arrays of neurons and the mechanisms which regulate the individual characteristics of these connections. Attainment of this goal requires, in our view, that we answer the following questions in detail: (1) How does an axon get from the array of origin to the topographically appropriate region of the target array? (2) Within the target region, what determines which and how many of the available neurons will form synaptic connections with a particular axon or group of axons? (3) How are specific features of the synaptic connections between cells in these arrays (such as location, number, and type of synaptic sites) attained?

For some time our laboratory has been investigating the anatomy and development of the visual system of the water flea *Daphnia magna* in an attempt to answer these questions. *Daphnia* is a suitable preparation for these sorts of studies for several reasons. The compound eye and optic ganglion are relatively small and contain together only about 600 cells that form an invariant and for the most part individually identifiable population of nerve cells. Moreover, the fact that *Daphnia* reproduce parthenogenetically and can therefore be maintained as an isogenic population permits us to carry out observations and experiments without needing to take into account possible effects of genetic differences among specimens.

We have addressed our questions mostly to the part of this system consisting of the array of photoreceptors in the compound eye, the array of laminar neurons in the optic ganglion, and the projection of optic axons from the eye to the lamina which connects these two arrays in a topographically ordered manner. Extensive analysis, using computer methods for the analysis of serial electron micrographs,[3–5] has allowed us to describe the cellular structure, synaptic connectivity, and development of the eye–lamina projection in great detail[6–8] and formulate some hypotheses about the mechanisms responsible for the formation of this projection.[7,9] In more recent work we have used [^{3}H]thymidine cell birthdating and electron microscopy to relate timing and order of final mitosis in the lamina to the timing and order of growth of optic axons into the lamina.[10] We have also conducted a series of experiments using UV radiation to delete or to delay the maturation of photoreceptors in order to change the spatial and temporal order of developmental events.[11–14] Our observations are described in Sections 2, 3, and 4 of this chapter; their implications are discussed in Section 5.

2. THE ADULT VISUAL SYSTEM

The single bilaterally symmetric compound eye of the branchiopod crustacean *D. magna* is about 200 μm in diameter (see Fig. 1a). Attachments from three pairs of muscles rotate the eye around three axes. Oscillations and saccades, as well as tracking movements of the eye, are prominent features of visual behavior.[15] There is, in addition, a median ocellus (or nauplius eye), located caudally with respect to the compound eye.

There are 22 ommatidia in the compound eye, 11 on each side of the midplane, each consisting of 8 photoreceptors and a lens. The total number of photoreceptors is therefore 176. The positions of the lenses (and hence the ommatidia) in the eye can be seen in the computer reconstruction shown in Fig. 1b. Within each ommatidium, the 8 photoreceptors are arranged in a highly stereotyped manner, forming a fused rhabdom with a rectangular cross-section (see Fig. 1c). The longer dimension of this rectangle is parallel to the midplane of the animal. Sections perpendicular to the axis of an ommatidium show that at any level only seven cells contribute microvilli to the rhabdom.[6] Serial section reconstructions, however, show that the rhabdomere of the eighth photoreceptor substitutes for one of the others about halfway along the long axis of the rhabdom. The microvilli are oriented in two orthogonal directions, parallel to the sides of the rectangle (see Fig. 1c).

The axons of the eight photoreceptors in each ommatidium travel in a fascicle to the optic lamina, making a 180° twist along the way. At the lamina each bundle forms a unit structure, the optic cartridge, with 5 laminar neurons. There are 22 cartridges in the lamina, 11 on each side of the midline, and hence a total of 110 laminar neurons. Six of the

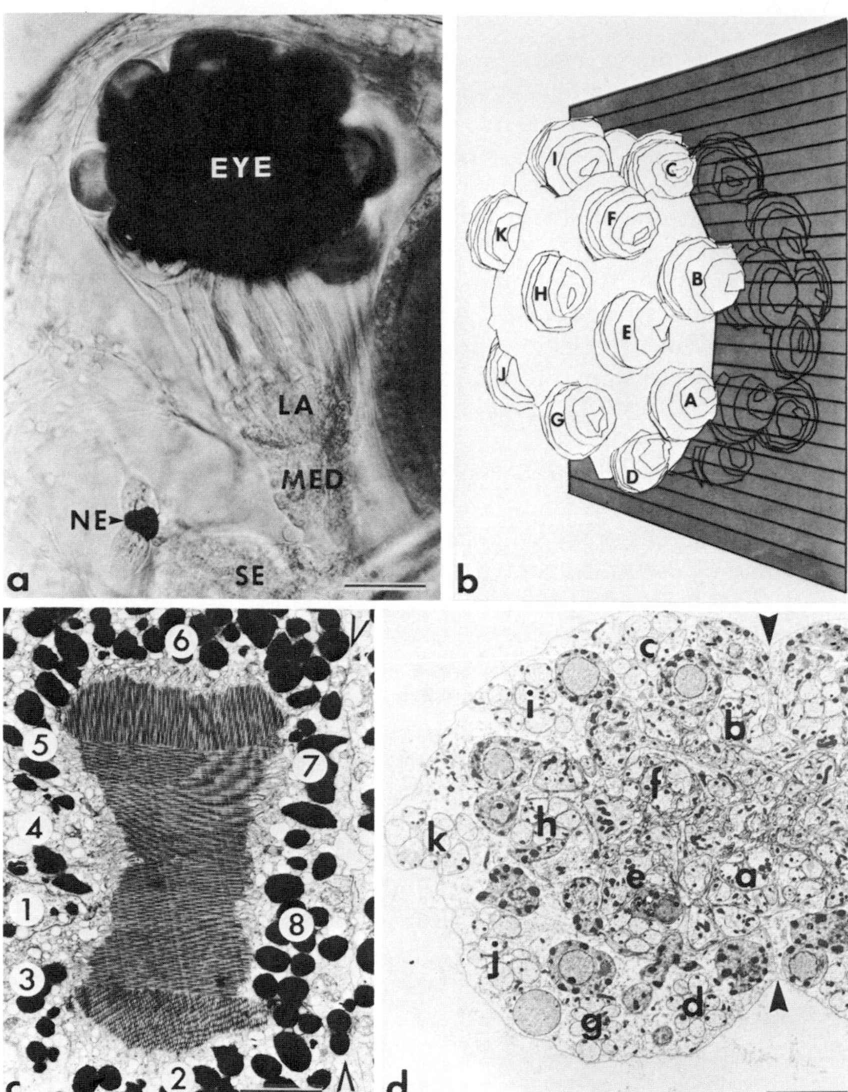

Figure 1. The adult visual system of *Daphnia magna*. Panel a is a light micrograph of the head of a living *Daphnia*. LA and MED are, respectively, the lamina and medulla of the optic ganglion. NE is the nauplius eye or median ocellus. SE is part of the supraesophageal ganglion. Dorsal is to the right. Scale bar, 50 μm. Panel b is a computer reconstruction of the surface of the compound eye from light-micrograph serial sections. The lettered structures are the 11 lenses of the left half of the eye. The gray sheet bisecting the eye is the midplane. The eye is rotated 30° to the right. Note that the arrangement of lenses is mirror symmetrical about the midplane. Dorsal is down. Panel c is an electron micrograph

photoreceptors make synapses with laminar cells in the anterior portion of the laminar neuropil, while two of the photoreceptors pass through to make contacts in a more posterior region. Each of the 5 laminar cells within a cartridge is unique with respect to its connectivity and shape. The photoreceptors are identifiable as well not only because of their positions in an ommatidium but also because of the shapes and connectivities of their terminals. The topographic order of the optic cartridges reflects the organization of the ommatidia in the eye (see Fig. 1d).

Both the photoreceptors and laminar cells make contacts with other neurons having their cell bodies in the next layer of the optic ganglion, the medulla. The total number of neurons in this layer is approximately 320. Some of these medullary neurons send axons down paired connectives (about 90 per connective) to higher centers in the supraesophageal ganglion, and some of these cells remain completely within the ganglion (about 70 per hemiganglion). There are also neurites in the optic ganglion whose cell bodies are located in the supraesophageal ganglion[16] (S. Sims, unpublished observations).

Within a resolution of a few microns, the positions of the cell bodies of photoreceptors and laminar cells and of their branches are conserved in animals of the same clone. Homologous cells on opposite sides of the midplane show bilateral symmetry. Finer details of the anatomy of the photoreceptors and laminar cells are more variable. For example, the overall synaptic connectivity is conserved, but the number of synaptic sites, the number of terminal branches, and the locations of synapses of a single cell varies. The amount of variation is as large from left to right in one animal as it is from animal to animal.[6]

Intracellular recordings from photoreceptors in the compound eye show that they are very similar to other microvillous invertebrate photoreceptors. These studies also show that there are at least two spectral sensitivity types (maximum sensitivities at about 450 nm and 580 nm).[17]

---

of a section perpendicular to an ommatidial axis through the rhabdom. Photoreceptor cell bodies are numbered according to a standard scheme. A photoreceptor in a given position around the rhabdom invariably has the same pattern of synaptic connections and the same orientation of microvilli. Photoreceptors may therefore be identified simply by knowledge of this position. The cell which produces the lead axon always becomes photoreceptor 1. The midline is to the right, indicated by the open arrowheads. Dorsal is down. Scale bar, 2 μm. Panel d is an electron micrograph of a transverse section at the top of the lamina. The letters are the standard naming scheme for cartridges. The photoreceptor axon bundle of any cartridge derives from the ommatidium with the same letter in panel b. The topographic order of the projection is evident. Since the lamina itself is curved, cartridges nearer the midline (closed arrowheads) are sectioned at a more posterior level than more lateral ones. Dorsal is down. Scale bar, 10 μm.

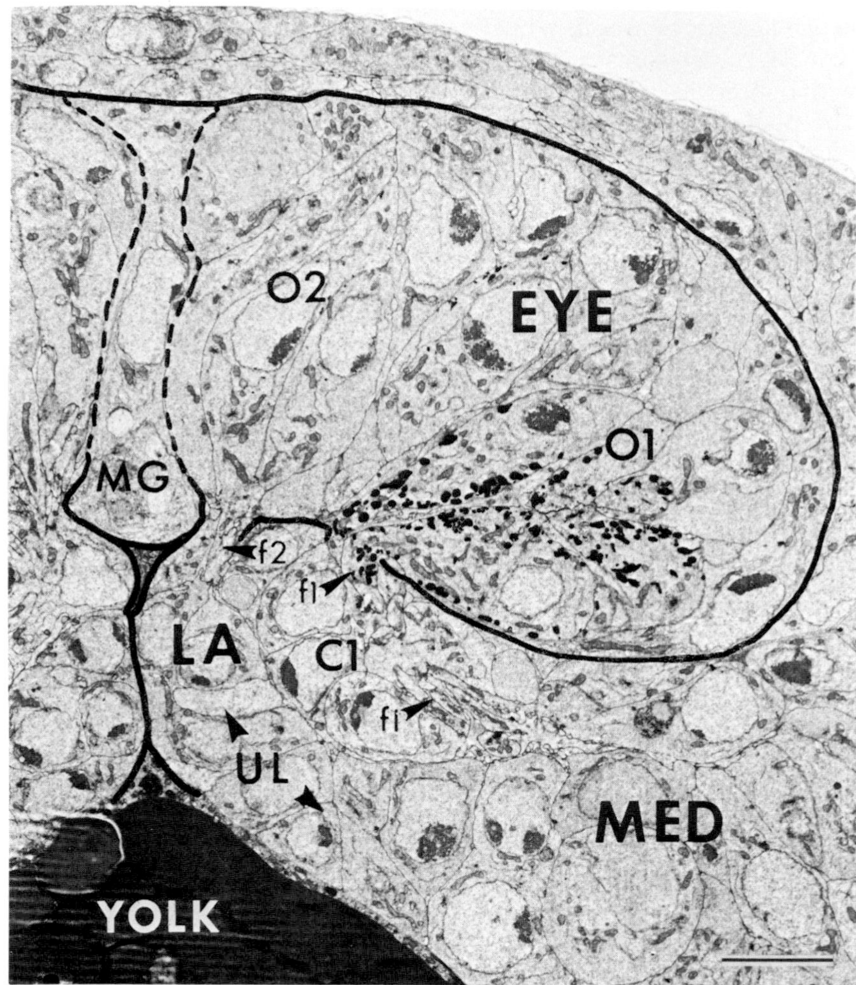

Figure 2. Electron micrograph of the visual system at 37 hr in development (22°C). This is a horizontal section through the eye, the lamina (LA) and the medulla (MED). This illustration shows only one side of these bilaterally symmetric structures. The midline runs down from anterior (top) to posterior through the midline glial palisade (MG), whose boundaries have been outlined with dashes for clarity, then through the sinus separating the two halves of the laminar anlage, and finally into the yolky region at the bottom of the micrograph. The boundary of the eye has also been drawn in for clarity. The posterior portion of that boundary, which separates the eye from the optic ganglion, is a sinus less than 1 μm in width and is too narrow to be easily resolved at this magnification. 01 and 02 are ommatidia. Notice that 01 contains a large number of screening pigment granules, while 02 contains very few granules of much smaller size. The axon bundle of 01 extends into the lamina (arrows f1), projecting to its cartridge C1. This axon bundle appears

Concomitant recording and dye-injection experiments reveal the location of these two types within the eye. As in other arthropods, *Daphnia* can make complex visual computations. There is evidence of wavelength discrimination,[18,19] polarization orientation,[20,21] and motion detection.[15,22,23]

3. DEVELOPMENT OF THE VISUAL SYSTEM

3.1. *General Aspects*

Development of parthenogenetic *Daphnia* embryos can be conveniently staged by time at constant temperature. Unless otherwise stated, the observations presented here refer to development at 24°C. Cell division begins shortly after the eggs are extruded from the ovaries into the dorsal brood chamber of the mother. Extrusion, which takes place 10–20 min after a molt, can be observed through the mother's transparent carapace and is taken as 0 hr of development. Embryos can be easily removed from the brood pouch at any time and will complete development normally *in vitro*. Animals enter the first postembryonic instar by about 55 hr of age. At that time they are free swimming and their gross morphological development is essentially complete. The timing of development is strongly dependent upon temperature. For example, decreasing the temperature to 22°C results in a 2- to 3-hr delay of developmental events occurring during the middle stages of embryogenesis.

The anlage of the compound eye is a curved, disk-shaped layer of cells situated anteriorly in the embryo, beneath the outer layer of ectoderm. Its boundaries become visible at about 25 hr of development. Immediately caudal and contiguous to the forming eye is the anlage of the optic ganglion (see Fig. 2). A narrow extracellular sinus separates the eye from the precursor cells of the optic lamina early in development (in the adult the separation of the eye and lamina is about 80 μm). A palisade of glial cells forms the midplane of the embryonic eye, bisecting it symmetrically. This glial palisade extends caudally to the optic lamina, dividing the anterior region of the optic ganglion anlage into left and right sides.

---

discontinuous only because of the plane of section. The fiber bundle from the medially positioned ommatidium 02 (arrow f2) has only recently reached the lamina and has yet to recruit its full complement of presumptive laminar cells and form a cartridge. Undifferentiated laminar cells (UL) are found adjacent to the midline. These cells or their immediate progeny will contribute to cartridges not yet formed. The scale bar at bottom right is 5 μm.

Before describing in detail some aspects of the development of the visual system, a brief overview will prove helpful. The photoreceptors of the eye are all postmitotic and in place before the embryo is 24 hr old (unpublished observations). For the next several hours there is little detectable morphological change in the eye anlage. At about 28 hr, as differentiated features begin to appear in the eye itself, the first ommatidial bundles grow toward the presumptive lamina and optic cartridge formation begins. Growth of ommatidial bundles into the laminar anlage spans about 10 hr. By that time mitotic activity has ceased in the lamina and is nearly complete in the medulla as well. Elaboration of neuropil continues at least until the first larval instar.

3.2. *The Compound Eye*

Various features of the differentiation of photoreceptors and ommatidia can be distinguished morphologically. Appearance of these features follows an invariant schedule for each ommatidium. The features, in their order of appearance, are elaboration of axons, formation of shielding pigment granules, increase in size of photoreceptors, association of photoreceptors with lens cells, and formation of a rhabdom.

The first evidence for morphological differentiation is found in the lateral margins of the eye anlage, among the photoreceptors that will make up the two most lateral ommatidia in the left and right halves of the adult eye (ommatidia J and K in Fig. 1b). At about 28 hr in development these photoreceptors begin to grow axons in a posterio-medial direction, with one photoreceptor in each ommatidium preceding the others, as described in Section 3.3.

Soon after axons begin to grow, shielding pigment granules (spg's) begin to appear within the cell bodies of the photoreceptors. These spg's grow both in number per cell and in average size (from <0.1 μm in diameter to about 1 μm in the adult), and are clearly visible in the live embryo by around 34 hr as two lateral bands of dark, particulate material in the region of the eye anlage.

Concomitant with the appearance of the previous features is an increase in the size of photoreceptors. This consists of both an elongation of the cells and an increase in their cross-sectional area. Association with lens cells occurs 4–5 hr after axon elaboration begins, with the formation of desmosomelike junctions between the base of the forming lens and the photoreceptors. The rhabdom begins to form at this location a few hours later (unpublished observations).

These events occur in more medial ommatidia at progressively later times in development, with those at the midline beginning to differentiate at about 38 hr of development, some 10 hr later than those most lateral.

3.3. *Development of the Eye–Lamina Projections*

The growth of optic axons is organized into an invariant temporal and spatial pattern.[7] Fibers from a single ommatidium grow out as a bundle and maintain this discrete organization within the optic nerve even when mature. By reconstructing many specimens from serial electron micrographs at a number of times throughout the course of development it has been possible to demonstrate that the details of bundle growth are the same for all ommatidia regardless of position within the eye. The only difference between developing ommatidia that we find is the time their axons begin to grow, which is correlated with their medio-lateral positions. The fiber bundles of the most lateral rank of ommatidia on each side of the eye reach the laminar anlage first, while fiber bundles from the medial rank reach the lamina last (see Fig. 3). (As previously mentioned, the lateral to medial sequence of fiber growth is just one aspect of a more general lateral to medial difference in ommatidial maturation stretching across either side of the developing eye. The factors that contribute to the establishment of this initial condition are not known.)

Within an ommatidial bundle one axon always extends first. This axon has a prominent growth cone and grows posteriorly along the midline glial surface into the laminar anlage and encounters embryonic laminar cells. We refer to this one as the lead axon. The other seven axons follow a short time later in a staggered sequence. Each of these appears to grow on the surface of the fiber(s) that came before it and exhibits a growth cone much smaller than that of the lead fiber. Desmosomes form between the fibers of a bundle and may serve to hold them together.[7]

The lead axon is elaborated by a cell which becomes photoreceptor R1 in each ommatidium; whether the order in which other photoreceptors elaborate their axons is invariant within an ommatidium is not known. These features are of interest when considering the determination of the fates of the target cells of these axons in the lamina and will be discussed in the concluding section.

The two most lateral fiber bundles grow at about the same time along the midplane, bound medially by the glial palisade and laterally by the extraocular space. More medially located bundles grow along the same route, but these are now bound laterally by earlier bundles already in place (see Fig. 3). Though bundles appear to use the midplane

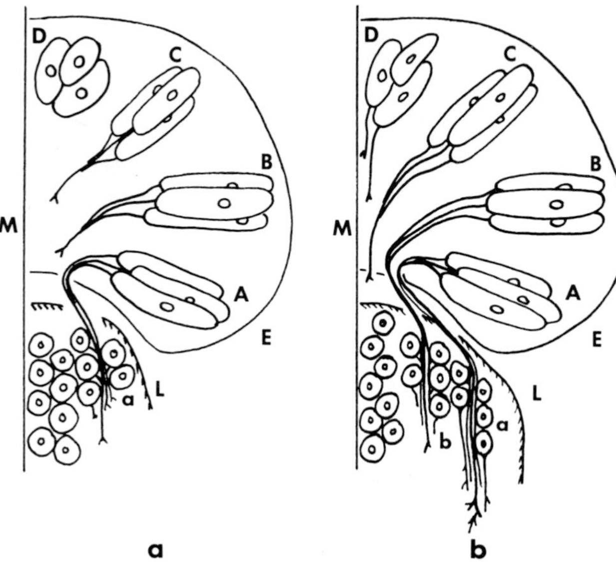

Figure 3. A schematic representation of the development of the eye–lamina projection at an early stage in its development (panel a) and several hours later (panel b). The drawings depict only one side of the eye and lamina in views perpendicular to the dorsoventral midplane (M). The other symbols used are E (developing eye); L (laminar rudiment); A,B,C,D (ommatidia) and a,b (laminar cartridges). Events pictured here for a single medio-lateral row of ommatidia are taking place in parallel in other rows. In panel a, the most lateral of the ommatidia, A, is developmentally the most advanced of the four while D is the least so. The axon bundle from ommatidium A has grown posteriorly along the midline glial palisade (which is not drawn in here, but refer to Fig. 2), has reached the lamina and recruited presumptive laminar neurons, forming cartridge a. The axon bundle from B, the medial neighbor of ommatidium A, follows the same route in its growth from the eye to the lamina. In panel b, the axon bundle from B has completed recruitment of five cells into cartridge b, while the older cartridge a has been laterally displaced. Cartridge a is also further along in its differentiation than b. Axon bundles from C and D have begun to grow but have not yet reached the lamina and contacted the undifferentiated cells near the midline.

glial surface as a substrate for growth, no permanent adhesion is formed since the more medial bundles displace those more lateral away from the midplane when they are added. Little is known concerning the problem of how the direction of bundle growth is controlled. Some observations from the results of UV microbeam deletion experiments do address this question and will be discussed in the section dealing with experimentally perturbed development. It can be seen from the foregoing account that ommatidial bundles sharing the same medio-lateral row on the same side of the eye enter the embryonic lamina sequentially at the same location (see Fig. 3).

3.4. *Recruitment of Laminar Cells into Cartridges*

When the lead axon of each ommatidial bundle arrives at the laminar anlage there ensues a stereotyped sequence of events resulting in the formation of a laminar cartridge.[7,8] As it enters the laminar region, a lead axon encounters a midline grouping of morphologically undifferentiated cells. Five cells are contacted sequentially by a lead axon. Which of the laminar neurons in a cartridge each of these five cells becomes can be predicted from the order in which they are contacted by the lead axon. As each cell is touched, it changes shape, temporarily wrapping around the lead axon and forming specialized contacts with it that include both desmosomes and a transient gap junction.[8] This process takes several hours. Following lead axon contact and the wrapping interaction, each of the laminar cells begins to grow a caudally directed process in association with the lead axon and those follower axons that have caught up in the interim. At any time after fiber contact the first cell to have been recruited shows the most morphological differentiation, while the last cell recruited into the cartridge shows the least. The bundle of what will eventually be 13 fibers (eight photoreceptor axons + five lamina cell neurites) will grow posteriorly and form the neuropil. Any of these growing processes may now show large growth cones, branches, and nascent synapses as laminar neuropil development begins.[24] During the course of cartridge formation the five laminar cell bodies, which originally were stacked in an anterio-posterior column, will move into a plane almost perpendicular to the midplane. To do this they also partially unwrap so that the five cell bodies together form a ring surrounding the bundle of optic axons. (This is essentially the adult configuration within a cartridge.)

As each fiber bundles completes recruitment, its cartridge is displaced laterally away from the midplane. At the same time it is surrounded everywhere but posteriorly by glial processes, which come to separate completed cartridges from each other but do not interdigitate between the elements of a cartridge until later, when local synaptogenesis is well underway. The midplane position is assumed by the next most medial ommatidial fiber bundle at that dorso-ventral position, together with the presumptive laminar neurons with which that bundle will interact (see Figure 3). The lateral displacement of cartridges is probably passive as there are no ultrastructural features present which would indicate active locomotion. One factor contributing to displacement may be the addition of new cells along the midline whose apparent source is the mitotically active region just posterior to the area where cells are recruited. The net result of the lateral displacements is to position the first cartridges to form at the lateral edge of the lamina and to leave the last cartridges to form at the midplane, producing the configuration that will be seen in the adult.

3.5. *Birthdates of Laminar Neurons*

The observations of laminar cell recruitment outlined above raise the question of whether there is any organization of the laminar cells prior to axon arrival. This question cannot be answered by anatomical analysis alone for two reasons. First, there are no visible boundaries separating the laminar and medullary rudiments; presumptive laminar and medullary cells cannot presently be distinguished from each other by morphological criteria. Thus, it is not possible to assess the number of available laminar precursors at any one time. Second, there is a lack of any overt cellular organization to indicate a segregation of presumptive laminar cells into separate groupings.

An approach to answering this question is to examine the birthdates of the laminar cells (the times of completion of their last round of DNA synthesis), to see if these bear any relationship to their fates or to the arrival times of the optic fiber bundles. If the laminar cells are born in a reproducible pattern, as it will be seen they are, we could exploit this by labeling the same group of cells in both normal and developmentally perturbed animals so that their respective fates can be followed.

In this study the birthdates of cells were defined as the earliest time during development at which they would repeatedly fail to label with tritiated thymidine. To do this, embryos were microinjected with label at a series of times, fixed when adult, and then processed for 1-μm serial autoradiography. 3-D computer reconstruction[4] and grain counting were used to determine the number and distribution of labeled laminar neurons. Embryos of the same age as those injected and usually from the same broods were fixed at the time of injection, to establish the stage of development of the eye–lamina projection.

The results of these experiments show that the cells of the lamina withdraw from the cell cycle in an orderly way that correlates with their prospective fate.[10] The first cells to become postmitotic are always found in cartridges at the lateral edge of the adult lamina, while the last cells to become postmitotic are located only in midline cartridges (see Fig. 4). When the number of laminar cells already born are compared with

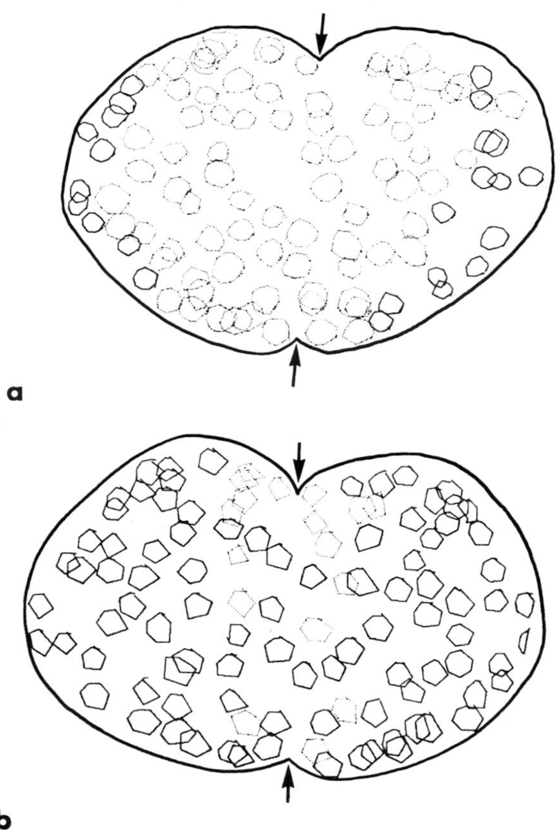

Figure 4. Computer-generated displays of reconstructions from serial sections of optic laminae from [^{3}H]thymidine-labeled specimens processed for autoradiography. The reconstruction of a specimen injected at 33 hr (22°C) and fixed when adult is shown in panel a; the reconstruction of a specimen injected at 40 hr and also fixed as an adult is shown in panel b. The views are transverse projections, looking posteriorly, with the dorsal surfaces toward the tops of the displays. Heavy outlines represent the boundary of the lamina while the arrows indicate the dorso-ventral midline. Each small contour is a cross-section of a laminar cell nucleus, indicating the position of that cell body. Solid contours indicate unlabeled nuclei; dotted contours indicate labeled nuclei. Nuclei were classified as unlabeled if the total number of grains over their nuclear profiles was less than 10% of maximal cell label in that specimen. Maximal cell label was defined as the mean grain count of the three most heavily labeled cells. In the specimen injected at 33 hr only lateral bands of cells had withdrawn from the cycle and are thus unlabeled. In the specimen injected at 40 hr most cells were postmitotic, and only a few near the midline are labeled.

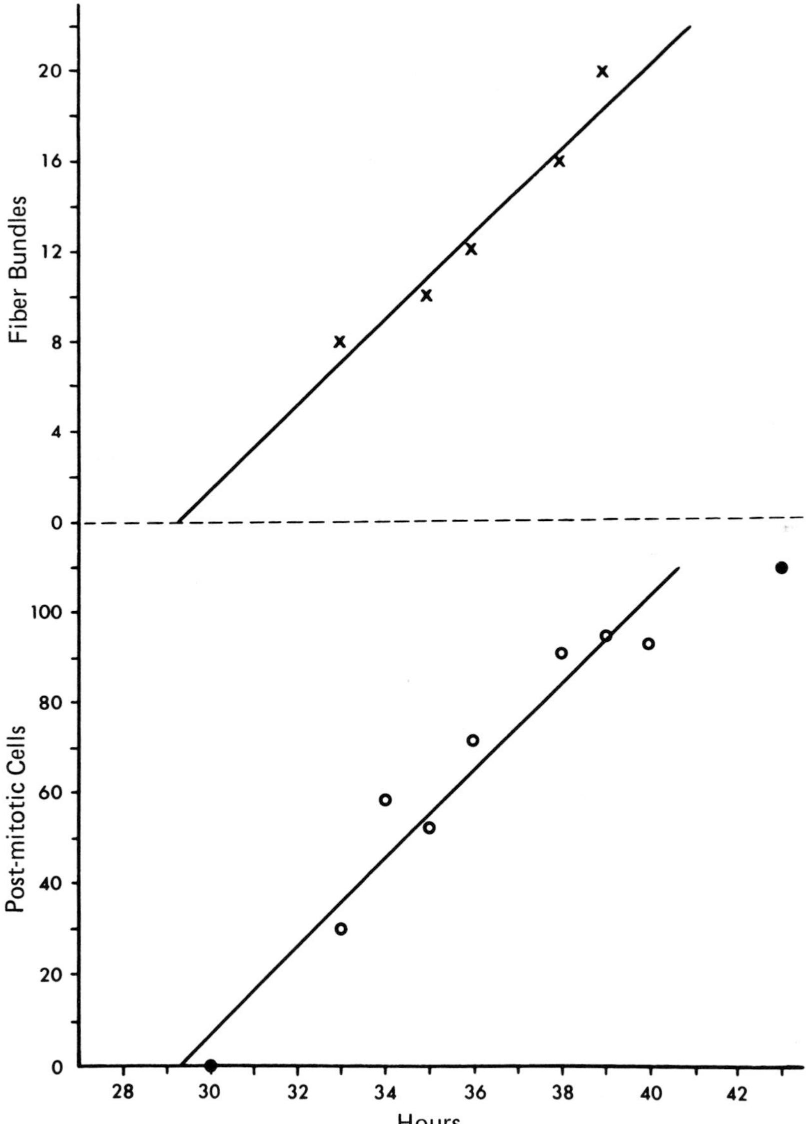

Figure 5. Photoreceptor axon bundle arrival at the lamina and laminar cell withdrawal from the cell cycle as a function of time in development. The total number of photoreceptor axon bundles present in the lamina (both left and right sides) is plotted in the top panel. Each point was obtained by a direct count of axon bundles from electron micrographs of a serially sectioned embryo. The line is a least-squares fit of the plotted points and has a slope of two axon bundles per hour (thus one bundle per side per hour). The number of postmitotic laminar neurons is plotted in the lower panel. Cells at a given position in

the number of optic fiber bundles that have reached the lamina by that time (Fig. 5), we find that these two processes occur at the same rate. By the same rate we mean that laminar cells withdraw from the cell cycle at an average rate of five cells per side per hour while fiber bundles add to that side at an average rate of one bundle per hour (there are five laminar cells in a cartridge). In addition, individual laminar cells become postmitotic not more than 2 hr (about the time it takes a lead fiber to contact five cells) prior to their interaction with an incoming fiber bundle.

We can also tentatively conclude that supply just matches demand in the sense that the number of presumptive laminar neurons available for recruitment at any one time is limited and corresponds to the number of fiber bundles newly arrived. This last conjecture depends heavily upon how we interpret the birthdate data, since it is possible that cells appear to be postmitotic shortly before their recruitment into a cartridge only because optic fiber contact inhibits further division of that particular cell. (The duration of the final laminar cell S phase, less than 3 hr, makes this latter interpretation difficult to rule out on the basis of the existing data alone.) Underlying this point is the question of whether the final division of these cells is determined by an autonomous mechanism or whether proliferation ceases as a result of external factors (e.g., an interaction with another cell or a response to a hormone). For that matter, a combination of both hypothetical mechanisms may be at work. More experiments are required before we can decide which of these possibilities determines the final number of presumptive laminar cells made. The interpretation and significance of the tight correlation between birthdates of target cells and fiber arrival into the target region will be discussed further in the concluding section.

4. EXPERIMENTAL PERTURBATIONS OF DEVELOPMENT

4.1. *Deletion of Photoreceptors*

In order to investigate further the nature of the conspicuous interaction between optic fiber bundles and laminar neurons, a series of

---

the lamina were defined as postmitotic when they consistently failed to label with [^{3}H] thymidine, though they showed heavy labeling at an earlier time. The filled circle indicates that all laminar neurons fail to label when [^{3}H]thymidine is injected into a 43-hr embryo. The line is a least-squares fit of the data points plotted as unfilled circles and has a slope of 10 cells per hour (thus five cells per side per hour). On the average, the number of cells becoming postmitotic is the number required for recruitment by newly arrived photoreceptor axon bundles.

photoreceptor deletion experiments were performed. The methodology used in these experiments has been reported elsewhere,[13] but can be summarized briefly.

A microbeam, whose source is a high-pressure mercury arc lamp, was used for deleting embryonic photoreceptors. The beam passes through a double-slit aperture of variable size whose image is focused on the embryonic eye in an orientation that avoids exposing the underlying optic ganglion anlage to the beam. By both adjusting the size of the slit and changing the duration of exposure to the UV beam, the extent of the resulting deletions can be varied. Ommatidia can be eliminated either completely or to different degrees. The number of photoreceptors killed by a given exposure can be reduced twofold by post-irradiating with longer-wavelength light.[13] This clearly demonstrated photoreactivation effect indicates that a primary site of the photo-induced lesion is DNA.[25] In adults, the large quantity of visual shielding pigment within the photoreceptors makes the use of a UV source impractical. Instead, an argon laser microbeam apparatus was used, and with this method cell death is due presumably to photocoagulation.

The first phase of these experiments involved deleting photoreceptors during development and analyzing the resulting effects in the lamina and medulla.[11,13] Irradiation of the eye was done at two distinct stages in development, either just before the first photoreceptor axon bundles reach the embryonic lamina (28–29 hr), which we shall refer to as stage A, or a short time after the last photoreceptor bundles have recruited laminar targets (42–44 hr), which we shall refer to as stage B. To follow the time course of photoreceptor degeneration, EM serial sections of animals fixed between 30 min and 5 hr after stage A irradiation were analyzed. Signs of cellular degeneration in the eye appear within 2 hr and are nearly gone by 5 hr. The fibers of irradiated photoreceptors appear to stop growing almost immediately so that the axons of dying cells do not reach the lamina. The time course of degeneration in the older group of irradiated embryos is similarly rapid.

Gross morphological analysis of adults where photoreceptors were deleted at either embryonic stage shows considerable reduction in the size of the lamina. Cell counts in serial reconstructions demonstrate that these reductions are due not only to the deficit in photoreceptor axons in the laminar neuropil but to a loss of laminar neurons as well. A plot of laminar cell numbers as a function of photoreceptor axon numbers (Fig. 6) shows that most points lie on or close to a line with slope 5/8, which is the normal photoreceptor : laminar neuron ratio. Thus, the loss of laminar neurons is generally proportional to the induced degeneration of photoreceptors. A markedly different result is found when photo-

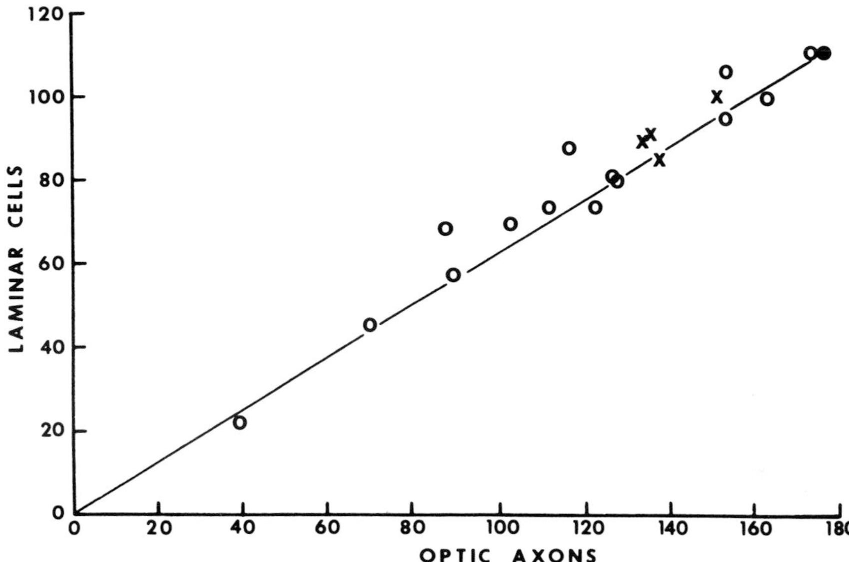

Figure 6. Results of embryonic photoreceptor deletions analyzed in adults. The total number of laminar neurons is plotted against the total number of photoreceptor axons that enter the lamina in adults previously irradiated at embryonic stage A (circles) or at stage B (Xs). The filled circle represents data from an unirradiated control. A line with slope $\frac{5}{8}$ has been drawn through the control so that deviations from the normal ratio of laminar cells to photoreceptor axons can be easily seen.

receptors are destroyed in adults, where all laminar neurons survive for some weeks after photoreceptors are deleted.

As shown in Fig. 6, individual cases can show a deviation from the normal ratio of laminar cells to photoreceptors. Several different types of cartridge aberrations can contribute to an *increase* in this ratio. Most commonly, there are cartridges with the normal complement of laminar cells associated with photoreceptor axon bundles of less than the normal number of eight axons. In those instances where photoreceptor bundles contain fewer than five axons, however, the number of cells found in these cartridges is also reduced, with typically the same number of laminar cells as axons. Occasionally cartridges contain six laminar cells (larger cartridges have never been observed), and in these instances the associated ommatidium may be made up of anywhere from six to eight cells. Cartridges with extra cells seem only to occur in eyes with extensive lesions.

Several phenomena contribute to a *decrease* in the laminar

cell: photoreceptor ratio. There are some cartridges with nearly all photoreceptors present but with a reduced number of laminar cells. The extreme case of a fiber bundle projecting into the lamina without any laminar cells associating with it to form a cartridge has been seen only once. In several cases where axons from two ommatidia have joined to form a single bundle there is a pronounced local surplus of photoreceptor axons. Atypical synaptic connections form between these photoreceptors and laminar cells of adjacent cartridges.[11] A more frequent instance of photoreceptors lacking associated laminar cells occurs in animals that have sustained large lesions at the midline. In these instances, some cells displaying differentiated features, including pigment granules and microvilli, fail to send axons to the lamina. The number of laminar cells in such specimens does not reflect the presence of these cells in the eye. UV-induced damage to the midline glial palisade is always correlated with these projectionless photoreceptors and may contribute to the failure of these cells to send fibers into the lamina.

Embryonic photoreceptor deletions can also result in decreased numbers of medullary cells. However, the effect on these higher-order neurons of the optic ganglion are strikingly different from the effects on the first-order cells of the lamina. Within the few percent error in counting, no changes in medullary cell number are observed when lesions to the eye are relatively small. With sufficiently large lesions to the eye (about 80% of the photoreceptors on one side), the number of medullary cells begins to show a decrease, but even complete destruction of the eye leaves a residual number (about 20%) of medullary cells surviving in the adult. The medulla appears relatively insensitive to eye lesions, showing both a very high threshold before cell reduction becomes apparent and a small number of cells which are fully independent of either the direct or indirect influence of the eye. Present knowledge of medullary development is insufficient to allow any attempt at a detailed analysis of these effects. However, important differences between the connections of medullary cells and laminar cells are worth pointing out. Most medullary cells connect to a number of laminar cartridges, and many either project to the supraesophageal ganglion or receive connections from that ganglion. The presence of these additional connections, which laminar cells lack at least during their initial development, may help explain the relative insensitivity of medullary cells to eye deletion.

Evidence concerning the existence of a trophic interaction between the eye and lamina would be incomplete unless one could account for the fate of the apparently missing cells and also delineate at what time during the life span of the dependent structure the trophism appears to be acting. The first of these tasks, which requires the exploration of three formal possibilities (cell death, failure of cells to proliferate, or cell migration away from their normal location) is experimentally the more difficult in this system. The second task, finding when the trophic function acts, is easier. Already established are the facts that laminar neurons will be missing in the adult if photoreceptor deletions are performed either before any of their axons reach the eye, or shortly (3–4 hr) after cartridge recruitment is complete. Deletions of photoreceptors in adults, however, do not result in the loss of laminar neurons, at least not over the course of several weeks, which is a large fraction of the average lifetime of *Daphnia*. The trophic influence of the eye on the lamina is not, therefore, a permanent feature, but is restricted to embryonic development.

In order to analyze the fate of laminar cells missing in the adult as a result of deletions of embryonic photoreceptors, small deletions were made in a large number of experimental animals which were then fixed at different times following irradiation. As mentioned earlier, in animals irradiated at stage A no signs of photoreceptor degeneration are observed in the laminar anlage. Dying cells, typified by their darkly staining, shrunken appearance in EM sections, and numerous smaller membrane-bound clumps of cellular debris, are found exclusively in the midline region of the lamina. They appear at any time from 15 to 25 hr after irradiation, which is 8–18 hr after the most medial laminar cells are normally born and recruited. Because cell death is scattered throughout this period, it is difficult to quantify, so that we cannot account for every cell that would normally be made. (Cell death is also occasionally observed in the lamina of control embryos during this period of time, but it is a rare event.) Still, we can conclude that at least a sizable fraction of the cells normally generated are produced when photoreceptors have already been deleted, but these extra cells subsequently die. At times before degeneration begins (up to 45 hr of age), medially located and unrecruited laminar cells show no signs of morphological differentiation, suggesting that in the absence of photoreceptor contact laminar cells are not triggered to begin to differentiate. The triggering function of the lead fiber interaction is also supported by experiments whose chief effect is to delay photoreceptor growth and will be discussed shortly.

When EM serial sections of animals irradiated at stage B are examined about 7 hr later, degenerating laminar cells are observed. Unlike the cell death occurring in animals irradiated at stage A, these cells have begun to differentiate and may be found in either lateral or medial positions in the lamina depending upon where the UV lesion was placed in the eye. This contrasts with the exclusively medial position of degenerating cells in the lamina of animals irradiated at stage A, and suggests that presumptive laminar cells never contacted by photoreceptors remain at the initial midline position. In normal embryos the last laminar cells to be made and recruited into cartridges are those at the midline (as demonstrated by the birthdate data and corroborated by the morphological analysis of development). This strongly suggests that it is always the last laminar cells to be made that degenerate as a result of stage A deletions.[12] The first laminar cells to withdraw from the cell cycle are normally recruited by the most lateral photoreceptor bundles, but when these lateral ommatidia are deleted at stage A, the next most medial photoreceptor bundles should instead pick up those cells. This shift in the normal connectivity between ommatidia and laminar neurons should occur along the entire medio-lateral extent of the laminar array. We strongly suspect that this is exactly what happens. Should this be the case, it demonstrates that the 1:1 projection of ommatidia onto laminar cartridges is solely a function of ordered ingrowth and cell–cell interactions and not a result of the recognition by photoreceptor axon bundles of the laminar cells of the particular cartridge to which they normally project. The postulated equivalence of presumptive laminar cells with respect to photoreceptor axon bundle recognition requires two further proofs. It must be shown that particular presumptive laminar cells are not systematically passed over by incoming axon bundles and also that they do not migrate elsewhere when they fail to be contacted by "correctly labeled" photoreceptor axons. The first possibility remains to be directly demonstrated. The second possibility seems unlikely inasmuch as extra cells are not found in the medulla, the only likely position where excess presumptive laminar cells which do not die might appear.

4.2. *Delay of Photoreceptor Differentiation*

The apparently time-dependent character of the development of the eye–lamina projection has prompted us to search for a method of delaying the ingrowth of photoreceptor axons in the lamina. Some results of the deletion experiments led us to believe that exposure to the UV microbeam caused delayed growth in some of the exposed photoreceptors under certain conditions, an effect we have explored in some detail in a recent series of experiments.[14]

In these experiments embryos were irradiated early in development, at a stage preceding the arrival of optic axons at the lamina (stage A mentioned above). Photoreceptors on one side of the eye were irradiated, those on the other serving as a built-in control. The exposure was selected to produce a situation where about 35 photoreceptors received a dosage of UV radiation sufficient to kill them. Postirradiation illumination with a fluorescent light source was then used to rescue about half of these photoreceptors; on the average, 16 photoreceptors were deleted under these conditions.

To analyze the development of rescued photoreceptors, groups of experimental and control animals were fixed at four different times ranging from 12 to 25 hr after irradiations were performed. The number of surviving photoreceptors was counted in either LM or EM series, while all analysis of structure in the lamina was done at the EM level.

A number of morphological features of photoreceptor cell bodies develop smoothly and progressively together as a function of age, as described in Section 3.2. These can be used as independent measures of the difference in degree of developmental advance of irradiated photoreceptors as compared with controls. By comparing the sizes of shielding pigment granules, their numbers, and the diameter of photoreceptor cell bodies it was possible to estimate the amount of delay in irradiated cells. Comparisons to cells at the same position on either the unirradiated side of the eye in these animals or in control animals yielded comparable estimates of delay which ranged from 2 to 8 hr in irradiated ommatidia examined at 42 hr of age. Delayed growth also extends to the crucial feature, the time of ingrowth of axons into the lamina. When the cartridges connected to delayed ommatidia were analyzed, they too showed a similar amount of delay, as judged by the number of lamina cells recruited at 42 hr. At later times, the extent of laminar cell morphological differentiation as measured by process elaboration was similarly delayed. These observations demonstrate that delay in photoreceptor development generally results in delayed arrival of photoreceptor axons into the lamina, which in turn results in similar amounts of delay in cartridge recruitment and laminar cell differentiation. We infer that laminar cell differentiation is triggered by photoreceptor axon contact.

The more complete picture of the photoreceptor–laminar cell interaction that emerges by combining the results of photoreceptor delays with morphological observation of normal development, cell birthdating, and the results of photoreceptor deletions can be listed as follows: (1) Laminar cells are triggered to differentiate morphologically, directly by photoreceptor fiber contacts. (2) Laminar cells remain capable of being triggered for as much as 8 hr following final division. (3) If fiber contact fails to occur within 10–15 hr after final laminar cell division, cell death ensues. (4) Even after laminar cells have been triggered to differentiate, disruption of the normal contacts between photoreceptor axons and laminar cells within the 5–10 hr will result in laminar cell death.

5. MECHANISMS FOR THE FORMATION OF THE EYE–LAMINA PROJECTION

The arrangement of repeating units in both the eye and the lamina, the tight spatiotemporal organization of development, and the results of delay, deletion, and birthdating experiments provide the basis for the following proposals to explain the construction of the optic projection in *Daphnia*:

1. The topographic order of the lamina is produced simply by the order of differentiation of ommatidia coupled with restrictions on where their axon bundles may grow.
2. Presumptive laminar cells are all equivalent before being contacted by optic axons.
3. At the laminar anlage the lead axon counts out five cells and claims them for its cartridge.
4. Within the cartridge further differentiation takes place because the individual photoreceptors instruct the naive laminar cells as to their adult fates.

An assumption underlying these proposals is that the prospective fates of individual photoreceptors are fixed prior to the arrival of their axons at the lamina. We base this assumption on the observation that the photoreceptor that extends the lead axon becomes R1 in each adult ommatidium, that the position of individual photoreceptors in an adult ommatidium is invariably the same, and that there is no evidence for rearrangement of cells in an ommatidium after the lead axon begins to grow.

5.1. *The Topographic Ordering of the Eye–Lamina Projection*

Our observations of the growth of optic axons show that the bundles from each ommatidium maintain their relative positions throughout development, growing sequentially to the target region in an invariant manner. The first two bundles on each side cross the narrow gap between the eye and lamina by growing on the surface of a column of glial cells which bridge this gap at the midline. Subsequent bundles, from ommatidia located more medially, grow to the lamina between the medial glial column and the bundles that precede them.

Two basic questions arise from these observations. The first is: How are relative positions maintained? One possible explanation is that mechanical constraints limit the available pathways along which axons can grow, and that the time when each bundle grows determines which pathway it will follow and thus which neighbors it will have as it arrives at the target region. A second possibility is that a bundle in some manner recognizes other bundles originating from neighboring ommatidia in the eye and actively pursues a pathway which maintains the same relative position. Our observations do not permit us to choose between these two alternatives at this time, but our ability to delay photoreceptor differentiation and axonal growth (see Section 4.2) suggests a possible experimental test. If we experimentally delay a bundle of axons, inverting the temporal order in which it grows with respect to its more medial neighbors, the first alternative predicts that the position of bundles should also be inverted at the target region. The other alternative predicts that the system will regulate so that the topographic ordering would not be affected by this type of perturbation. Preliminary results (E. R. Macagno, unpublished observations) in two embryos treated in this manner indicate that the first alternative is probably correct (see also Chapter 7).

The second basic question raised by our observations is: How do optic axons determine the direction they will grow? The observation that some photoreceptors fail to send axons to the lamina when the midline glial cell column is partially destroyed by UV radiation suggests that this substrate is necessary for optic axons to find the target region, but it doesn't explain why axons grow posteriorly rather than in other directions. One possibility, since the gap between the eye and laminar anlage is very narrow (less than 1 μm) early in development, is that the lead axons from the first two lateral bundles do a small amount of exploration on the surface of the midline cells, until they touch the target region and grow into it (Chapter 5). Again mechanical constraints, as well as the fact that photoreceptors extend axons only from their basal surface near the lamina, could explain this result, but other explanations are equally possible. For example, a direction could be encoded on the surface of the midline cells, or the axons could be sensing an attractive gradient in the antero-posterior direction (see Chapter 6).

Another feature of optic axon growth in *Daphnia* bears further discussion. The axons originating in a single ommatidium grow together as a fascicle, the lead axon with its prominent growth cone preceding the other seven axons with their very reduced growing tips. Although photoreceptors from adjacent ommatidia lie in close apposition we have never found, in hundreds of observations of normal embryos and adults, a case where axons from one ommatidium join the bundle of another ommatidium. Although different times of outgrowth could explain this observation for ommatidia lying in a medio-lateral row, it cannot explain it for ommatidia lying in a dorso-ventral row, since these extend axons at about the same time. It would appear that axons from an ommatidium can only follow each other (or at least the lead axon), were it not for some observations in animals with experimental photoreceptor deletions. We have found a few instances where the remaining axons from a partially deleted ommatidium have merged with the axons of an adjacent ommatidium to form a single fascicle. A possible interpretation for this effect is that the partial deletion of an ommatidium destroyed its lead axon and the remaining axons joined those following an adjacent lead axon. Thus, we can suggest as a hypothetical rule that axons will follow the lead axon from their ommatidium exclusively unless it is deleted, in which case they can switch allegiance to a neighboring one. The morphological differences between growing tips of follower axons and lead axons may be a structural expression of the differences in the growth mechanisms acting in each type.

Another characteristic feature of the adult projection is that each ommatidial bundle twists by 180° as it travels from the eye to the lamina. This rotation is in opposite directions on the left and right of the midline. How these rotations are achieved during development has yet to be determined. It is possible to distinguish between rotation of the ommatidium, a twist of a fascicle prior to laminar cell contact, and a rotation of the entire cartridge after contact has been made. Rotation of the cartridge may be a feature of the rearrangement of laminar cell bodies from a column into a ring.

5.2. *The Equivalence of Target Cells*

When growing axons reach their target region, interaction with target cells and synapse formation follow. Depending on the system studied, initial interactions may cover areas far broader than those where permanent connections are actually made, and connections may actually shift gradually in time.[26] Our results in *Daphnia* suggest strongly that the group of presumptive laminar cells selected by each bundle of photoreceptor axons is composed of those available at the position where axons enter the target region, rather than a prespecified set. When ommatidia are deleted, other axon bundles appear to recruit the target cells normally destined to be the targets of the deleted group. Moreover, we have found no indications that the lead axons of ommatidial bundles engage in a broad search for targets, nor have we seen any transient interactions with presumptive target cells other than those which lead to permanent associations. This apparent equivalence of groups of target cells is contrary to the chemospecificity model first proposed by Sperry[1] as a result of his observations of regeneration of the retino-tectal projection in fish and amphibia. No direct proof of a special affinity between certain axons and particular target neurons exists in any system, and a lively debate about the validity of this hypothesis persists (e.g., pro: Gottlieb and Glaser[27]; con: Horder and Martin[28]).

Whereas our data support the suggestion that the group of laminar cells forming a particular optic cartridge can be recruited to form any other cartridge, it does not provide any direct evidence that would allow us to decide whether the fate of each cell within a cartridge is determined prior to recruitment. It is possible, therefore, that growing optic axons recognize their respective synaptic targets within each group of five cells, predetermined to become one of the five adult cells in the cartridge. An alternative explanation is that the five cells in a group are all equivalent before being contacted by a bundle of optic axons, their fates being decided by the order and manner in which they interact with the axons, and perhaps with each other as well. Support for this notion stems from the observation of an invariant position and arrangement of the elements of an adult cartridge, since we might expect some variability in these features if axons need only recognize specific synaptic targets, regardless of their exact position. In addition, the fates of the laminar cells correlate directly with the order in which they are touched by the lead axon during recruitment. This would imply, if the cells have predetermined fates, that their relative positions on the midline before recruitment are rigidly determined. Furthermore, since they are normally postmitotic for 2 hr or less before being contacted by a lead axon, the assembly of these cells into a stereotyped order must be either very rapid or a consequence of geometrically precise clonal divisions. These phenomena are not apparent morphologically. Thus, although the evidence is quite indirect, we favor the notion that the fates of target cells within a cartridge group are not predetermined but are achieved through interactions with other elements of the cartridge after recruitment. An experimental test of this idea is to delete single immature laminar cells prior to recruitment. If the cell fates are predetermined, then we would expect that any one of the five neurons could be missing in an adult cartridge.

Further indirect evidence supporting this suggestion is provided by observations in animals where eye irradiation has produced a relative excess of optic axons at some locations in the lamina. Such a situation occurs, for example, when a bundle fails to recruit its own set of targets. In such instances laminar cells from adjacent cartridges form additional processes which receive synapses from the extra bundle of axons. A similar behavior is found when bundles fuse to form cartridges with more than eight optic axons. Therefore, the structure of laminar neurons changes in response to unusual arrangements of optic axons, supporting the hypothesis that optic axons influence the shape and synaptic connectivity of laminar cells.

5.3. *The Nature of the Interaction between Optic Axons and Laminar Cells*

The optic axon–laminar cell interaction has several features. The first, and most clearly defined, is the triggering of laminar cell differentiation by the initial contact with optic axons. The evidence for this stems from both cell deletion experiments, which show that laminar cells fail to initiate differentiation if they are not contacted, and from experiments where optic axon growth is delayed, which indicate that laminar cell differentiation is delayed until axons arrive at a later than normal time. Failure of target cells to differentiate under similar experimental conditions has also been reported to occur in the grasshopper visual system.[29] The results of delay experiments also indicate that there is an extended period over which differentiation can be triggered.

Several developmental roles can be proposed for the triggering action of the photoreceptor axons. First, it provides a mechanism for insuring that the maturation of axons and target cells is temporally coordinated, which may play an important role in the attainment of a particular pattern of synaptic connectivity. Second, it is a means for recruiting a group of target cells from the general pool available to other incoming optic axons. Third, it insures that only the required number of target cells differentiate; those lacking the contact interaction degenerate. It should be pointed out that the relative amount of cell death observed normally in *Daphnia* is much less than in vertebrates, where significant percentages of the initial cell populations degenerate[30] (see Chapter 9).

A second property of the interaction is to ensure target cell survival, since deletion of embryonic axons, even after laminar cell differentiation has started, leads to the degeneration of the embryonic target cells which are deprived of optic axon association. Thus an extended dependence of laminar cells on optic axons exists. The fact that embryonic photoreceptors without laminar connections can persist into the adult shows that this dependence is not reciprocal. Moreover, the dependence is limited in time, since adult laminar neurons survive the deletion of their optic inputs.

Although the mechanism that mediates the dependence of the lamina on the embryonic eye is unknown, it is clear that photoreceptors whose axons never exit the eye do not increase the number of laminar cells that survive. Thus, the mechanism cannot involve a freely diffusing trophic factor which acts at some distance from the eye. Additional evidence against a simple diffusion mechanism comes from eye lesions that are extensive but strictly unilateral. In these instances the overall laminar cell:photoreceptor ratios of either side can be accounted for independently of each other. Furthermore, small lesions to the eye result in very local aberrations in the lamina. These observations together with the morphological description of development argue that close contact is necessary to the trophic function.

A third function of the interaction between growing optic axons and laminar cells suggested by our observations is to determine the number of target cells per bundle of axons. The observation of a tight correlation between the number of laminar cells withdrawing from the cell cycle and the number required for recruitment by incoming axons at any particular time suggests the possibility that five cells are recruited by each bundle because only five are available at the appropriate time. If this were true, however, we would predict that if more cells are made available we should find cartridges formed with more than five laminar cells. Such a situation should exist when photoreceptor deletions leave a number of cells unrecruited, but we seldom find cartridges with more than five cells in irradiated *Daphnia*, the exception being a few cartridges with six target cells in animals with very extensive damage to the eye. The interpretation of these observations as evidence against availability as the determining factor for the number of cells per cartridge is not, however, the only one possible. An alternative interpretation is that the proliferation of target cells is somehow controlled by the rate of recruitment and that photoreceptor deletions lead to an underproduction of target cells, thus still limiting the number available. This is probably not the case, however, since cell death in the lamina is a prominent feature of development in animals with photoreceptor deletions. Furthermore, target cell proliferation is generally thought to be independent of afferent innervation[31]. Among invertebrates the observations of Nordlander and Edwards[32] on the butterfly optic ganglion demonstrate that mitosis in the lamina is completed before optic axons arrive, ruling out an effect of the latter on laminar cell proliferation. Anderson[29] reports that mitotic divisions continue in an apparently normal fashion in the locust optic lamina after removal of the growth zone of the eye. We have at present no direct evidence for or against the existence of an effect on laminar cell proliferations in *Daphnia*, but the very tight correlation between optic axon arrival at the target region and withdrawal of target neurons from the cell cycle is suggestive of an effect of the former on the latter and merits further investigation.

We are left with the hypothesis that optic axons know how to count to five when they recruit targets. How this counting is achieved is unknown, but it is of interest to note that this number does not appear to be determined simply by the number of axons in an ommatidial bundle. We have found cases where partial deletions of ommatidia reduce the number of axons from 8 to 7, 6, or 5, and cases where bundle fusions lead to fascicles with 9–14 axons. In all these cases cartridges are formed with the normal number of five target cells. In general, ommatidia with fewer than 5 axons are found to make cartridges with fewer than five laminar cells; however, we do not know if this is because fewer were recruited or because some degenerated for lack of an appropriate level of trophic factor. We conjecture, therefore, that it is the lead axon which, in the process of sequentially touching undifferentiated laminar cells, counts to five.

The proposals we have discussed here are addressed only to the formation of eye–lamina connections. Connections made by medullary cells, many of which associate with more than one optic cartridge, represent a further level of complexity. This development may require different mechanisms than those we have suggested to explain our present observations.

6. REFERENCES

1. Sperry, R. W., 1963, Chemoaffinity in the orderly growth of nerve fiber patterns and connections, *Proc. Natl. Acad. Sci. U.S.A.* **50:**703.
2. Gottlieb, D. I., and Cowan, W. M., 1972, Evidence for a temporal factor in the occupation of available synaptic sites during development of the dentate gyrus, *Brain Res.* **41:**452.
3. Levinthal, C., Macagno, E. R., and Tountas, C., 1974, Computer aided reconstruction from serial sections, *Fed. Proc. Fed. Am. Soc. Exp. Biol.* **33:**2336.
4. Macagno, E. R., Levinthal, C., and Sobel, I., 1979, Three-dimensional computer reconstruction of neurons and neuronal assemblies, *Ann. Rev. Biophys. Bioeng.* **8:**323.
5. Sobel, I., Levinthal, C., and Macagno, E. R., 1980, Special techniques for the automatic computer reconstruction of neuronal structures, *Ann. Rev. Biophys. Bioeng.* **9:**347.
6. Macagno, E. R., Lo Presti, V., and Levinthal, C., 1973, Structure and development of neuronal connections in isogenic organisms: Variations and similarities in the optic system of *Daphnia magna*, *Proc. Natl. Acad. Sci. U.S.A.* **70:**56.
7. Lo Presti, V., Macagno, E. R., and Levinthal, C., 1973, Structure and development of neuronal connections in isogenic organisms: Cellular interactions in the development of the optic lamina of *Daphnia*, *Proc. Natl. Acad. Sci. U.S.A.* **70:**433.

8. Lo Presti, V., Macagno, E. R., and Levinthal, C., 1974, Structure and development of neuronal connections in isogenic organisms: Transient gap junctions between growing optic axons and lamina neuroblasts, *Proc. Natl. Acad. Sci. U.S.A.* **71**:1098.
9. Levinthal, F., Macagno, E. R., and Levinthal, C., 1976, Anatomy and development of identified cells in isogenic organisms, *Cold Spring Harbor Symp. Quant. Biol.* **40**:321.
10. Flaster, M., and Macagno, E., 1980, Correlation between cell birthdates and synaptic connectivity in a neuronal array, *Neurosci. Abstr.* **6**:410.
11. Macagno, E. R., 1977, Abnormal synaptic connectivity following UV-induced cell death during *Daphnia* development, in: *Cell and Tissue Interactions* (J. W. Lash and M. M. Burger, eds.), pp. 293–309, Raven Press, New York.
12. Macagno, E. R., 1978, Mechanism for the formation of synaptic projections in the arthropod visual system, *Nature (London)* **275**:318.
13. Macagno, E. R., 1979, Cellular interactions and pattern formation in the development of the visual system in *Daphnia magna* (Crustacea, Branchiopoda). I. Trophic interactions between retinal fibers and laminar neurons, *Dev. Biol.* **73**:206.
14. Macagno, E. R., 1981, Cellular interactions and pattern formation in the development of the visual system in *Daphnia magna* (Crustacea, Branchiopoda). II. Induced retardation of optic axon ingrowth results in a delay in laminar neuron differentiation, *J. Neurosci.* **1**:945.
15. Frost, B. J., 1975, Eye movements in *Daphnia pulex, J. Exp. Biol.* **62**:175.
16. Macagno, E. R., and Levinthal, C., 1975, Computer reconstruction of the cellular architecture of the *Daphnia magna* optic ganglion, in: *Proceedings, Electron Microscopy Society of America* (G. W. Bailey, ed.), pp. 284–285, Clayton's Publishing Division, Baton Rouge, LA.
17. Schehr, R., and Macagno, E. R., 1979, Physiological properties of photoreceptors in the compound eye of *Daphnia magna, Neurosci. Abstr.* **5**:806.
18. Heberdey, R. F., 1948, Das Unterscheidungsvermogen von *Daphnia* fur Helligkeiten farbiger Lichter, *Z. vgl. Physiol.* **31**:89.
19. Young, S., 1974, Directional differences in the colour sensitivity of *Daphnia magna, J. Exp. Biol.* **61**:261.
20. Baylor, E. R., and Smith, F. E., 1953, The orientation of cladocera to polarized light, *Am. Nat.* **87**:97.
21. Waterman, T. H., 1981. Polarization sensitivity, in: *Handbook of Sensory Physiology,* vol. VII/6B (H. Autrum, ed.), pp. 283–469, Springer-Verlag, New York.
22. Ringelberg, J., Flik, B. J. G. and Buis, R. C., 1975, Contrast orientation in *Daphnia magna, Neth. J. Zool.* **25**:454.
23. Stavn, R. H., 1970, The application of the dorsal light reaction for orientation in water currents by *Daphnia magna strauss, Z. Vgl. Physiol.* **70**:349.
24. Lo Presti, V. C., 1974, The development of the eye-lamina neural connections in *Daphnia magna*: A serial section electron microscopic study, Ph.D. dissertation, Columbia University.
25. Cook, J. S., 1970, Photoreactivation in animal cells, *Photophysiology* **5**:191.
26. Gaze, R. M., Keating, M. J., and Chung, S. H., 1974, The evolution of the retinotectal map during development in *Xenopus, Proc. R. Soc. London* **185**:301.
27. Gottlieb, D. I., and Glaser, L., 1980, Cellular recognition during neural development, *Ann. Rev. Neurosci.* **3**:303.
28. Horder, T. J., and Martin, K. A. C., 1978, Mophogenetics as an alternative to chemospecificity in the formation of nerve connections, *Symp. Soc. Exp. Biol.* **32**:275.
29. Anderson, H., 1978, Postembryonic development of the visual system in the locust,

Schistocerca gregaria. I. Patterns of growth and developmental interactions in the retina and optic lobe, *J. Embryol. Exp. Morphol.* **45**:55.

30. Cowan, W. M., 1979, Selection and control in neurogenesis, in: *The Neurosciences: Fourth Study Program* (F. O. Schmitt and F. G. Worden, eds.), pp. 59–80, The MIT Press, Cambridge, MA.
31. Jacobson, M., 1978, *Developmental Neurobiology*, 2nd ed., Plenum Press, New York.
32. Nordlander, R. H., and Edwards, J. S., 1969, Postembryonic brain development in the monarch butterfly *Danaus plexippus*. II. The optic lobes, *Wilhelm Roux Arch. Entwicklungsmech. Org.* **163**:197.

9

Cell Death in Neuronal Development

Regulation by Trophic Factors

DARWIN K. BERG

1. INTRODUCTION

Neuronal death has been identified as a widely occurring phenomenon in the development of the vertebrate nervous system. More than half of the cells initially present in such populations as the motoneuron pool of the spinal cord and neurons of autonomic and sensory ganglia disappear during embryonic development. The number of surviving neurons appears to depend on the amount of target tissue available for innervation by the neurons. Removal of the target tissue prior to the period of cell death causes nearly all of the neurons to die subsequently, while transplantation of additional tissue to the embryo to serve as a potential target for the neurons permits more neurons to survive through the normal die-off period.

Current interpretation of these observations suggests that an oversupply of neurons is produced early in development and that the target tissue allows only the number of neurons necessary for complete innervation to survive. Such target-based regulation would insure an economical matching of pre- and postsynaptic populations with respect

DARWIN K. BERG · Department of Biology, University of California, San Diego, La Jolla, CA 92093.

to size. Furthermore, it has been proposed that the dependence of neuronal survival on the target tissue might serve as a means of correcting "errors" during innervation: neurons which projected to inappropriate targets or were unable to contact their intended targets would simply not survive. If neuronal survival is related to synaptic specificity, however, it would require that the influence of the target be specific, namely, that only neurons of the appropriate type could be supported by the corresponding target.

Two proposals have commonly been advanced to account for the correlation between neuronal survival and target tissue. The first is that the neurons compete for a limited number of synaptic sites provided by the target (see Chapter 10). If a neuron were denied the opportunity to form and maintain a synapse, its developmental program would become disrupted and lead to degeneration. The second is that the neurons become dependent on diffusible components supplied in limiting amounts by the target tissue. The components, termed trophic factors, would be preferentially available to neurons which form close contacts or synapses with the target tissue.

Exploration of the second model has drawn attention to nerve growth factor (NGF), the only known substance which appears to function as a trophic factor for regulating neuronal survival. NGF has been purified to homogeneity and displays many of the properties expected for a target-derived component that acts on sensory and sympathetic neurons (see Chapter 6). The credibility and significance of the trophic factor model in neuronal development would be much enhanced by the identification of additional components which served as putative trophic factors for other neuronal populations. Characterization of such components would also indicate whether trophic factors contribute to specificity during synaptogenesis, that is, whether different classes of targets produce different trophic factors, each specific for the neurons destined to innervate that target class.

This review will first take up the question of neuronal cell death during development *in vivo* and will examine the major findings about how survival is influenced by manipulation of the target tissue normally innervated by the neurons. As a possible way of accounting for target influences on neuronal survival, evidence supporting the role of NGF as a trophic factor will then be summarized briefly. Both topics have been covered more extensively elsewhere in a number of excellent articles.[1–9] The major focus of the present review will be a discussion of new evidence from cell culture for the existence of factors different from NGF that influence the survival, growth, and development of parasympathetic neurons. Studies identifying factors that promote the survival and development of other neuronal populations will be discussed as well. The references have been selected to illustrate specific points and to serve as guides to the literature; they are not meant to be inclusive.

2. NEURONAL CELL DEATH

Hamburger and Levi-Montalcini[10] first demonstrated the importance of neuronal death during normal development in the nervous system. They found that large-scale degeneration of neurons occurs in chick cervical and thoracic dorsal root ganglia around embryonic days 5 and 6. Subsequent work has shown that neuronal death occurs in many populations both in the peripheral and central nervous systems during development and that it can claim 30–80% of the neurons initially present. Examples include motoneurons in the frog,[11] chick,[12] mouse,[13] and monkey[14]; dorsal root ganglion (DRG) neurons in frog[15] and opossum[16]; neurons in the chick trochlear and isthmo-optic nuclei,[17,18] the mesencephalic nucleus of the trigeminal nerve,[19] Hofmann's nucleus,[20] and the optic tectum;[21] and neurons in the mouse oculomotor nucleus.[22] Cell death during normal development has also been demonstrated either directly or indirectly for numerous other neuronal populations.[9] Only one published account documents an absence of cell death for an identified neuronal population, the pontine nuclei of the chick, during their development.[23] Naturally occurring cell death usually takes place during a restricted time period, as in the case of the chick ciliary ganglion where half of the neurons are lost between embryonic days 8 and 14[24] (Fig. 1).

A number of studies have shown that removal of the synaptic target tissue in the embryo causes massive cell death in the neuronal population innervating the tissue. Studies of the trochlear nucleus by Cowan and Wenger[17] and of frog motoneurons by Prestige[25] were the first to demonstrate that cell death induced by removal of the target tissue follows the same time course as does naturally occurring cell death. These observations indicated that as development progresses, the neurons acquire a dependence on the target tissue for continued survival. Competition among the neurons for a limited amount of target tissue or substance produced by the target tissue might then account for the naturally occurring cell death.[10,25]

The proposal that neuronal survival depends on interactions with the target tissue is consistent with findings on the time course of innervation of the target. The period of cell death in the chick ciliary ganglion coincides with the time when the iris can first be activated by

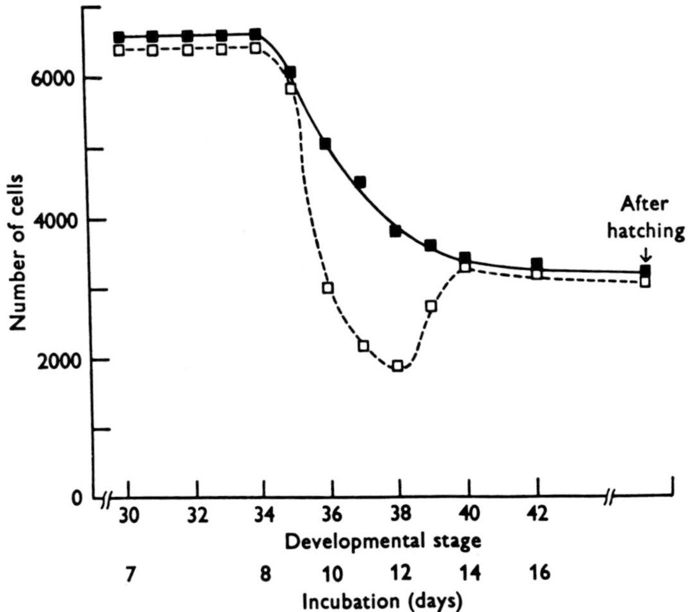

Figure 1. Comparison of the number of transmitting ganglion cells with total cell number in the embryonic chick ciliary ganglion. Total number of cells per ganglion (filled squares) declines monotonically to approximately 50% of the original number between stages 34 and 40. During the same stages, the number of transmitting cells (open squares; total number of cells times percent transmission) drops to a minimum of 2000 and returns to approximately 3000. (From Landmesser and Pilar.[24])

stimulation of the ciliary nerve.[24] Hamburger[26] observed a similar correlation between neuronal death in the chick motor column and the first signs of functional neuromuscular transmission.

Direct support for the competition model comes from studies of the effect of additional target tissue on naturally occurring cell death: supernumerary limbs increase the number of surviving motoneurons in frog,[27] and transplantation of an additional eye in the chick increases the number of surviving neurons in both the accessory oculomotor nucleus[28] and the trochlear and isthmo-optic nuclei.[29] Similar results have been obtained in a number of other studies, but in many cases the observed reduction in cell death was less than expected given the amount of additional target available.[9] The grafted tissue may not have been able to interact with the neurons as effectively as did the normal target because of its position, damage, or interaction with adjacent tissues.

The competition model is further supported by evidence that neurons lost through naturally occurring cell death are not preprogrammed to die. Pilar *et al.*[30] used selective axotomy to remove about two-thirds of the neurons present in the chick ciliary ganglion prior to the period of normal death. Of the remaining neurons, more survived than would have done so otherwise, and some of the surviving neurons innervated target tissue normally supplied exclusively by neurons removed by the axotomy.

However, the hypothesis that neuronal survival is limited by the availability of target tissue has been recently challenged by the work of Lamb.[31] Frogs with bilaterally innervated hind limbs were produced by amputating one hind limb bud and disrupting the dorsal midline barriers so that both contralateral and ipsilateral motoneuron populations could innervate the remaining limb. In this case it was reported that the number of surviving motoneurons (combining right and left sides) was about twice that supported by the limb in unoperated control animals or in animals having either a limb bud amputated or the dorsal midline disrupted but not both. These results were interpreted as refuting the hypothesis that the limb normally limits the number of surviving neurons. While others have pointed out important reservations about the interpretation as presented,[9,32] clearly the observation is of interest and deserves follow-up.

Cell death does not reflect failure of the neuron to extend an axon to the target tissue. Counts of individual axons in the ventral root suggest that all motoneurons, including those that subsequently die, extend axons to the periphery prior to the period of cell death.[33,34] Likewise, chick ciliary ganglion neurons all appear to extend axons into the ganglionic nerves prior to the period of neuron death in the ganglion.[35] Retrograde labeling of neurons by injecting horseradish peroxidase (HRP) into the target tissue confirms that the axons have reached the target. Thus all of the neurons in the isthmo-optic nucleus of the chick can be labeled by HRP injections into the eye prior to the period of cell death, though 60% of the neurons in the nucleus later die normally.[36] The HRP technique permitted the same conclusion for motoneurons in the chick.[34] It has not been determined, however, whether neurons that fail to survive ever form functional synaptic contacts on target cells.

The possibility that functional synaptic contacts may mediate the influence of the target tissue on neuronal survival has been investigated recently by several laboratories. The approach taken has been to maintain chronic pharmacological blockade of synaptic transmission to the target tissue during the normal period of cell death and then determine the effect on neuronal survival. Pittman and Oppenheim[37,38] produced chronic paralysis of chick embryos with drugs such as *d*-tubocurarine or botulinum toxin and found that the treatment significantly increased the number of motoneurons present after the normal period of cell death (Fig. 2). The drug treatment did not increase the number of motoneurons present if initiated after the die-off period, and did not prevent death of motoneurons if the limb bud was amputated. Extended neuronal survival has also been reported for frog motoneurons[39] and for neurons in the trochlear nucleus of duck[40] following chronic application of α-bungarotoxin to maintain neuromuscular blockade. It will be important to determine whether the decreased cell death is accompanied by maturation of the neurons, or whether the drug treatment simply arrests the neurons at a developmental stage in which they have not yet become dependent on the target tissue. The fact that limb bud amputation prevents the drug treatment from extending neuronal survival,[38] together with preliminary observations on the surviving neurons,[9] argues against a block in maturation as the primary drug effect. However, one study using α-bungarotoxin injections to obtain extended survival of motoneurons reports that the mean soma size was significantly less than that of motoneurons in control animals at the same stage.[39]

One interpretation of these results is that the neurons normally compete for the opportunity to form synapses and that synapse formation is necessary for neuronal survival.[35,37,38] It is known that chronic neuromuscular blockade permits hyperinnervation of the muscle[41–43]

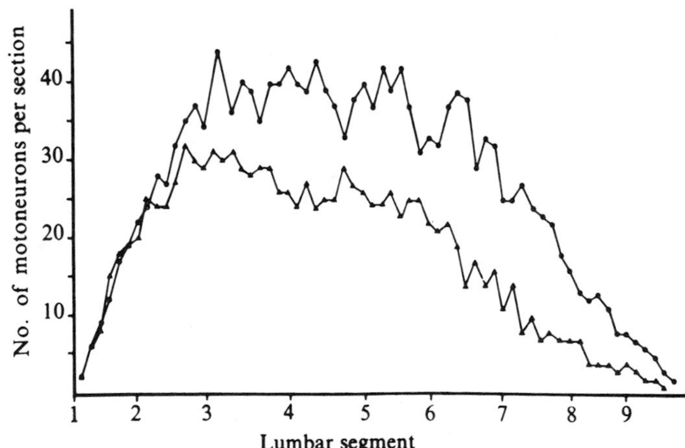

Figure 2. Motoneuron counts in the right lateral motor column in lumbar segments 1–9 of 16-day control (triangles) and curare-treated (circles) chick embryos. Counts for every 10th section represented. Note the increased cell number in segments 3–9 for curare-treated embryos. Motoneuron distribution after botulinum toxin treatment is basically the same as that after curare. (From Pittman and Oppenheim.[37])

(see Chapter 10). Accordingly, in the present studies the drug treatment may have increased survival by enabling synapses to be formed by neurons that would not otherwise have done so.

The results can also be explained by neuronal dependence on a trophic factor supplied by the target tissue. The factor might be transferred to neurons only at points of synaptic contact. Alternatively, synaptic transmission might normally serve to down-regulate the levels of factor produced by the target. The drug treatment would then cause abnormally high levels of factor to be available for neurons.

Two main hypotheses have emerged concerning the function of target regulation of neuronal survival. The first argues that such regulation acts as an economical mechanism for insuring that each target cell becomes innervated. One might debate, however, the economy of a mechanism that results in the destruction of over half of the neurons initially present. The second proposal is that the regulation contributes to synaptic specificity and removes inappropriate synaptic connections.[44] Available evidence does not support the latter possibility, at least with respect to whole target tissues. Thus motoneurons appear to project to the appropriate target muscles even before the period of cell death.[45–47] Furthermore, neurons which are rescued from cell death by chronic pharmacological blockade of synaptic input to the target tissue appear to extend axons to the same targets as do neurons which normally survive the die-off period.[9,40] However, cell death does remove the few neurons in the isthmo-optic nucleus of the chick that have aberrant locations or connections.[36] It is also conceivable that cell death influences the specificity of synaptic connections within a particular target, e.g., to produce a smooth topographic correlation between neurons and target cells.[9] To understand the function of cell death in the formation of the nervous system, it will very likely be necessary to know much more about its mechanism and regulation.

3. NERVE GROWTH FACTOR

The only identified component which appears to act as a trophic factor for regulating neuronal survival is NGF. It was discovered when a mouse sarcoma transplanted into a chick embryo was found to release a diffusable agent that dramatically increased the size of sympathetic and spinal ganglia.[48–50] It was subsequently identified as NGF and was found to be present in a number of tissues including snake venom and the submaxillary glands of male mice, where it is stored in high concentrations. NGF has been purified to homogeneity[51–53] and can be isolated either in a 7S complex with a molecular weight of about 140,000 and three kinds of subunits, or in a 2.5S form. The NGF activity of the 7S form is associated with the β subunit, which is a dimer composed of two polypeptide chains, each having a molecular weight of 13,259. The 2.5S form of NGF is identical with the β subunit except for the absence of nine amino acids from one of the two polypeptide chains.[7,54]

The significance of NGF for neuronal development was appreciated early on when it was found that injection of anti-NGF antiserum into neonatal mice resulted in the selective destruction of the sympathetic nervous system.[55,56] Though the antiserum did not induce comparable changes in sensory ganglia, it has been found in rat that anti-NGF antiserum blocks the development of a subpopulation of DRG neurons containing substance P.[57] DRG neurons are clearly sensitive to NGF: the most common bioassay for NGF activity relies on NGF-induced extension of neurites from DRG explants in culture. Furthermore, DRG axons have been shown to respond chemotactically to the component: when confronted with a gradient of NGF, they turn toward the NGF source[58,59] (see Chapter 6).

NGF displays many of the properties predictable for a target-derived trophic factor that acts on sympathetic and DRG neurons. It is necessary for the survival and development of sympathetic and DRG neurons in dissociated cell culture.[60,61] Sympathetic neurons can be maintained in cell culture by NGF even when it is supplied exclusively to the neurite terminals.[62] *In vivo* NGF can be taken up with a high degree of specificity by nerve terminals of sympathetic and DRG neurons and transported in a retrograde manner to the cell soma; other types of neurons do not accumulate NGF in this fashion.[63–65] Systemic application of NGF increases the survival of sympathetic[66] and DRG neurons[67] during normal development *in vivo*. Degenerative changes in the ganglion after postganglionic axotomy can be prevented or reversed by administration of NGF.[64,68–70] A nice example is provided by the studies of Purves and his collaborators, who showed that postganglionic axotomy of the superior cervical ganglion in adult guinea pig causes depression of synaptic transmission and loss of synaptic contacts on the ganglionic neurons.[71,72] Anti-NGF antiserum administered systemically mimics the effects of axotomy, while chronic application of NGF in pellet form partially reverses the effects.

Finally, if target tissues supply NGF as a trophic factor to sustain sympathetic and DRG neurons then NGF should at least be present in, though not necessarily confined to, the tissues innervated by those neurons. Although early results with immunological assays suggested that NGF was widespread among vertebrate tissues, a better appreciation for the complexities of the immunological assay has led to the disturbing conclusion that NGF is currently undetectable in many peripheral tissues.[7] The high concentrations of NGF found in some tissues such as male mouse salivary gland remain a physiological mystery.

A possible resolution to the question of why the targets appear to lack NGF comes from a recent report by Ebendal *et al.*[73] They found that normal rat iris tissue lacked NGF activity, but when the iris was transferred to organ culture or denervated *in vivo,* it quickly developed NGF activity. These results suggest that innervation may regulate the levels of trophic factor produced by the target tissue. In addition to being economical, such regulation might serve to maintain factor output at the minimum level necessary to sustain the innervation while being inadequate to attract or maintain additional innervation. Further studies on the distribution of NGF and its regulation by cell–cell interactions will likely be very important for models proposing NGF as a trophic factor. The properties of NGF have been extensively reviewed recently.[3–5,7,8]

4. PARASYMPATHETIC NEURONS

Chick ciliary ganglion neurons in culture have recently become a promising system for identifying target-derived trophic factors that act on parasympathetic neurons (see Chapter 3 for another interesting use of this system). Several assays have been used to characterize active components in tissue extracts and culture media conditioned by non-neuronal cells that influence the neurons. Neurite extension, short- and long-term neuronal survival, and growth and development of neurons can all be measured by assays similar to those performed previously with sympathetic and sensory neurons, which led to the purification and characterization of NGF. Current application of these different assays to ciliary ganglion neurons, however, suggests that more than one kind of factor exists and that the factors have different effects on parasympathetic neurons.

4.1. *Neurite Extension*

Helfand *et al.*[74] first showed that chick ciliary ganglion neurons could be grown in dissociated cell culture. By using a culture substratum coated with polyornithine and a culture medium conditioned by heart cells, they found that 10–15% of the neurons initially present in the ganglion could survive in cell culture for 24 hr and could extend neurites under such conditions. The material in the conditioned medium responsible for the survival and neurite extension was clearly different from NGF: purified NGF did not substitute for the conditioned medium, anti-NGF antiserum did not block the effect of the conditioned medium, and the conditioned medium contained little if any NGF, as judged by its ability to compete for NGF binding sites on sensory ganglion cells.[75]

Collins[76–78] extended the observations of Helfand and co-workers on neurite extension. He found that an active component in heart-conditioned medium (HCM) could absorb to the polyornithine and that it probably stimulated neurite extension by modifying the culture substratum.[76,79] The absorbed material acted very rapidly, causing most ciliary ganglion neurons in such cultures to initiate an axon within the first hour. The absorbed material was not adequate to sustain neuronal survival: neuronal degeneration was widespread after 12–15 hr when neurons were grown in unconditioned medium on a polyornithine substrate previously absorbed with the neurite factor. These observations may also account for a previous report that the active component(s) in HCM could not be absorbed to the polyornithine substrate[74]; presumably the authors did not look for such a rapid response.

Similar results have been obtained by Varon and his collaborators. They also found that HCM contained a component that stimulates neurite extension by ciliary ganglion neurons in culture, and that the component could be absorbed to polyornithine substrata.[80] They termed the component neurite-promoting factor (NPF). A wide range of cell types can produce material with the properties of NPF in cell culture,[81] including apparently the ciliary ganglion itself when maintained in culture as an explant.[82] Moreover, NPF-like material from several representative sources was found to induce neurites from a number of neuronal populations of peripheral origin, including parasympathetic, sympathetic, and sensory ganglia, but was ineffective on most neurons tested from the CNS.

Ebendal[83] has described an activity released from embryonic chick heart tissue in explant culture that stimulates the growth of neurites from chick ciliary, sympathetic, sensory, and Remak ganglia in explant culture. Assayed on ciliary ganglia, the material cannot be replaced with mouse NGF and is not inactivated by anti-mouse NGF antiserum. Gel filtration studies with heart tissue extracts indicated that the material responsible for eliciting neurite extension had an approximate molecular weight of 40,000.[84]

It is not yet clear whether a family of active components is revealed by these studies or whether different cell types produce the same component that induces neurite extension. It has been suggested that factors such as NPF, secreted by a variety of cell types, might construct extracellular matrices guiding neurites to their proper destinations.[79,82,83] The significance of such components for neuronal development, however, is difficult to evaluate based solely on *in vitro* studies. For example, NPF is apparently ineffective on a collagen substratum in culture[80] even though ciliary ganglion neurons can extend neurites and survive on collagen.

4.2. *Neuronal Survival*

Nishi and Berg[85] first demonstrated that all of the neurons present in embryonic ciliary ganglia, including neurons that would die *in vivo*, could survive and develop in cell culture when grown under proper conditions. Dissociated neurons were prepared from 8-day embryonic chick ciliary ganglia, just prior to the initiation of the die-off period *in vivo*. The neurons were grown either with skeletal myotubes[85] or alone on a collagen-coated substratum with culture medium conditioned by heart cells and supplemented with chick embryo extract.[86] In both kinds of cultures about 7000 surviving neurons were obtained per ganglion used to prepare the initial cell suspension. No significant decrease in the number of surviving neurons was observed over a 2-week period in culture (Fig. 3a). Autoradiographic experiments with [^{3}H]thymidine labeling excluded the possibility that neuronal cell division had occurred.[87] Since the ciliary ganglion in 8-day chick embryos only contains about 7000 neurons,[24] it was possible to conclude that both the choroid and the ciliary neuron populations from the ganglion must have survived in cell culture. Furthermore, the neurons (ca. 50%) in each population which would have died *in vivo* between embryonic days 8 and 14 were rescued by the culture conditions. Similar results have been obtained by Tuttle *et al.*,[88] who found that all of the neurons could survive for weeks in cell culture on collagen-coated substrata with culture medium containing chick embryo extract.

These observations raised the possibility that the enriched culture medium contained components derived from the target tissue of parasympathetic neurons that were required for survival of the neurons *in vivo*, where the components would normally be present only in limiting amounts. Alternatively, the abnormally high level of neuronal survival in cell culture might have reflected a "maintenance" of the neurons in a premature state, i.e., a state characteristic of neurons in ciliary ganglia prior to the die-off period when they have not yet developed a dependence on information from the target tissue. To assess this possibility, several aspects of neuronal development were examined.

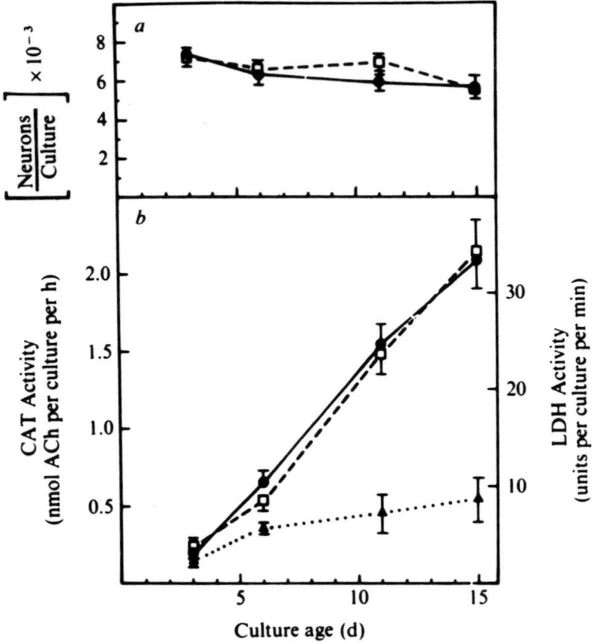

Figure 3. Survival and development of ciliary ganglion neurons in culture. Ciliary ganglion neurons from 8-day-old embryos were grown either with skeletal mytotubes or alone with HCM. At the indicated times, cultures were counted for neurons and assayed for CAT and LDH activity. Each point represents the mean ± S.E. for 7–10 cultures taken from two to five different cell platings. Neurons grown alone are indicated by the open squares; neurons grown with myotubes, the filled circles; LDH activity for neurons grown alone, the filled triangles. (From Nishi and Berg.[86])

Choline acetyltransferase (CAT) activity and high-affinity choline uptake were measured as properties of cholinergic development. Levels of CAT activity increased substantially during the 2-week period in culture for ciliary ganglion neurons grown either alone or with skeletal myotubes (Fig. 3b). The increases in CAT levels reflected specific development since they were much larger than the net growth of the neurons during the same period. Net growth was estimated by following the levels of lactate dehydrogenase (LDH), a common cytoplasmic enzyme. At the end of the 2-week period, the amount of CAT activity per neuron was substantially larger[86] than that estimated for ciliary ganglion neurons at the end of the die-off period *in vivo*.[89] Tuttle *et al.*[88] also observed a large increase in CAT levels for ciliary ganglion neurons grown in cell culture. The neurons express a sodium-dependent high-affinity uptake mechanism for choline in cell culture[90] as they do *in vivo*.[91] The high-affinity uptake mechanism can be used to label the neurons with [^{3}H]choline metabolites and then can be combined with autoradiographic procedures to demonstrate that most, if not all of the neurons, have acquired the uptake mechanism for choline[90] (Fig. 4).

When grown with skeletal myotubes, ciliary ganglion neurons readily formed functional cholinergic synapses on the muscle.[85] Stimulation of a neuron with an extracellular electrode elicited postsynaptic potentials in a nearby myotube that could be detected with intracellular recording (Fig. 5). The elicited responses represented cholinergic synaptic transmission since they could be reversibly abolished in the presence of 50 μg/ml *d*-tubocurarine. Intracellular stimulation of presynaptic neurons often evoked postsynaptic responses adequate to stimulate action potentials in the post synaptic muscle cell.[85] Using this procedure it was possible to estimate that at least 70% of the neurons had innervated at least one myotube when examined at 1–2 weeks in culture.[85] Recently evidence has also been obtained for cholinergic synaptic transmission between ciliary ganglion neurons either grown alone or with myotubes in culture, indicating that the neurons can innervate each other under these conditions.[92,93]

The studies on cholinergic development and synapse formation by the neurons suggest that they can progress beyond developmental stages which *in vivo* characterize the die-off period. This, together with the fact that all of the neurons initially present in the ganglion can exhibit long-term survival in cell culture, provides some assurance that

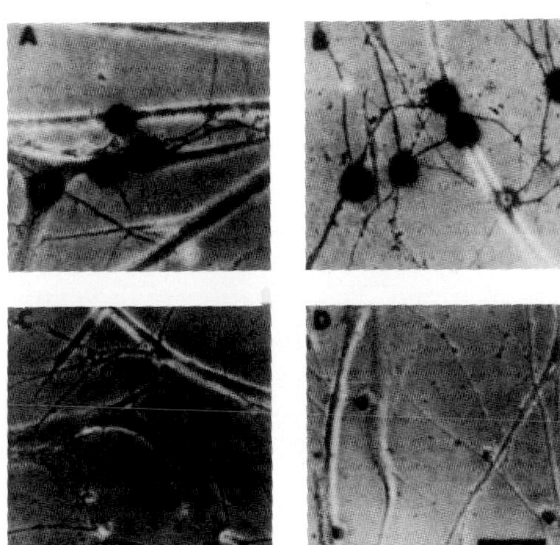

Figure 4. Choline labeling in ciliary ganglion neuron–myotube cultures. Eight-day-old cultures were incubated for 1 hr in 1 μM [^{3}H]choline, "chased" for 30 min in 1 mM choline, and processed for autoradiography. (A) Standard conditions showing labeled neurons. (B) Labeled neurons plus one very lightly labeled neuron. Less than 1% of the neurons fell in this latter category. (C) Addition of 10 μM hemicholinium-3. (D) Replacement of Na^+ by Li^+. Calibration bar: 75 μm. (From Barald and Berg.[90])

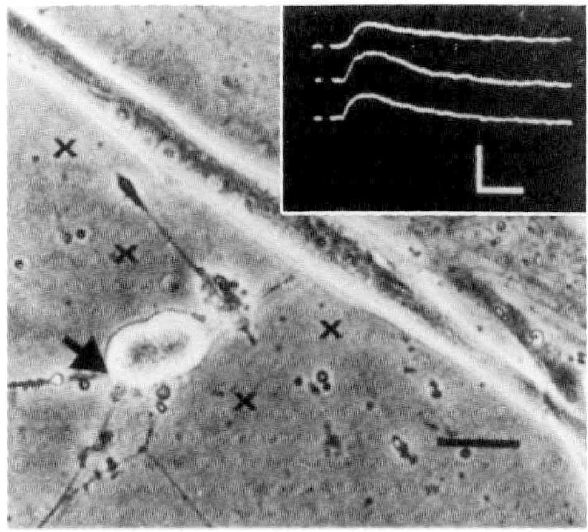

Figure 5. Synaptic potentials in a muscle evoked by extracellular stimulation of a ciliary ganglion neuron. Two closely associated neurons are shown, at least one of which extends a process to the muscle fiber. Stimulation with an extracellular electrode at the point indicated by the arrow repeatedly elicited synaptic potentials in the muscle cell. No responses were obtained when stimulation was applied at the points indicated by X. The neurons, prepared from 8-day embryos, had been maintained in culture for 8 days. Calibration bar: 30 μm. Inset: Oscilloscope tracings of repeated synaptic potentials evoked in the muscle cell. The break in the traces indicates the stimulus artifact. Muscle resting potential: –70 mV. Calibration bars: vertical, 4 mV; horizontal, 10 msec. (From Nishi and Berg.[85])

the culture system can be used to identify components required by parasympathetic neurons for survival and development *in vivo.*

Several laboratories have used a short-term assay to characterize the components in conditioned media and in tissue extracts that enhance the survival of ciliary ganglion neurons in dissociated cell culture. The number of surviving neurons is usually determined after a 24 hr period in the medium to be tested.[94] With this assay it was found that soluble extracts prepared from embryonic chick eye tissue had much higher levels of activity than did extracts from other chick tissues.[94] The activity appeared to be developmentally regulated in the eye in that it increased more rapidly with embryonic age than did the total amount of protein recovered in the extract.[95] Efforts to purify the active material using the short-term assay, however, yielded mixed results: about 85% of the activity was lost when the eye extract was concentrated by Amicon filtration and fractionated by gel filtration; no increase in specific activity was obtained. Fractionation of the extract by ion exchange chromatography on DEAE-cellulose combined with Amicon filtration produced a fourfold increase in the specific activity of the recovered material with a 50% loss of total activity. The gel filtration studies indicated an apparent molecular weight for the active material in crude extracts of about 40,000.[96]

Using the short-term assay for neuronal survival, Bonyhady *et al.*[97] have identified active components in extracts of ox cardiac muscle. Gel filtration studies suggested an apparent molecular weight of about 20,000 for one of the components. Additional fractionation of the extract was limited by poor recoveries of the active components. The short-term assay was also used to identify activities in conditioned media obtained from heart and skeletal muscle cultures that stimulated neuronal survival, but purification of the actitivies was not reported.[80,98]

The short-term assay has the obvious advantage of being quick. Its disadvantage is that it may not be specific. Components which serve only to promote adhesion of the neurons to the culture substratum or which temporarily "buffer" the neurons against a hostile environment in culture would score as trophic factors in the short-term assay. Accordingly, as with the neurite extension factors, it will be necessary to examine the role of such components *in vivo* in order to assess their significance for neuronal development. This requirement holds, of course, for any putative trophic factor identified and purified by an *in vitro* assay, but it becomes especially important when the original assay is relatively nonspecific. At present the best evidence for the biological significance of active components revealed by the short-term assay is that extracts prepared from eye tissue, which contain all of the normal synaptic targets of the neurons, have the highest levels of activity.[94]

4.3. *Regulation of Long-Term Development*

Recently a different culture approach has been taken to identify target-derived trophic factors that regulate survival and development of ciliary ganglion neurons.[99] In this case, control conditions were first established to permit the long-term maintenance of the neurons in the absence of tissue extracts or conditioned media. Neurons in the control conditions were used to define "basal levels" of growth and development over the test period. Trophic factors were then sought by testing extracts prepared from embryonic eye tissue for activities which stimulated growth and development beyond the basal levels. This approach lessened the chances of mistakenly isolating components which did not influence neuronal survival *in vivo,* but only compensated for some negative feature of the initial culture procedure, such as facilitating neuronal repair after dissociation of the ganglia to produce the original cell suspension, permitting adhesion of the neurons to the culture substratum, or counteracting toxic materials present in the basic culture medium.

Two modifications of the culture procedure permitted long-term maintenance of the neurons without extracts or conditioned media. The first was the use of fibroblast material to coat the collagen substratum.

Nonneuronal cells have previously been shown to produce microexudate material in culture which remains firmly attached to the culture surface and increases the adhesion of neurons and neuronal processes to the substratum.[100,101] Accordingly, fibroblasts were grown to confluency and then lysed and removed with distilled water before adding the neurons. The second modification was the addition of KCl to the culture medium to increase the concentration of K^+ to 25 mM. Elevated K^+ concentrations have been found to enhance survival and development for a number of neuronal populations in culture.[102–106] The combination of these two conditions permitted the survival of nearly all of the neurons present in the ganglion for a period of at least 3 weeks in cell culture.[99] Neuron size showed little change over the 3-week period, and CAT levels remained low.

The mechanism by which the modified conditions permit long-term maintenance is unclear. Possibly the fibroblasts provide a threshold level of a required trophic factor.[78,80,81,101] Alternatively, the conditions may simply enhance attachment of neurons to the substratum while maintaining them in a relatively immature state. In any case, the conditions provide a useful control for identifying components which stimulate neuronal growth and development.

Eye tissue was chosen as a potential source of stimulatory factors because it includes all of the normal synaptic target tissues for ciliary ganglion neurons. Extracts prepared from embryonic eye tissue produced a substantial increase in the development of CAT activity compared with control conditions (Fig. 6). Titration experiments over an 11-day test period indicated that the extract also stimulated general neuronal growth, as reflected by increased levels of LDH activity (Fig. 7).

Fractionation of the eye extract by gel filtration through a P200 column resolved two stimulatory components which had different effects on the neurons (Fig. 8). One component, with an apparent molecular weight of about 20,000, stimulated neuronal growth, as indicated by increased LDH levels, higher rates of protein synthesis, and larger neuronal somata size.[99] The material, referred to as growth-promoting activity (GPA), had no effect on the levels of CAT activity per neuron. The second component, with an apparent molecular weight of about 50,000, stimulated cholinergic development, as reflected by increased levels of CAT activity per neuron, but had no effect on neuronal growth. The second component was referred to as CAT-stimulating activity (CSA). Small and variable amounts of GPA and CSA-like material were also recovered in the excluded volume of the column, perhaps representing aggregated material, while a small amount of CSA-like material was sometimes recovered in the completely included volume of the

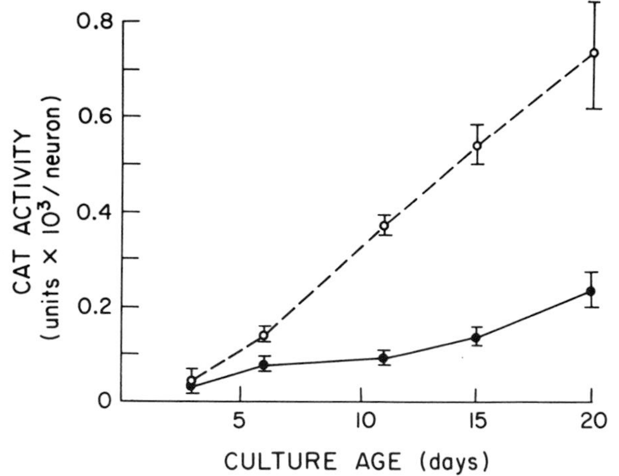

Figure 6. Stimulation of CAT levels per neuron by eye extract. Ciliary ganglion neurons were grown on substrata coated with fibroblast material and fed with simple medium containing 25 mM K^+ (basal conditions) (filled circles) or the same medium supplemented with 5% (vol/vol) eye extract (open circles). Cell counts and CAT assays were performed on the same cultures. Values represent the mean of 4–18 cultures pooled from three to nine experiments; bars indicate the S.E. (From Nishi and Berg.[99])

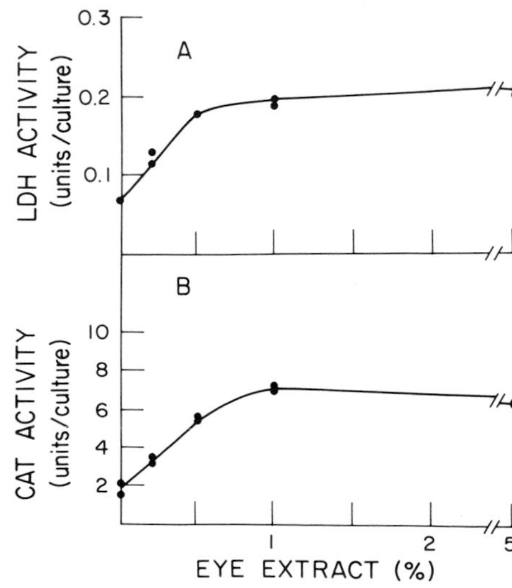

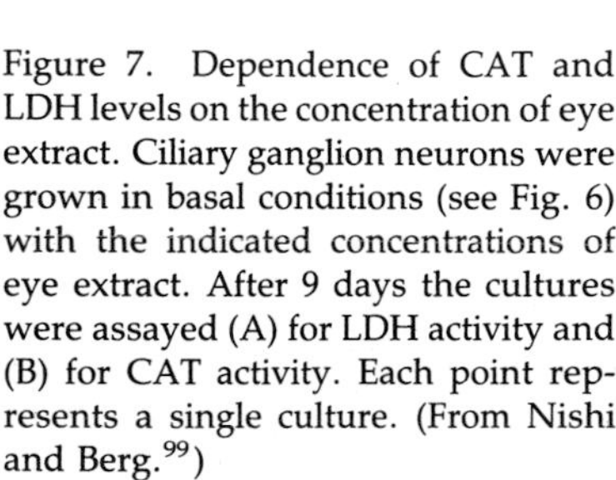
Figure 7. Dependence of CAT and LDH levels on the concentration of eye extract. Ciliary ganglion neurons were grown in basal conditions (see Fig. 6) with the indicated concentrations of eye extract. After 9 days the cultures were assayed (A) for LDH activity and (B) for CAT activity. Each point represents a single culture. (From Nishi and Berg.[99])

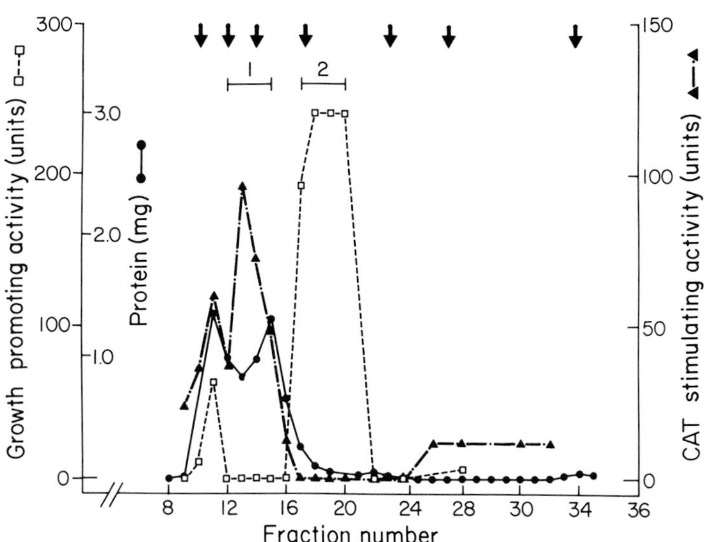

Figure 8. Fractionation of eye extract by gel filtration. Embryonic chick extract (3 ml) was applied to a Bio Gel P200 column (105 ml; 1.8 × 35 cm) equilibrated with phosphate-buffered saline solution at 4°C. Fractions (3 ml) were collected, measured for protein, and tested for effects on ciliary ganglion neurons by growing cultures in basal conditions supplemented with diluted aliquots from the fractions, and then assaying the cultures for LDH activity, CAT activity, and the number of surviving neurons. To calculate units of stimulatory activity, cultures were also grown in a range of eye extract concentrations (0.5% vol/vol) and assayed for CAT and LDH activities to construct a "dose–response" curve. Column fraction dilutions were chosen to yield responses estimated to be in the linear range of the assay; actual volumes assayed were the same in all cases. A unit of GPA was defined as the amount of stimulation necessary to produce half the maximum increment in LDH levels caused by eye extract; a unit of CSA was defined in the same way with respect to CAT levels. The horizontal bars indicate fractions pooled for CSA (Pool 1) and GPA (Pool 2). The arrows from left to right indicate the elution positions for blue dextran (200,000), human transferin (80,000), ovalbumin (40,000), soybean trypsin inhibitor (26,000), cytochrome c (13,500), α-bungarotoxin (8000), and [^{3}H]choline chloride (140). The elution position of blue dextran marks the void volume of the column, while [^{3}H]choline chloride indicates the completely included volume. (From Nishi and Berg.[99])

column as well (Fig. 8). Total recoveries of GPA and CSA from the column were quite good (ca. 75%) and paralleled recovery of total protein from the column.

GPA was able to drive the neurons to the same maximum rate of growth as that induced by unfractionated eye extract, suggesting that no other components in the extract were necessary for the effect (Fig. 9). GPA had no effect on CAT levels per neuron under these conditions. A different pattern emerged with CSA. CSA stimulated development

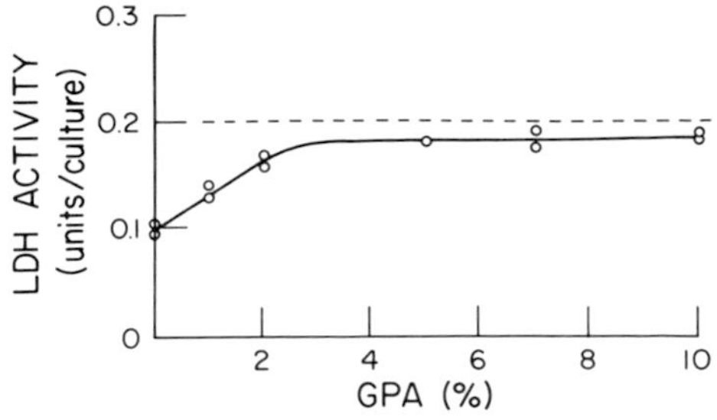

Figure 9. Dependence of LDH levels on GPA concentration. Ciliary ganglion neurons were grown in basal conditions with the indicated concentrations (vol/vol) of GPA (Pool 2, Fig. 8) for 9 days and then assayed for LDH activity. Each point represents a single culture. The dotted line indicates the level of LDH activity obtained with 5% (vol/vol) eye extract. Cultures receiving 0 and 10% GPA were also assayed for CAT activity and were found to have equivalent amounts. (From Nishi and Berg.[99])

of CAT activity, but not to the same extent as did eye extract (Fig. 10). The reason for this was suggested by an examination of the cultures: neurons grown in CSA without GPA were much smaller than neurons grown in eye extract. Presumably the response of the neurons to CSA was restricted by their reduced overall capacity. This was demonstrated by comparing the levels of CAT-specific activity (CAT/LDH) for neurons grown in CSA, GPA, and the two together (Table I). While CSA alone promotes the highest level of CAT-specific activity, GPA clearly has a permissive effect with respect to CAT induction: GPA allows higher levels of CAT total activity to be achieved in CSA, even though the resulting specific activity is lower than for CSA alone because of the increased neuronal size caused by the GPA.

The effects of GPA and CSA on neurons were usually tested in culture conditions with elevated K^+ levels. The high K^+ concentrations were not necessary, however, for the effects of either GPA or CSA. Each component produced a significant stimulation even in culture medium with normal levels of K^+ (5.6 mM) when compared to the high K^+

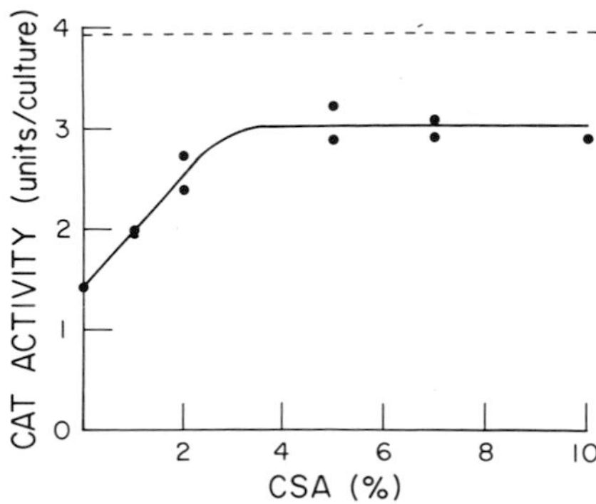

Figure 10. Dependence of CAT levels on CSA concentration. Ciliary ganglion neurons were grown in basal conditions with the indicated concentrations (vol/vol) of CSA (Pool 1, Fig. 8) for 9 days and then assayed for CAT activity. Each point represents a single culture. The dotted line indicates the level of CAT activity obtained with 5% (vol/vol) eye extract. Cultures receiving 0 and 10% CSA were also assayed for LDH activity and were found to have equivalent amounts. (From Nishi and Berg.[99])

Table I. Effects of GPA and CSA on Specific Activities of CAT[a]

Supplement	CAT activity (units)	LDH activity (units)	Specific activity (CAT/LDH)
Eye extract	6.65	0.205	32.4
	6.30	0.192	32.8
GPA	1.97	0.170	11.6
	2.51	0.182	13.8
CSA	3.07	0.047	65.3
	3.91	0.050	78.2
GPA + CSA	5.57	0.172	32.4
	6.50	0.182	35.7
	6.70	0.190	35.3

[a] Neurons were grown for 9 days in basal conditions with the indicated supplements at 5% (vol/vol). CAT and LDH activities were measured on the same cultures and are shown as total units per culture. Values represent individual cultures from the same experiment.

control conditions.[99] NGF (0.15 μg/ml) was unable to substitute for either GPA or CSA.

The results obtained with GPA and CSA on ciliary ganglion neurons suggest an interesting parallel to the much better understood system provided by sympathetic neurons. Studies with rat superior cervical gangion neurons demonstrate that NGF stimulates survival and growth of the neurons but does not influence the choice of neurotransmitter to be synthesized.[107,108] A different component, present in culture medium conditioned by various types of nonneuronal cells, induces the neurons to undergo cholingeric development instead of the normal noradrenergic development.[109] Conceivably, GPA and CSA play similar roles for parasympathetic neurons, though too little is known about their mechanisms of action and their specificities to allow further comparison at present.

One curious feature of GPA action is that it stimulates overall neuronal growth, as reflected in LDH levels, rates of protein synthesis, and soma volume, but does not increase levels of CAT activity per neuron. It is possible that in the absence of CSA, the expression of CAT activity by the neurons is limited by a step that is not influenced by GPA. Alternatively, CAT activity in the absence of CSA may be confined to a subpopulation of neurons that is not responsive to GPA.

The results summarized in this section represent a first step toward characterizing the effects of GPA and CSA. It will be important to purify the activities to determine how many components are involved, which tissues produce the components, and which neuronal populations respond to them. Information of this kind should help clarify the significance of these components for neuronal development *in vivo*, and indicate whether they are in fact target-derived trophic factors which play a role in neuronal survival.

5. OTHER GANGLIONIC NEURONS

Though NGF may serve as a trophic factor for sympathetic and DRG neurons, an increasing body of evidence indicates that other components can also act as trophic agents for these neurons. A number of studies have described trophic activities in a variety of tissue extracts and conditioned culture media that can stimulate neurite extension or neuronal survival for DRG or sympathetic neurons in culture.[81,83,84,110–118]

Several lines of evidence suggest that these more recently identified components are different from NGF. In most studies anti-NGF antiserum was used to demonstrate that the trophic activity of the component was not blocked by the antiserum. Though useful as a test, the immunological approach by itself is not wholly convincing in cases where the putative trophic factor and the NGF against which the antiserum was raised were obtained from different species. As Harper and Thoenen[7] point out, NGFs from different species may have very different crossreactivities with an antiserum. Another line of evidence differentiating newly studied trophic activities from NGF is the demonstration of a difference in neuronal responses, as seen, for example, in the rate or extent of neurite elongation.[117,118] Perhaps most convincing are experiments in which the trophic activities are shown to be additive with the effects of NGF or in which the activities affect neurons that are insensitive to NGF.

Thoenen and his collaborators have carried out an interesting series of experiments on factors governing the survival and development of DRG neurons. They demonstrated that culture medium conditioned by the glioma cell line C-6 (GCM) permits the survival of DRG neurons in dissociated cell culture that would not have survived when supplied with NGF alone.[111–112] When cultures are prepared with DRG neurons from 8- or 10-day-old chick embryos, nearly all of the neurons present survive through the 48-hr test period in the combined presence of NGF and GCM. Many fewer neurons live this long in cultures supplied with either NGF or GCM alone; furthermore, the sum of the surviving neurons in NGF cultures and GCM cultures is substantially less than in cultures supplied with both NGF and GCM. Apparently some fraction of the neurons initially requires both sources of trophic activity. Few DRG neurons prepared from older embryos, e.g., day 16, survive when applied only with NGF, but nearly all survive in the presence of GCM. Rat brain extract can substitute for the GCM. These observations not only suggest that the active components in GCM and rat brain extract are clearly different from NGF, but also indicate that either DRG neurons express changing trophic requirements during development or the ganglion includes neuronal subpopulations with requirements for different trophic factors. These results are not in conflict with the findings of Hamburger *et al.*,[67] who showed that repeated injections of NGF prolonged the survival of many ventrolateral cells and nearly all dorsomedial cells that would have died in thoracic spinal ganglion 18 and brachial spinal ganglion 15 of young chick embryos. Some neurons degenerated in each population even with the NGF injections, and substantial numbers of ventrolateral neurons degenerated at late times. Though these experiments have provided the first evidence that ventrolateral neurons are responsive to NGF *in vivo*, they also leave open the possibility that some DRG neurons respond to other factors as well, especially at later times during development.

Sympathetic neurons also appear to be responsive to several kinds of factors in cell culture. NGF, GCM, and chick HCM were compared for their effects on the survival and development of chick sympathetic neurons in dissociated cell culture.[113] The effects of saturating amounts of NGF, GCM, and HCM on survival of neurons prepared from 12-day chick embryos were roughly additive, suggesting that they acted on different neuronal subpopulations. By examining neuronal survival from different age embryos, it was found that the responses of the total population in culture appeared to change (Fig. 11). NGF and GCM each permitted the survival of over a third of the neurons from 12-day embryos while HCM supported about 5%. NGF supported about a third of the neurons from 14-day embryos, GCM over half, and HCM about 10%. For neurons from 18-day embryos NGF had little effect, while GCM permitted survival of about 40% and HCM supported over half of the neurons. It remains to be determined whether the neurons change their requirements for trophic factors during development (e.g., neurons requiring NGF at first become dependent on HCM instead later) or whether different subpopulations of neurons are being rescued by the different agents in culture. A difference in the effects of NGF and HCM was also indicated by assays of CAT and tyrosine hydroxylase (TH) activity in the cultures. Cultures of sympathetic neurons from 12-day

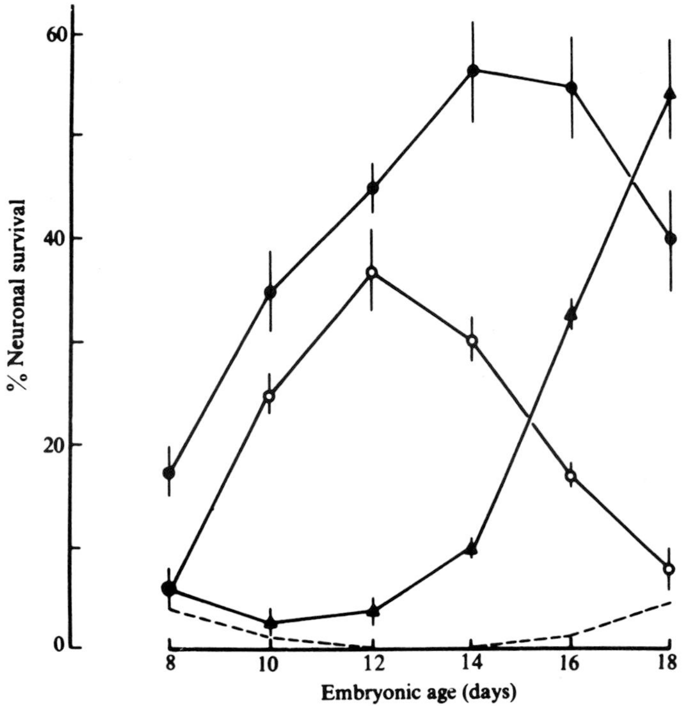

Figure 11. Different requirements for survival factors by subpopulations of chick sympathetic neurons. Neurons were dissociated from paravertebral sympathetic ganglia taken from chicks of embryonic ages shown. After preplating, 5000–8000 neurons were plated on poly-DL-ornithine. Neuronal survival was estimated between days 2 and 5 after the start of culture, and it was confirmed that the percentage of neuronal survival did not decrease significantly on two subsequent days. The dashed line shows the low basal levels of neuronal survival without added factors. The increased neuronal survival seen in control cultures of neurons from 8- and 18-day-old chicks is a consequence of the slower death rate of the younger cells, and of the presence of more nonneuronal cells which support neurons in the cultures from older embryos. Parallel cultures were set up with supplements of: 5 ng/ml NGF (open circles), GCM plus 500 ng/ml NGF antibodies (filled circles), and HCM plus 500 ng/ml NGF antibodies (filled triangles). Results are expressed as percentages of surviving neurons ± S.E. (n = 3). (From Edgar *et al.*[113])

embryos had low levels of CAT activity and high levels of TH activity (CAT/TH = 0.36) when maintained with NGF for 48 hr. Cultures receiving HCM had high levels of CAT and low levels of TH (CAT/TH = 6.07), while CAT and TH levels in cultures receiving both agents were nearly additive. Again, a significant question raised by these studies is whether NGF and HCM select for the survival of different subpopulations of sympathetic neurons in culture or whether they induce different enzyme patterns.[113]

Coughlin *et al.*[117] have examined the effects of a partially purified component from mouse HCM on the extension of neurites and the development of CAT and TH activities by mouse sympathetic ganglion explants in culture. HCM was fractionated by stepwise elution from a DEAE-Bio Gel A column and then concentrated by ultrafiltration through a PTHK millipore filter with an exclusion limit of 10^5 daltons. The recovered material stimulated the rapid extension of neurites by sympathetic ganglia. It also caused a major increase in TH activity, a small increase in CAT activity, and no change in total protein associated with the ganglia over a 4-day period. The partially purified material enhanced the survival of mouse submandibular neurons, mouse nodose neurons, and chick DRG neurons in dissociated cell culture as well, but it had little effect, if any, on mouse DRG neurons. A quite different pattern of survival among the same populations was obtained with NGF. The fractionated material was inactivated by trypsin or by boiling for 5 min but was not significantly affected by incubation at 60° for 30 min. Further fractionation of the material will be necessary to determine whether a single component acts both on sympathetic and on parasympathetic and sensory neurons, or whether the partially purified material contains a number of components, each specific for a different neuronal population.

These studies provide promising leads in the identification of new trophic factors for ganglionic neurons. It seem likely that the survival and development of individual neuronal populations are guided by the interplay of a number of such components rather than by a single target-derived factor.

6. CNS NEURONS

6.1. *Spinal Cord Neurons*

Survival and development of motoneurons in the spinal cord *in vivo* are clearly dependent on interactions with the periphery. Giller *et al.*[119] examined the effects of muscle cells on mouse spinal cord neurons in cell culture to determine if the muscle provided components that influenced the fate of motoneurons. CAT activity was measured as a marker for the development of motoneurons since they represent the major known population of cholinergic neurons in the spinal cord. It was found that spinal cord cells grown with muscle produced 10 times as much CAT activity in a 3-week period as did spinal cord cells grown alone. Using silver-staining to identify neurons in the cultures, they concluded that the large difference in CAT levels could not be accounted for by the small difference in neuronal survival between the two kinds of cultures. This, together with other observations, led them to suggest that the muscle stimulated cholinergic development of surviving neurons rather than having increased the "plating efficiency" or long-term survival of cholinergic neurons in culture. This conclusion cannot be held without reservation, however, since it was not possible to distinguish cholinergic neurons from other neuronal populations in the heterogeneous cultures. Neuronal cell counts would not have revealed large differences in small subpopulations.

Later experiments demonstrated that the muscle effect could be communicated through the medium by diffusable factors. Culture medium conditioned by contact with muscle cells stimulated development of CAT activity in spinal cord cultures.[120] No increase was observed for glutamic acid decarboxylase (GAD) activity in spinal cord cells grown with muscle, suggesting that the muscle effect on spinal cord cells might be specific for cholinergic neurons. The muscle effect showed some species specificity: culture medium conditioned by mouse or rat muscle induced high CAT levels, but medium conditioned by chick muscle had no stimulatory effect.[121] Similarly, specificity was found for the responding cell type: muscle-conditioned medium stimulated CAT levels in cell cultures prepared from spinal cord and from medulla but not from midbrain or from cortex. In contrast, little specificity was found for the tissue source of the stimulatory component: enhanced CAT levels were obtained with conditioned media from muscle, heart, kidney, and liver cell cultures. The active component in the conditioned medium was stable to moderate heat (20 min at 58°), was nondialyzable, and was retained by filters having an exclusion limit of 50,000 daltons.[120]

Dribin and Barrett[122] have used rat spinal cord explants to identify a component in muscle-conditioned medium that stimulated the outgrowth of neurites in culture. Some general features of the component were similar to those of the mouse factor that stimulated development of CAT activity in cultures of spinal cord cells. The component was stable to moderate heat (30 min at 58°); it was retained by filters with an exclusion limit of 10,000 daltons; and it was produced and released into the culture medium by a range of cell types including muscle, fibroblast, and lung.

Experiments with chick spinal cord cells in long-term culture failed to reveal a dependence on muscle-derived components for cholinergic development. Levels of CAT activity were only slightly higher in cultures of spinal cord and muscle cells than in cultures of spinal cord cells alone.[123] The relative rates of [^{3}H]acetylcholine synthesis by the intact cells, using [^{3}H]choline as a precursor, were consistent with the relative levels of CAT activity for the two kinds of cultures. Replacing the chick embryo extract in the culture medium by fetal calf serum[119,120] also failed to reveal a significant dependence on muscle-derived components for cholinergic development. Possibly species differences are involved. Chick spinal cord neurons may not require muscle-derived components to undergo the initial states of cholinergic development. Alternatively, chick muscle may release very little stimulatory material into the culture medium,[121] while chick spinal cord cells may produce adequate levels of required components in culture.[123]

6.2. *Identified Populations*

A serious limitation of most CNS culture systems for studying putative trophic factors is that the cultures are usually heterogeneous with respect to cell types. The cultures normally contain a large number of neuronal cell types in addition to several types of nonneuronal cells.[124] Cellular heterogeneity makes it difficult to distinguish trophic effects on neuronal development from those affecting neuronal survival for the subpopulation of interest. Cellular heterogeneity also raises the possibility of cellular interactions mediating the effects of the putative trophic factor.

Two general approaches have been explored for coping with cellular heterogeneity in CNS cultures. The first involves the development of cell-specific markers for distinguishing different neuronal cell types. Initial efforts focused on the types of neurotransmitters characteristic of different neurons. For spinal cord cultures, high-affinity GABA uptake was used to identify a subpopulation of neurons that excluded cholinergic neurons.[125] High-affinity choline uptake was used to distinguish the neuronal population that included cholinergic neurons.[126] Immunohistochemical assays using antibodies prepared against specific neurotransmitter synthesizing enzymes such as CAT[127] and GAD[128,129] have also been used to stain discrete neuronal populations *in situ*. Such procedures may prove useful for distinguishing different neuronal populations in culture as well. Recently monoclonal antibodies directed against cell surface components have been used to distinguish different cellular classes in heterogeneous CNS cultures.[130,131] Monoclonal antibodies specific for subpopulations of neurons are also possible,[132–134] and will provide powerful tools for examining the developmental requirements of neurons in culture. Monoclonal antibodies have already been used to distinguish different neuronal populations during development (see Chapter 3).

Another method of identifying discrete neuronal populations is to label the neurons *in vivo*, prior to transferring them to cell culture. Bennett *et al.*[135] have used retrograde transport of HRP injected into the hind limb of a developing chick embryo to label the motoneurons supplying the muscle. In a preliminary account they report that the labeled neurons can subsequently be identified in cell culture, and that survival of the labeled neurons for a 2-day period in culture requires the presence of skeletal-muscle-conditioned medium. Medium conditioned by smooth muscle or by kidney cells apparently will not substitute.[135] It was not clear whether the dependence on muscle-conditioned medium was unique to the labeled neurons or whether all spinal cord neurons in the cultures displayed a similar dependence.

The second general approach to dealing with CNS heterogeneity in cell culture has been to simplify the cellular composition of the cultures. Cultures enriched in motoneurons have been produced by applying cell fractionation techniques to suspensions of embryonic spinal cord cells[136,137] or by selecting for nondividing cells from very early embryos.[138]

Banker and Cowan[139,140] selected the fetal hippocampus as a source of neurons for study in cell culture, in part because of its simple composition. Pyramidal cells constitute the major neuronal cell type *in vivo* at early times, and careful histological and birth-dating experiments demonstrated that they were the major neuronal cell type present in culture as well. When hippocampal neurons were grown in the presence of hippocampal explants, a substantial fraction of the dissociated neurons (20–30%) survived for a 2-week period.[139] Subsequent work has shown that culture medium conditioned by astroglial cells can support the survival and maintenance of hippocampal neurons in dissociated cell culture.[141]

7. CONCLUSIONS

Recent studies in cell culture have provided evidence for several putative trophic factors in addition to NGF. For ciliary ganglion neurons components have been identified in tissue extracts and in culture media conditioned by nonneuronal cells that stimulate neurite extension, long-term survival, cholinergic development, and overall growth. At least two components are involved, and they appear to be different from NGF. Studies with sympathetic and DRG neurons reveal a similar pattern: several components in addition to NGF stimulate the survival and development of the neurons. Results with spinal cord cells and hippocampal neurons suggest that trophic factors may also be identified for CNS neurons.

The discovery of components which stimulate neuronal survival and development in cell culture represents, of course, only a beginning toward identifying trophic factors. It will be important to purify the factors to compare their properties and determine the range of cell types responsive to individual components. It will also be important to determine which tissues produce the components and under what conditions. Finally, it will be crucial to confirm the effects of the components *in vivo*.

Evidence for the existence of trophic factors should not be allowed to obscure the importance of other events in regulating neuronal survival and development. It would seem likely that in most cases regulation is achieved by the complex interplay of a number of influences such as synaptic input, local tissue interactions, and synapse formation, in addition to diffusible trophic factors from the target tissue.

Acknowledgments

I wish to thank Dr. Ronald Oppenheim for providing me with a copy of his review chapter on cell death in the nervous system[9] prior to publication; it was very useful in preparing the section on neuronal cell death. I also want to thank Dr. Susan Kirkpatrick for editorial comments. Grant support was provided by the National Institutes of Health (NS 12601).

8. REFERENCES

1. Cowan W. M., 1973, Neuronal death as a regulative mechanism in the control of cell number in the nervous system, in: *Development and Aging in the Nervous System* (M. Rockstein, ed.), pp. 19–41, Academic Press, New York.
2. Cowan, W. M. 1978, Aspects of neural development, *Int. Rev. Physiol.* **17**:149.
3. Jacobson, M., 1978, *Developmental Neurobiology*, Plenum Press, New York.
4. Varon, S. S., and Bunge, R. P., 1978, Trophic mechanisms in the peripheral nervous system, *Ann. Rev. Neurosci.* **1**:327.
5. Bradshaw, R. A., 1978, Nerve growth factor, *Ann. Rev. Biochem.* **47**:191.
6. Hamburger, V., 1980, Trophic interactions in neurogenesis: A personal historical account, *Ann. Rev. Neurosci.* **3**:269.
7. Harper, G. P., and Thoenen, H., 1980, Nerve growth factor: Biological significance, measurement, and distribution, *J. Neurochem.* **34**:5.

8. Green, L. A., and Shooter, E. M., 1980, The nerve growth factor: Biochemistry, synthesis, and mechanism of action, *Ann. Rev. Neurosci.* **3**:353.
9. Oppenheim, R. W., 1981, Neuronal cell death and some related regressive phenomena during neurogenesis: A selective historical review and progress report, in: *Studies in Developmental Neurobiology: Essays in Honor of Viktor Hamburger,* (W. M. Cowan, ed.), pp. 74–133, Oxford University Press, New York.
10. Hamburger, V., and Levi-Montalcini, R., 1949, Proliferation, differentiation and degeneration in the spinal ganglia of the chick embryo under normal and experimental conditions, *J. Exp. Zool.* **111**:457.
11. Hughes, A., 1961, Cell degeneration in the larval ventral horn of *Xenopus laevis, J. Embryol. Exp. Morphol.* **9**:269.
12. Levi-Montalcini, R., 1950, The origin and development of the visceral system in the spinal cord of the chick embryo. *J. Morphol.* **86**:253.
13. Harris, A. E., 1969, Differentiation and degeneration in the motor horn of foetal mouse, *J. Morphol.* **129**:281.
14. Bodian, D., 1966, Spontaneous degeneration in the spinal cord of monkey foetuses, *Bull. Johns Hopkins Hosp.* **119**:217.
15. Prestige, M. C., 1965, Cell turnover in the spinal ganglia of *Xenopus laevis* tadpoles, *J. Embryol. Exp. Morphol.* **13**:63.
16. Hughes, A., 1973, The development of dorsal root ganglia and ventral horns in the opossum: A quantitative study, *J. Embryol. Exp. Morphol.* **30**:359.
17. Cowan, W. M., and Wenger, E., 1967, Cell loss in the trochlear nucleus of the chick during normal development and after radical extirpation of the optic vesicle, *J. Exp. Zool.* **164**:265.
18. Cowan, W. M., and Wenger, E., 1968, Degeneration in the nucleus of origin of the preganglionic fibers to the chick ciliary ganglion following early removal of the optic vesicle, *J. Exp. Zool.* **168**:105.
19. Rogers, L. A., and Cowan, W. M., 1973, The development of the mesencephalic nucleus of the trigeminal nerve in the chick. *J. Comp. Neurol.* **147**:291.
20. Dubey, P. N., Kadasane. D. K., and Gosavi, V. S., 1968, The influence of the peripheral field on the morphogenesis of Hofmann's nucleus major of chick spinal cord, *J. Anat.* **102**:407.
21. Cantino, D., and Sisto-Daneo, L., 1972, Cell death in the developing optic tectum, *Brain Res.* **38**:13.
22. Zilles, D., and Wingert, F., 1973, Quantitative studies on the development of the fresh volumes and the number of neurons of the *N. oculomotorii* of white mice during ontogenesis, *Brain Res.* **56**:63.
23. Armstrong, R. C., and Clarke, P. G. H., 1979, Neuronal death and the development of the pontine nuclei and inferior olive in the chick, *Neurosci.* **4**:1635.
24. Landmesser, L., and Pilar, G., 1974, Synaptic transmission and cell death during normal ganglionic development, *J. Physiol.* **241**:737.
25. Prestige, M. C., 1967, The control of cell number in the lumbar ventral horn during the development of *Xenopus laevis* tadpoles, *J. Embryol. Exp. Morphol.* **18**:359.
26. Hamburger, V., 1975, Cell death in the development of the lateral motor column of the chick embryo, *J. Comp. Neurol.* **160**:535.
27. Hollyday, M., and Hamburger, V., 1976, Reduction of the naturally occurring motor neuron loss by enlargement of the periphery, *J. Comp. Neurol.* **170**:311.
28. Narayanan, C. H., and Narayanan, Y., 1978, Neuronal adjustments in developing nuclear centers of the chick embryo following transplantation of an additional optic primordium, *J. Embryol. Exp. Morphol.* **44**:53.

29. Boydston, W. R., and Sohal G. S., 1979, Grafting of additional periphery reduces embryonic loss of neurons, *Brain Res.* **178**:403.
30. Pilar, G., Landmesser, L., and Burstein, L., 1980, Competition for survival among developing ciliary ganglion cells, *J. Neurophysiol.* **43**:233.
31. Lamb, A. H., 1980, Motoneurone counts in *Xenopus* frogs reared with one bilaterally-innervated hindlimb, *Nature (London)* **284**:347.
32. Purves, D., 1980, Neuronal competition, *Nature (London)* **287**:585.
33. Prestige, M. C., and Wilson, M. A., 1972, Loss of axons from ventral roots during development, *Brain Res.* **41**:467.
34. Chu-Wang, I.-W., and Oppenheim, R. W., 1978, Cell death of motoneurons in the chick embryo spinal cord. II. A quantitative and qualitative analysis of degeneration in the ventral root, including evidence for axon outgrowth and limb innervation prior to cell death, *J. Comp. Neurol.* **177**:59.
35. Pilar, G., and Landmesser, L., 1976, Ultrastructural differences during embryonic cell death in normal and peripherally deprived ciliary ganglia, *J. Cell Biol.* **68**:339.
36. Clarke, P. G. H., and Cowan, W. M., 1976, The development of the isthmo-optic tract in the chick, with special reference to the occurrence and correction of developmental errors in the location and connections of isthmo-optic neurons, *J. Comp. Neurol.* **167**:143.
37. Pittman, R., and Oppenheim, R. W., 1978, Neuromuscular blockade increases motoneurone survival during normal cell death in the chick embryo, *Nature (London)* **271**:364.
38. Pittman, R., and Oppenheim, R. W., 1979, Cell death of motoneurons in the chick embryo spinal cord. IV. Evidence that a functional neuromuscular interaction is involved in the regulation of naturally occurring cell death and the stabilization of synapses, *J. Comp. Neurol.* **187**:425.
39. Olek, A. J., 1980, Effects of α and β-bungarotoxin on motor neuron loss in *Xenopus* larvae, *Neurosci.* **5**:1557.
40. Creazzo, T. L., and Sohal, G. S., 1979, Effects of chronic injections of α-bungarotoxin on embryonic cell death, *Exp. Neurol* **66**:135.
41. Jansen, J. D. S., Lømo, T., Nicolaysen, K., and Westgaard, R. H., 1973, Hyperinnervation of skeletal muscle fibers: Dependence on muscle activity, *Science* **181**:559.
42. Jansen, J. K. S., and Van Essen, D. C., 1975, Re-innervation of rat skeletal muscle in the presence of α-bungarotoxin, *J. Physiol.* **250**:651.
43. Cangiano, A., Lømo, T., Lutzemberger, L., and Sveen, O., 1980, Effects of chronic nerve conduction block on formation of neuromuscular junctions and junctional AChE in the rat, *Acta Physiol. Scand.* **109**:283.
44. Hughes, A., 1965, A quantitative study of the development of the nerves in the hind-limb of *Eleutherodactylus martinicensis*, *J. Embryol. Exp. Morphol.* **13**:9.
45. Landmesser, L., and Morris, D. G., 1975, The development of functional innervation in the hind limb of the chick embryo, *J. Physiol.* **249**:301.
46. Landmesser, L., 1978*a*, The distribution of motoneurones supplying chick hind limb muscles, *J. Physiol.* **284**:371.
47. Landmesser, L., 1978*b*, The development of motor projection patterns in the chick hind limb, *J. Physiol.* **284**:391.
48. Bueker, E. D., 1948, Implantation of tumors in the hindlimb field of the embryonic chick and developmental response of the lumbosacral nervous system, *Anat. Rec.* **102**:369.
49. Levi-Montalcini, R., and Hamburger, V., 1951, Selective growth-stimulating effects

of mouse salivary glands on the sympathetic system of mammals, *J. Exp. Zool.* **116:**321.
50. Levi-Montalcini, R., and Hamburger, V., 1953, A diffusible agent of mouse sarcoma producing hyperplasia of sympathetic ganglia and hyperneurotization of the chick embryo, *J. Exp. Zool.* **123:**233.
51. Cohen, S., 1959, Purification and metabolic effects of a nerve growth-promoting protein from snake venom, *J. Biol. Chem.* **234:**1129.
52. Varon, S., Nomura, J., and Shooter, E. M., 1967, The isolation of the mouse nerve growth factor protein in a high molecular weight form, *Biochem.* **6:**2202.
53. Varon, S., Nomura, J., and Shooter, E. M., 1968, Reversible dissociation of the mouse nerve growth factor protein into different subunits, *Biochem.* **7:**1296.
54. Greene, L. A., Varon, S., Piltch, A., and Shooter, E. M., 1971, Substructure of the subunit of mouse 7S nerve growth factor, *Neurobiology* **1:**37.
55. Levi-Montalcini, R., and Cohen, S., 1960, Effects of the extract of the mouse salivary glands on the sympathetic system of mammals, *Ann. N.Y. Acad. Sci.* **85:**324.
56. Levi-Montalcini, R., 1964, Growth control of nerve cells by a protein factor and its antiserum, *Science* **143:**105.
57. Otten, U., Goedert, M., Mayer, N., and Lembeck, F., 1980, Requirement of nerve growth factor for development of substance P-containing sensory neurones, *Nature(London)* **287:**158.
58. Gundersen, R. W., and Barrett, J. N., 1979, Neuronal chemotaxis: Chick dorsal-root axons turn toward high concentrations of nerve growth factor, *Science* **206:**1079.
59. Gundersen, R. W., and Barrett, J. N., 1980, Characterization of the turning response of dorsal root neurites toward nerve growth factor, *J. Cell Biol.* **87:**546.
60. Levi-Montalcini, R., and Angeletti, P., 1963, Essential role of the nerve growth factor in the survival and maintenance of dissociated sensory and sympathetic embryonic nerve cells *in vitro, Dev. Biol.* **7:**653.
61. Greene, L. A., 1977, Quantitative *in vitro* studies on the nerve growth factor (NGF) requirement of neurons, *Dev. Biol.* **58:**106.
62. Campenot, R. B., 1977, Local control of neurite development by nerve growth factor, *Proc. Natl. Acad. Sci. U.S.A.* **74:**4516.
63. Hendry, I. A., 1976, Control in the development of the vertebrate sympathetic nervous system, *Rev. Neuroscience* **2:**149.
64. Thoenen, H., and Schwab, M. E., 1978, Physiological and pathophysiological implications of the retrograde axonal transport of macromolecules, *Adv. Pharmacol. Chemother.* **5:**37.
65. Brunso-Bechtold, J. D., and Hamburger, V., 1979, Retrograde transport of nerve growth factor in chicken embryo, *Proc. Natl. Acad. Sci. U.S.A.* **76:**1494.
66. Levi-Montalcini, R., and Angeletti, P. U., 1968, Nerve growth factor, *Physiol. Rev.* **48:**534.
67. Hamburger, V., Brunso-Bechtold, J. K., and Yip, J. W., 1981, Neuronal death in the spinal ganglia of the chick embryo and its reduction by nerve growth factor, *J. Neurosci.* **1:**60.
68. Hendry, I. A., 1975*a*, The retrograde trans-synaptic control of the development of cholinergic terminals in sympathetic ganglia, *Brain Res.* **86:**483.
69. Hendry, I. A., 1975*b*, The response of adrenergic neurones to axotomy and nerve growth factor, *Brain Res.* **94:**87.
70. Aloe, L., Mugnaini, E., and Levi-Montalcini, R., 1975, Light and electron microscopic studies on the excessive growth of sympathetic ganglia in rats injected daily from birth with 6-OHDA and NGF, *Arch. Ital. Biol.* **113:**326.

71. Purves, D., 1975, Functional and structural changes of mammalian sympathetic neurones following interruption of their axons, *J. Physiol.* **252:**429.
72. Njå, A., and Purves, D., 1978, The effects of nerve growth factor and its antiserum on synapses in the superior cervical ganglion in the guinea-pig, *J. Physiol.* **277:**53.
73. Ebendal, T., Olson, L., Seiger, A., and Hedlund, K.-O., 1980, Nerve growth factors in the rat iris, *Nature (London)* **286:**25.
74. Helfand, S. L., Smith, G. A., and Wessells, N. K., 1976, Survival and development in culture of dissociated parasympathetic neurons from ciliary ganglia, *Dev. Biol.* **50:**541.
75. Helfand, S. L., Riopelle, R. J., and Wessells, N. K., 1978, Non-equivalence of conditioned medium and nerve growth factor for sympathetic, parasympathetic, and sensory neurons, *Exp. Cell Res.* **113:**39.
76. Collins, F., 1978*a*, Induction of neurite outgrowth by a conditioned-medium factor bound to the culture substratum, *Proc. Natl. Acad. Sci. U.S.A.* **75:**5210.
77. Collins, F., 1978*b*, Axon initiation by ciliary neurons in culture, *Dev. Biol.* **65:**50.
78. Collins, F., 1980, Neurite outgrowth induced by the substrate associated material from nonneuronal cells, *Dev. Biol.* **79:**247.
79. Collins, F., and Garrett, J. E., Jr., 1980, Elongating nerve fibers are guided by a pathway of material released from embryonic nonneuronal cells, *Proc. Natl. Acad. Sci. U.S.A.* **77:**6226.
80. Adler, R., and Varon, S., 1980, Cholinergic neuronotrophic factors. V. Segregation of survival- and neurite-promoting activities in heart-conditioned media, *Brain Res.* **188:**437.
81. Adler, R.,Manthorpe, M., Skaper, S. D., and Varon, S., 1981, Polyornithine-attached neurite-promoting factors (PNPFs). Culture sources and responsive neurons, *Brain Res.* **206:**129.
82. Adler, R., and Varon, S., 1981, Neuritic guidance by polyornithine-attached materials of ganglionic origin, *Dev. Biol.* **81:**1.
83. Ebendal, T., 1979, Stage-dependent stimulation of neurite outgrowth exerted by nerve growth factor and chick heart in cultured embryonic ganglia, *Dev. Biol.* **72:**276.
84. Ebendal, T., Belew, M., Jacobson, C.-O., and Porath, J., 1979, Neurite outgrowth elicited by embryonic chick heart: Partial purification of the active factor, *Neurosci. Lett.* **14:**91.
85. Nishi, R., and Berg, D. K., 1977, Dissociated ciliary ganglion neurons *in vitro*: Survival and synapse formation, *Proc. Natl. Acad. Sci. U.S.A.* **74:**5171.
86. Nishi, R., and Berg, D. K., 1979, Survival and development of ciliary ganglion neurons grown alone in cell culture, *Nature (London)* **277:**232.
87. Nishi, R., 1980, Studies on chick ciliary ganglion neurons developing in cell culture, Ph.D. dissertation, University of California, San Diego.
88. Tuttle, J. B., Suszkiw, J. B., and Ard, M., 1979, Long-term survival and development of dissociated parasympathetic neurons in culture, *Brain Res.* **183:**161.
89. Chiappinelli, V., Giacobini, E., Pilar, G., and Uchimura, H., 1976, Induction of cholinergic enzymes in chick ciliary ganglion and iris muscle cells during synapse formation, *J. Physiol.* **257:**749.
90. Barald, K. F., and Berg, D. K., 1979*a*, Ciliary ganglion neurons in cell culture: High affinity choline uptake and autoradiographic choline labeling, *Dev. Biol.* **72:**15.
91. Suszkiw, J. B., and Pilar, G., 1976, Selective localization of a high affinity choline uptake system and its role in ACh formation in cholinergic nerve terminals, *J. Neurochem.* **261:**133.

92. Margiotta, J. F., and Berg, D. K., 1981, Evidence for synaptic transmission between ciliary ganglion neurons in cell culture, *Soc. Neurosci. Abstr.* **7**:596.
93. Margiotta, J. F., and Berg, D. K., 1982, Functional synapses are established between ciliary ganglion neurons in culture, *Nature (London)*, in press.
94. Adler, R., Landa, K. B., Manthorpe, M., Varon, S., 1979, Cholinergic neuronotrophic factors: Intraocular distribution of trophic activity for ciliary neurons, *Science* **204**:1434.
95. Landa, K. B., Adler, R., Manthorpe, M., and Varon, S., 1980, Cholinergic neuronotrophic factors. III. Developmental increase of trophic activity for chick embryo ciliary ganglion neurons in their intraocular target tissues, *Dev. Biol.* **74**:410.
96. Manthorpe, M., Skaper, S., Adler, R., Landa, K., and Varon, S., 1980, Cholinergic neuronotrophic factors: Fractionation properties of an extract from selected chick embryonic eye tissues, *J. Neurochem.* **34**:69.
97. Bonyhady, R. E., Hendry, I. A., Hill, C. E., and McLennan, I. S., 1980, Characterization of a cardiac muscle factor required for the survival of cultured parasympathetic neurons, *Neurosci. Lett.* **18**:197.
98. Bennett, M. R., and Nurcombe, V., 1979, The survival and development of cholinergic neurons in skeletal muscle conditioned media, *Brain Res.* **173**:543.
99. Nishi, R., and Berg, D. K., 1981, Two components from eye tissue that differentially stimulate the growth and development of ciliary ganglion neurons in cell culture, *J. Neurosci.* **1**:505.
100. Schubert, D., 1977, The substrate attached material synthesized by clonal cell lines of nerve, glia, and muscle, *Brain Res.* **132**:337.
101. Hawrot, E., 1980, Cultured sympathetic neurons: Effects of cell-derived and synthetic substrata on survival and development, *Dev. Biol.* **74**:136.
102. Scott, B. S., 1977, The effects of elevated potassium on the time course of neuron survival in cultures of dissociated dorsal root ganglia, *J. Cell. Physiol.* **91**:305.
103. Phillipson, O., and Sandler, M., 1975, The influence of NGF, potassium depolarization and dibutyryl (cyclic) AMP on explant cultures of chick sympathetic ganglia, *Brain Res.* **90**:273.
104. Lasher, J., and Zagon, R., 1972, The effect of potassium on neuronal differentiation in cultures of dissociated newborn rat cerebellum, *Brain Res.* **41**:482.
105. Bennett, M. R., and White, W., 1979, The survival and development of cholinergic neurons in potassium-enriched media, *Brain Res.* **173**:549.
106. Chalazonitis, A., and Fischbach, G. D., 1980, Elevated potassium induces morphological differentiation of dorsal root ganglionic neurons in dissociated cell culture, *Dev. Biol.* **78**:173.
107. Patterson, P. H., and Chun, L. L. Y., 1977*a*, The induction of acetylcholine synthesis in primary cultures of dissociated rat sympathetic neurons. I. Effects of conditioned medium, *Dev. Biol.* **56**:263.
108. Patterson, P. H. and Chun, L. L. Y., 1977*b*, The induction of acetylcholine synthesis in primary cultures of dissociated rat sympathetic neurons. II. Developmental aspects, *Dev. Biol.* **60**:473.
109. Patterson, P. H., 1978, Environmental determination of autonomic neurotransmitter functions, *Ann. Rev. Neurosci.* **1**:1.
110. Ebendal, T., Jordell-Dylberg, A., and Soderstrom, S., 1978, Stimulation by tissue explants on nerve fibre outgrowth in culture, *Zoon* **6**:235.
111. Barde, Y.-A., Lindsay, R. M., Monard, D., and Thoenen, H., 1978, New factor released by cultured glioma cells supporting survival and growth of sensory neurons, *Nature* **274**:818.

112. Barde, Y.-A., Edgar, D., and Thoenen, H., 1980, Sensory neurons in culture: Changing requirements for survival factors during embryonic development, *Proc. Natl. Acad. Sci. U.S.A.* **77:**1199.
113. Edgar, D., Barde, Y.-A., and Thoenen, H., 1981, Subpopulations of cultured chick sympathetic neurons differ in their requirements for survival factors, *Nature* (*London*) **289:**294.
114. Lindsay, R. M., 1979, Adult rat brain astrocytes support survival of both NGF-dependent and NGF-insensitive neurons, *Nature* (*London*) **282:**80.
115. Lindsay, R. M., and Tarbit, J., 1979, Developmentally regulated induction of neurite outgrowth from immature chick sensory neurons (DRG) by homogenates of avian or mammalian heart, liver and brain, *Neurosci. Lett.* **12:**195.
116. Varon, S., Skaper, S. D., and Manthorpe, M., 1981, Trophic activities for dorsal root and sympathetic ganglion neurons in media conditioned by Schwann and other peripheral cells, *Dev. Brain Res.* **1:**73.
117. Coughlin, M. D., Bloom, E. M., and Black, I. B., 1981, Characterization of a neuronal growth factor from mouse heart-cell-conditioned medium, *Dev. Biol.* **82:**56.
118. Riopelle, R. J., and Cameron, D. A., 1981, Neurite growth promoting factors of embryonic chick-ontogeny, regional distribution, and characteristics, *J. Neurobiol.* **12:**175.
119. Giller, E. L., Jr., Schrier, B. K., Shainberg, A., Fisk, H. R., and Nelson, P. G., 1973, Choline acetyltransferase activity is increased in combined cultures of spinal cord and muscle cells from mice, *Science* **182:**588.
120. Giller, E. L., Jr., Neale, J. H., Bullock, P. N., Schrier, B. K., and Nelson, P. G., 1977, Choline acetyltransferase activity of spinal cord cell cultures increased by co-culture with muscle and by muscle-conditioned medium, *J. Cell Biol.* **74:**16.
121. Godfrey, E. W., Schrier, B. K., and Nelson, P. G., 1980, Source and target cell specificities of a conditioned medium factor that increases choline acetyltransferase activity in cultured spinal cord cells, *Dev. Biol.* **77:**403.
122. Dribin, L. B., and Barrett, J. N., 1980, Conditioned medium enhances neuritic outgrowth from rat spinal cord explants, *Dev. Biol.* **74:**184.
123. Berg, D. K., 1978, Acetylcholine synthesis by chick spinal cord neurons in dissociated cell culture, *Dev. Biol.* **66:**500.
124. Fischbach, G. D., and Nelson, P. G., 1977, Cell culture in neurobiology, in: *Handbook of Physiology. Section 1: The Nervous System,* vol. 1, part 2 (J. M. Brookhart and V. B. Mountcastle, eds.), pp. 719–774, American Physiological Society, Bethesda, MD.
125. Farb, D. H., Berg, D. K., and Fischbach, G. D., 1979, Uptake and release of [^{3}H] aminobutyric acid by embryonic spinal cord neurons in dissociated cell culture, *J. Cell Biol.* **80:**651.
126. Barald, K. F., and Berg, D. K., 1979*b*, Autoradiographic labeling of spinal cord neurons with high affinity choline uptake in cell culture, *Dev. Biol.* **72:**1.
127. Cozzari, C., and Hartman, B. K., 1980, Preparation of antibodies specific to choline acetyltransferase from bovine caudate nucleus and immunohistochemical localization of the enzyme, *Proc. Natl. Acad. Sci. U.S.A.* **77:**7453.
128. Barber, R. P., and Saito, K., 1976, Light microscopic visualization of GAD and GABA-T in immunocytochemical preparations of rodent CNS, in: *GABA in Nervous System Function* (E. Roberts, T. N. Chase, and D. B. Tower, eds.), pp. 113–132, Raven Press, New York.
129. Wood, J. G., McLaughlin, B. J., and Vaughn, J. E., 1976, Immunocytochemical localization of GAD in electron microscopic preparation of rodent CNS, in: *GABA*

in Nervous System Function (E. Roberts, T. N. Chase, and D. B. Tower, eds.), pp. 133–148, Raven Press, New York.

130. Raff, M. C., Brockes, J. P., Fields, K. L., and Mirsky, R., 1979, Neural cell markers: The end of the beginning, *Progr. Brain Res.* **51**:17.
131. Raff, M. C., Fields, K. L., Hakomori, S.-I., Mirsky, R., Pruss, R. M., and Winter, J., 1979, Cell-type-specific markers for distinguishing and studying neurons and the major classes of glial cells in culture, *Brain Res.* **174**:283.
132. Barnstable, C. J., 1980, Monoclonal antibodies which recognize different cell types in rat retina, *Nature (London)* **286**:231.
133. Chun, L. L. Y., Patterson, P. H., and Cantor, H., 1980, Preliminary studies on the use of monoclonal antibodies as probes for sympathetic development, *J. Exp. Biol.* **89**:73.
134. Zipser, B., and McKay, R., 1981, Monoclonal antibodies distinguish identifiable neurons in the leech, *Nature (London)* **289**:549.
135. Bennett, M. R., Lai, K., and Nurcombe, V., 1980, Identification of embryonic motoneurons *in vitro*: Their survival is dependent on skeletal muscle, *Brain Res.* **190**:537.
136. Berg, D. K., and Fischbach, G. D., 1978, Enrichment of spinal cord cell cultures with motoneurons, *J. Cell Biol.* **77**:83.
137. Schnaar, R. L., and Schaffner, A. E., 1981, Separation of cell types from embryonic chicken and rat spinal cord: Characterization of motoneuron-enriched fractions, *J. Neurosci.* **1**:204.
138. Masuko, S., Kuromi, H., and Shimada, Y., 1979, Isolation and culture of motoneurons from embryonic chicken spinal cords, *Proc. Natl. Acad. Sci. U.S.A.* **76**:3537.
139. Banker, G. A., and Cowan, W. M., 1977, Rat hippocampal neurons in dispersed cell culture, *Brain Res.* **126**:397.
140. Banker, G. A., and Cowan, W. M., 1979, Further observations on hippocampal neurons in dispersed cell culture, *J. Comp. Neurol.* **187**:469.
141. Banker, G. A., 1980, Trophic interactions between astroglial cells and hippocampal neurons in culture, *Science* **209**:809.

10

Neuromuscular Synapse Elimination

Structural, Functional, and Mechanistic Aspects

DAVID C. VAN ESSEN

1. INTRODUCTION

It is well known that synaptic connections are established with a high degree of specificity during the development of the nervous system. Nonetheless, the pattern of connections at early stages of neurogenesis differs from that in the adult in several important respects. Two major phases of reorganization are now recognized to be common to the maturation of many parts of the nervous system. In the first phase there is widespread neuronal death, which generally occurs around the time of synapse formation. Neuronal death appears to be primarily a mechanism for adjusting the number of cells in a given structure to the number of target cells available and secondarily a mechanism for eliminating cells which have aberrant connections[1,2] (see Chapter 9). The second phase of reorganization involves extensive remodeling of synaptic connections without attendant cell death. In some parts of the nervous system the majority of synapses initially formed are subsequently eliminated.[1–3] Although many unanswered questions pertain to the functional significance of synapse elimination, it is a basic phenomenon in neurogenesis and is deserving of careful scrutiny.

DAVID C. VAN ESSEN · Division of Biology 216–76, California Institute of Technology, Pasadena, CA 91125.

The present article is concerned with synapse elimination at the mammalian neuromuscular junction. It is no accident that this is the preparation in which synapse elimination has been studied most intensively. The attributes of physical accessibility and simplicity of organization, which have made the neuromuscular junction the best-studied synapse in the adult nervous system, have made it equally advantageous for developmental studies. A particularly attractive feature of mammalian skeletal muscle is the uniformity of the adult innervation pattern, in which there is only one synaptic input to each muscle fiber. This indicates that the mechanisms for regulating the number of synaptic contacts are highly refined and makes the system particularly suitable as a model for understanding the factors controlling the fate of synapses.

The emphasis in this article will largely reflect my own research interests, but I hope as well to provide a reasonably broad perspective by discussing various aspects of neuromuscular synapse elimination that have been pursued in other laboratories. The presentation is organized in three parts. The first is a description of basic aspects of polyneuronal innervation and its subsequent elimination. Major considerations include questions of where the excess inputs are located, how extensive they are, and over what time course they are removed. The second part deals with experiments aimed at revealing the mechanisms underlying synapse elimination. Some clues about mechanisms have been obtained from descriptive analyses of normal development; additional clues have come from a variety of experimental perturbations. Particular emphasis is placed on the question of what factors might provide some synapses with an advantage over others in the competition for survival. The third part contains a discussion of models and possible molecular mechanisms for synapse elimination. An argument is developed that the occurrence of polyneuronal innervation and its subsequent elimination can be accounted for in terms of mechanisms already known or strongly suspected to be operative during the initial formation and stabilization of synapses. This model is then compared to other models that have been proposed, in which additional factors or interactions are invoked to explain how synapses are eliminated.

2. GENERAL FEATURES OF POLYNEURONAL INNERVATION AND SYNAPSE ELIMINATION

2.1. *Dual Basis of Multicomponent End-Plate Potentials*

Although classical neuroanatomists remarked on the presence of multiple inputs to individual muscle fibers in developing mammalian muscle,[4,5] their observations attracted scant attention until recently. Current interest in this topic was sparked by Redfern's observation, reported in 1970,[6] that multiple inputs to neonatal muscle fibers can be readily detected using intracellular recording techniques. In brief, he found that graded nerve stimulation elicited multiple, discrete components of the end-plate potential (e.p.p.) in neonatal rat muscle fibers that were partially curarized in order to block postsynaptic action potentials. The different e.p.p. components had similar time courses, indicating that they arose from nearby sites. Redfern suggested that the multicomponent e.p.p.'s most likely reflected polyneuronal innervation of a single end-plate on each fiber. Subsequent studies have confirmed that polyneuronal innervation indeed occurs in neonatal muscles.[7–9] In addition, it is now known that electrical coupling between muscle fibers occurs early in development and persists for a significant time after innervation takes place.[10] This gives rise to a second class of multicomponent e.p.p.'s in which some components arise indirectly, by way of coupling between fibers. Electrical coupling disappears more rapidly than does polyneuronal innervation, but determination of their relative importance at any given stage requires careful consideration of several factors.

In the rat intercostal muscle Dennis *et al.*[10] showed that electrical coupling between muscle fibers is common from the time the muscle forms around embryonic day 14 until birth a week later. During this period many fibers have e.p.p. components with markedly different time courses. They also demonstrated that e.p.p. components arising indirectly could be recognized by their slow time course. Whether all slow e.p.p. components reflect indirect inputs is unclear, however, as it is difficult to exclude the possibility of occasional distant inputs, lacking cholinesterase, on the fiber being assayed.

The incidence of physiologically detectable coupling in the rat intercostal muscle declines rapidly around the time of birth,[10] and in the soleus muscle no coupling at all was detected at early postnatal ages.[7] However, it is important to note that during the first postnatal week many muscle fibers are organized into small clusters, with the individual fibers in a cluster not being easily resolvable in conventional light-microscopic sections.[11,12] Coupling among the fibers within a cluster may persist after that between adjacent clusters has disappeared. In such case one might expect to see e.p.p. components with different time courses, although the degree of heterogeneity would be rather small if synapses were close together within a cluster. In any event, the muscle fiber clusters disappear by the end of the first postnatal week,[11,12] at which time multicomponent e.p.p.s are still widespread.[7,9,10,12]

The evidence for genuine polyneuronal innervation of single end-plates comes from a number of complementary physiological and anatomical observations. First, the upper limit for the separation between inputs is about 30–50 μm, based on the fact that all components of the e.p.p. can be desensitized in parallel by focal acetylcholine iontophoresis.[7] Second, there is only one cholinesterase-positive end-plate on each muscle fiber,[7,13] and all components of the e.p.p. are enhanced by the cholinesterase blocker, prostigmine.[7] Third, end-plates in neonatal, but not adult, muscles are innervated by multiple preterminal axons.[7,9,14] The possibility that the multiple preterminal axons derive from a single parent axon farther back in the motor nerve has not been ruled out on anatomical grounds. However, it is made very unlikely by the physiological observation of a large-scale tension overlap, revealed by comparing the summed tension produced by sequential stimulation of ventral root filaments with the maximal tension generated by direct muscle stimulation.[7,8,12]

To summarize, the innervation of developing rat skeletal muscle can be divided into three major stages. In the first stage, which occurs prenatally, both polyneuronal innervation and electrical coupling are extensive. In the second stage, which occurs mainly postnatally, coupling has disappeared and polyneuronal innervation is widespread but declining. It remains to be determined whether the transition between these stages involves a persistence of localized coupling within fiber clusters after the loss of coupling between neighboring clusters. In the third stage the mature state of single innervation is reached.

Polyneuronal innervation of neonatal muscle fibers has been found in a variety of muscles from several mammalian species. These include four different muscles in the rat, six in the rabbit, and one in the cat.[6–10,12,14,15] Since no muscles have been found which lack polyneuronal innervation at birth, it is reasonable to conclude that the phenomenon is a widespread, perhaps universal, feature of mammalian neuromuscular development. Polyneuronal innervation also occurs in developing muscles of lower vertebrates; the principal differences in comparison to the mammalian system are that the innervation pattern in many muscles is distributed rather than focal, and that a substantial degree of polyneuronal innervation often persists even in adult muscles.[9,16]

2.2. *Time Course of Synapse Elimination*

The loss of synaptic inputs at the neuromuscular junction begins around the time of birth and continues into the early postnatal period. It is important to know the timing of synapse elimination in some detail, both as baseline data for experimental manipulations of the elimination process and as a basis for understanding how maturation occurs in muscles of different types and in different parts of the body. Figure 1 shows the time course of elimination of polyneuronal innervation in the rat soleus muscle as assessed by the incidence of multicomponent e.p.p.'s in partially curarized muscles.[7] The first singly innervated fibers do not appear until postnatal day 9. After this there is a sharp decline in polyneuronal innervation, and at day 15 fewer than 10% of the fibers have multiple inputs. Synapse elimination begins well before day 9, though, as the incidence of fibers having three or more inputs declines during the first postnatal week. Based on observations of average motor unit sizes at various ages,[7] it is likely that the process is underway within

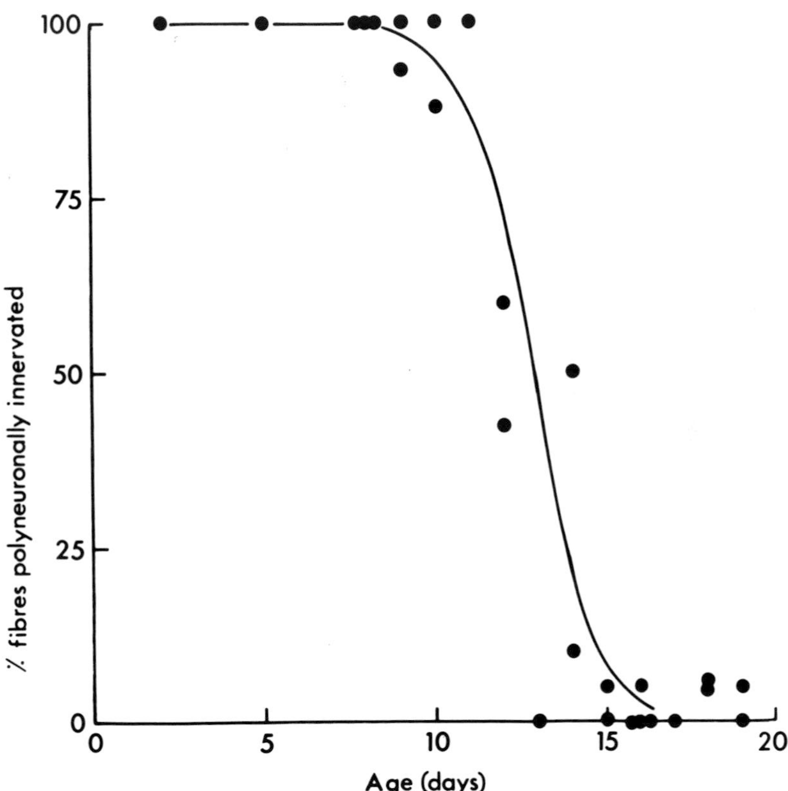

Figure 1. Time course of synapse elimination in the rat soleus muscle. Each data point indicates the percentage of polyneuronally innervated muscle fibers in a muscle of the indicated age. Determinations were based on the incidence of multicomponent e.p.p.'s detected with intracellular recordings from at least 20 muscle fibers in a partially curarized muscle. (From Brown *et al.*[7])

a few days after birth and may even begin prenatally. It is also noteworthy that a low degree of polyneuronal innervation persists for at least a few days beyond day 15. Whether substantial reorganization occurs during this late phase of synapse elimination remains to be determined (see section 3.4.1).

The timing of synapse elimination has been examined in three other muscles in the rat. In two of these, the lumbrical muscle[12] and the diaphragm,[17] the time courses are indistinguishable from that in the soleus. In intercostal muscles, however, synapse elimination occurs significantly earlier, with nearly all polyneuronal innervation having disappeared by the 10th postnatal day.[10] The peak level of polyneuronal innervation in intercostal muscles occurs over a several-day period from embryonic day 16, only a few days after neuromuscular synapses have begun to form, to day 19, just 2 days before birth. This plateau may represent a clear separation between the period in which synapses are formed and that in which they are eliminated. Alternatively, it may represent a time in which both processes are going on at equal rates. It is difficult to envision experiments which would clearly distinguish between these possibilities.

Given the relatively synchronous loss of synapses found in several different rat muscles, we were initially surprised to find much more heterogeneity in the timing of synapse elimination in various muscles from the rabbit.[15] For example, synapse elimination in the diaphragm precedes that in the soleus by about a week in the rabbit, as illustrated in Fig. 2. The first singly innervated fibers appear prenatally in the rabbit diaphragm, and synapse elimination is nearly complete by the end of the 1st postnatal week. In contrast, singly innervated fibers do not appear until around postnatal day 5 in the soleus, and the loss of remaining multiple inputs occurs mainly during the 2nd postnatal week. There are also significant differences in the rate of synapse elimination, with the peak rate in the soleus being more than twice that in the diaphragm.

In order to see whether the time course of synapse elimination is related in any systematic fashion to the type of muscle or its position in the body, we studied four other muscles in the rabbit.[15] The time course in the extensor digitorum longus (EDL), a fast muscle, is very similar to that in the soleus, a slow muscle, indicating that the timing is not closely related to muscle contractile properties. There is a tendency for synapse elimination to occur sooner in muscles situated in the rostral half of the body. The correlation is not a perfect one, though, and it seems likely that the position of a muscle in the body is not the only factor influencing the time course of synapse elimination.

One of the important conclusions to be drawn from these experi-

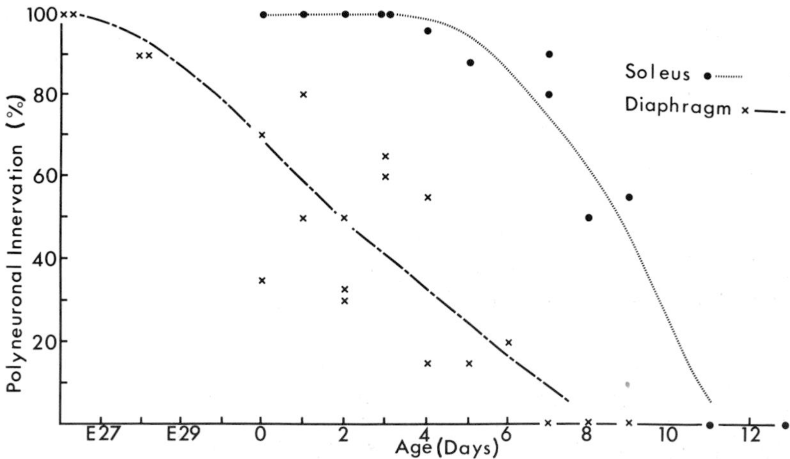

Figure 2. Time course of synapse elimination in the soleus muscle (filled circles) and diaphragm (crosses) of the rabbit. As in the preceding figure each data point indicates the percentage of polyneuronally innervated fibers detected by intracellular recordings from a single muscle. (From Bixby and Van Essen.[15])

ments is that the asynchrony of synapse elimination in muscles from various parts of the body argues against the process being initiated or controlled by some systemic influence, hormonal or otherwise. Rather, it is likely that maturation of neuromuscular connections involves a more specific set of interactions between each muscle and the motor neurons supplying it.

2.3. *Numbers of Motor Neurons, Muscle Fibers, and Synapses*

A variety of questions naturally arise concerning the quantitative aspects of polyneuronal innervation. How much redundancy of inputs is there in any given muscle, does this vary from one muscle to another, and do all fibers in a muscle pass through a stage of excess innervation? Is the loss of polyneuronal innervation associated with any change in the number of motor neurons supplying the muscle or in the number of muscle fibers receiving innervation?

It is well known that a large-scale loss of motor neurons occurs during normal development in vertebrates,[1,2] and this raises the question of whether the loss of neuromuscular synapses might simply be a consequence of cell death in the spinal cord. This seems unlikely in view of evidence that cell death is restricted to the period shortly after initial synaptic contacts are made, in mammals[18] as well as in lower vertebrates.[1,2] More direct evidence comes from counts of motor axons at different postnatal ages. In the rat we found no detectable change in the number of motor axons supplying the soleus muscle during the first two postnatal weeks, when most synapse elimination takes place.[7] Similarly, we found no postnatal loss of myelinated fibers in the soleus nerve of the rabbit, suggesting that postnatal death of motor neurons does not occur in this species either.[15]

The question of whether there are postnatal increases in the number of muscle fibers has proven more difficult to resolve, as some investigators have reported large increases[19,20] and others have reported no significant change.[21,22] Ontell and Dunn[11] have shown that some of these discrepancies are attributable to difficulties in recognizing small myotubes in neonatal muscles. They found that in the rat EDL the number of muscle cells (myotubes and muscle fibers) remains nearly constant after birth but that many myotubes are satellites of larger fibers and are not easily recognizable at the light microscopic level. In the soleus muscle of rats there is at most a 50% increase in muscle cell number after the 3rd postnatal day,[23] and the increase may be considerably less than this given the problems with neonatal fiber counts. In the neonatal rabbit and cat it is easier to identify muscle cells in the light microscope. We found no postnatal increase at all for the rabbit soleus,[15] nor was any increase found for the kitten soleus or flexor hallucis longus.[24] However, this conclusion clearly does not apply to all muscles, as Betz *et al.*[12] found that the number of muscle cells identifiable at the EM level in rat lumbrical muscles nearly doubles after birth.

The extent of polyneuronal innervation in any given muscle can be assessed in any of several ways, e.g., by determining the average number of e.p.p. components after partial curarization, by determining the tension overlap from stimulation of individual motor units, and by counting the average number of preterminal axons to each end-plate visible in silver-stained sections. Significant uncertainties are associated with each type of measurement; nevertheless, when more than one approach has been applied to muscles of the same age, the estimates have been in reasonably good agreement.[7,8,12,14,25–27] Estimates of the peak level of polyneuronal innervation range from around two to three synapses per fiber for the extensor digitorum longus and pronator teres in the rabbit[15] and the lumbrical muscle of the rat[12] to four to five synapses per fiber for soleus muscles in the rat[7] and rabbit.[28] Thus, there appears to be some variability in peak levels of polyneuronal innervation. In all muscles examined, the great majority of muscle fibers pass through a stage of polyneuronal innervation, although in some muscles a significant percentage of fibers becomes singly innervated before birth.

Another important aspect of the postnatal reorganization of neuromuscular connections concerns the alterations in size of motor units, i.e., the number of synapses made by individual motor neurons. The magnitude of these changes obviously depends not only on the number of redundant synapses to be removed from a muscle, but also on the number of new synapses that must be established in the event that new muscle fibers are added to the muscle. At one end of the spectrum are muscles such as the soleus muscle of the rat and rabbit, in which there is little postnatal increase in fiber number, and on average each motor neuron loses about 80% of its synapses.[7,28] At the opposite end of the spectrum is the lumbrical muscle of the rat, in which the loss of polyneuronal innervation is nearly balanced by the postnatal addition of muscle fibers, and there is only a small decrease in average motor unit size.[12]

2.4. *A "Critical Period" for Neuromuscular Synapse Elimination?*

It is well established that in the visual system there is a critical period in early postnatal development during which abnormal experience can lead to major alterations in connections within the visual cortex.[29,30] It is natural to wonder whether a similar critical period might regulate the susceptibility of neuromuscular synapses to being eliminated. If this were so, one would expect synapses in adult muscle to be resistant to elimination. Of course, this is difficult to test in a completely normal adult mammalian muscle because the absence of polyneuronal innervation prevents the opportunity for competitive interactions between synapses. There are several ways to obtain polyneuronal innervation of adult muscle fibers, however, and hence to address this issue directly.

One means of obtaining polyneuronal innervation in the adult is to denervate a muscle, cross-innervate it in an ectopic location, and allow reinnervation by the original nerve. Under such circumstances muscle fibers become dually innervated and can remain so indefinitely.[31] However, the stability of this dual innervation does not result from its occurrence in adult muscle, but rather from the spatial segregation of the persisting inputs. Even in early postnatal muscles dual innervation can persist when the inputs are widely separated.[7] Conversely, when multiple inputs are close to one another in adult muscle, synapse elimination can in fact take place. This has been shown for the multiple innervation that takes place through the foreign nerve in cross-innervated muscle,[32,33] for the reinnervation that takes place after crushing the original nerve,[34] and for the regression of sprouts after reinnervation of a partially denervated muscle.[35]

These results provide clear evidence that synapse elimination can occur in adult mammalian muscle. It could be argued, however, that such interactions are limited to situations in which the synapses undergoing elimination are immature. Thus, a critical period, if it existed, would be related to the age of the synapses, not of the muscle as a whole. To evaluate this possibility it is of interest to know whether situations exist in which fully mature, normally functioning synapses can be eliminated. We therefore implanted a foreign nerve directly over the synaptic region of adult rat soleus muscles.[36] The foreign nerve thus obtained access to the original end-plates, where it could compete directly with synapses made by the soleus nerve, rather than being forced to induce new end-plates in an ectopic region if it were to innervate successfully. In those cases in which the foreign nerve remained situated over the end-plate region and grew directly into the muscle, cross-innervation of original end-plate sites took place consistently, albeit to only a small degree in any particular muscle. About half of the cross-innervated fibers in our sample had lost their inputs from the original nerve. This can be seen using both anatomical techniques (Fig. 3) and physiological techniques (Fig. 4). It might be suggested that the foreign nerve was able to take over because of irritation or denervation associated with the surgical procedure. However, control experiments involving implantation of a resected piece of nerve over the soleus muscle did not induce any detectable transient denervation of muscle fibers. Moreover, we did not see significant innervation by the foreign nerve at ectopic sites, which should have occurred if transmission through the original nerve had been disrupted. We conclude, therefore, that mature end-plates occupied by normally functioning synapses can be cross-innervated by a foreign nerve and that in many instances the original input can be eliminated altogether.

These observations suggest that the timing of synapse elimination during normal development does not reflect the existence of a critical period *per se*, since the mechanisms for both the establishment of polyneuronal innervation and its subsequent removal persist into adulthood. Clearly there are major differences in the dynamics of neuromuscular interactions in adult vs. immature animals; as will be argued more explicitly in section 4.2, however, these differences may be quantitative rather than qualitative.

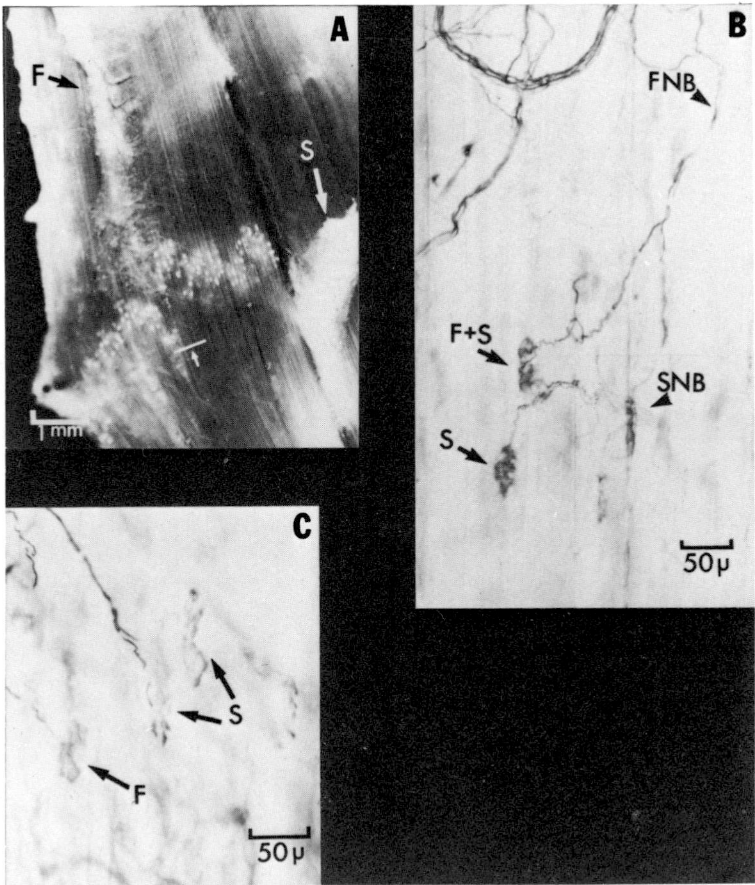

Figure 3. Displacement of original nerve synapses by a foreign nerve transplanted onto the end-plate region of adult skeletal muscle. (A) An adult rat soleus muscle stained for acetylcholinesterase and photographed with dark-field illumination, so that end-plates appear as bright spots. A foreign nerve (F) had been transplanted over a region close to the end-plate band 6 weeks prior to the final experiment. Foreign axons grew over a substantial portion of the muscle but reached the original end-plate band only in the narrow strip indicated by the white bar with arrow. Contractions elicited by foreign nerve stimulation were restricted to this same narrow strip. No ectopic deposits of acetylcholinesterase were found, indicating that foreign synapses were made only in the original end-plate band. (B, C) Silver-stained preparations taken from different muscles and showing foreign innervation of soleus nerve end-plates. In B, a foreign nerve branch (FNB) and an intramuscular branch of the soleus nerve (SNB) both innervate a single end-plate (F + S). Also visible is another end-plate innervated only by the soleus nerve (S). In C, several end-plates are visible, two of which are innervated only by the soleus nerve (S) and one of which is innervated only by the foreign nerve (F). (From Bixby and Van Essen.[36])

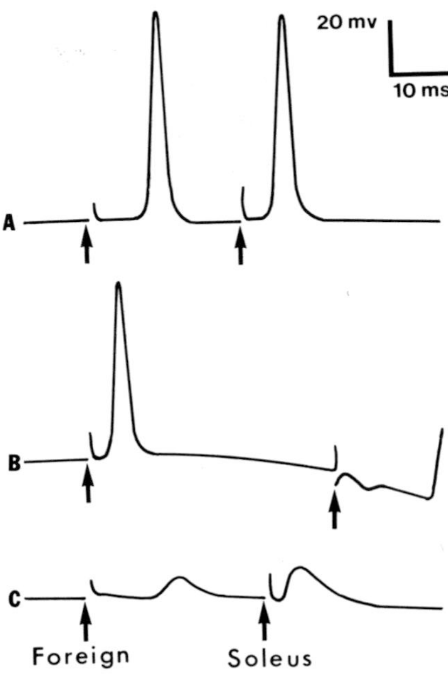

Figure 4. Intracellular recordings from foreign-innervated muscle fibers. (A) Recording from a fiber receiving suprathreshold inputs from both foreign and original nerves. (B) Recording from a fiber receiving inputs only from the foreign nerve. (C) Recording from a fiber responding with a subthreshold e.p.p. to stimulation of either the foreign or the original nerve. (From Bixby and Van Essen.[36])

3. MECHANISMS UNDERLYING SYNAPSE ELIMINATION

3.1. *Morphological Changes*

The transition from polyneuronal to single innervation involves the physical removal of redundant synapses, and it is obviously important to know exactly what sequence of morphological changes takes place during this process. One question of particular interest is whether a synapse persists for any significant period after functional transmission has ceased. Another is whether synapses are eliminated by a mechanism involving casting off and subsequent degeneration of a terminal or by one involving retraction into the parent axon.

The possibility of intact but nonfunctional inputs in immature muscle has been studied by comparing the incidence of multiple inputs detected histologically, using silver or zinc iodide–osmium stains, with those detected physiologically, using intracellular recording techniques. As mentioned already, there is general agreement that the two methods reveal a similar time course of synapse elimination. On the other hand, O'Brien *et al.*[26] reported a low incidence of multiaxonal innervation in histological sections of rat soleus muscle taken at an age (day 16) when they detected no multiple inputs physiologically. They suggested that this represents a stage at which synapses are intact but nonfunctional. However, it was previously shown[7] that a significant level of polyneuronal innervation can be detected physiologically at day 16 and beyond (see Fig. 1), suggesting that the physiological estimates of O'Brien *et al.* may have been spuriously low. A more detailed comparison of anatomical and physiological indices of polyneuronal innervation by Brown *et al.*[27] revealed no significant differences in time course, and they concluded that synapse removal probably coincides with the cessation of functional transmission and is certainly delayed by no more than a day.

The question of whether synapse elimination is associated with the degeneration of synapses or their retraction has been the subject of several recent studies. Korneliussen and Jansen[37] originally reported an absence of degenerating profiles in their EM study of neuromuscular synapses in the early postnatal rat soleus, and they suggested that synapse elimination involves retraction of terminals. In contrast, Rosenthal and Taraskevitch[17] reported a surprisingly high incidence of degenerating profiles in the neonatal rat diaphragm.

In order to resolve this question it is important to know what the expected incidence of degenerating profiles would be, if this is the mechanism by which synapses are removed. Bixby[38] found that the terminal degeneration produced by axotomy in the neonatal rabbit diaphragm occurs over a relatively brief time interval, beginning 6–8 hr after nerve transection, and is largely complete 15–20 hr later. Using this information, along with data concerning the rate at which synapse elimination occurs in the rabbit diaphragm[15] and estimates of the fraction of a polyneuronally innervated end-plate occupied by an individual terminal, Bixby estimated that degeneration would be seen in at least 2% of sections through end-plates if this were the sole mechanism of elimination. Since no signs of degeneration were seen in his sample of hundreds of sections through end-plates, it is likely that retraction is the predominant mode by which excess neuromuscular synapses are removed. Further evidence supporting the retraction hypothesis comes from observations at both the light- and electron-microscopic level of processes suggestive of retraction bulbs.[25,39] The principle argument against the retraction hypothesis is the observation of degenerating profiles in the neonatal rat diaphragm[17]; however, the reported incidence of such profiles was much higher than would be predicted on the basis of known rates of synapse elimination[17,25] and axotomy-induced degeneration,[38,39] and it is thus likely that these profiles resulted instead from rapid degradative changes after tissue isolation.

3.2. *Dynamic State of Synapses*

Recent studies on the neuromuscular junction have led to two important insights pertaining to the stability of synaptic connections. One is that the stability of the synapse is linked to the presence of an extracellular "scaffold" responsible for inducing and maintaining the characteristic specializations on both the presynaptic and postsynaptic sides. The other is that the interaction between the presynaptic terminal and this scaffold is evidently a dynamic one, with an ongoing sprouting and regression of processes continuing even in the mature state.

The presence of something akin to a synaptic scaffold can be inferred from the stability of various end-plate features in muscle that has been denervated or cross-innervated at ectopic sites. These features include end-plate acetylcholinesterase,[31,40–42] acetylcholine receptors,[31,43] and receptivity to innervation.[31,42] Evidence pointing to the extracellular nature of this scaffold has come from an ingenious series of experiments by McMahan and his collaborators. They have obtained evidence that synaptic basal lamina can induce both normal-looking presynaptic terminals in the absence of muscle[44,45] and, in separate experiments, normal distributions of junctional folds and end-plate acetylcholine receptors in the absence of the nerve.[46] It remains unclear whether the same basal lamina components are involved in both presynaptic and postsynaptic inductive interactions. What is most important in the present context is that the synaptic basal lamina retains its specialized properties for a significant period in the absence of nerve or muscle and hence can be regarded as providing a stable scaffold, albeit not necessarily a permanent one. As a matter of terminology, the term *scaffolding* will be used for the particular constituents in or near the basal lamina which serve as markers for pre- and postsynaptic differentiation; *scaffold* will be used to refer to the complete array of these constituents as they occur at any particular end-plate.

In view of the apparent stability of the synaptic scaffold, evidence suggestive of a dynamic state of the presynaptic terminal becomes of particular interest. Several histological studies have revealed significant imperfections in the alignment of pre- and postsynaptic elements in both immature and adult muscles. For example, Fig. 5 shows an electron micrograph of a synaptic region in a neonatal rabbit diaphragm in which the junctional folds characteristic of the end-plate region are apposed either by vacant regions (asterisk) or Schwann cell profiles (arrow). Of course, such a misalignment might be attributable either to a regression of the presynaptic terminal or to an overextended induction of the junctional folds. It seems likely that presynaptic retraction is at least partly

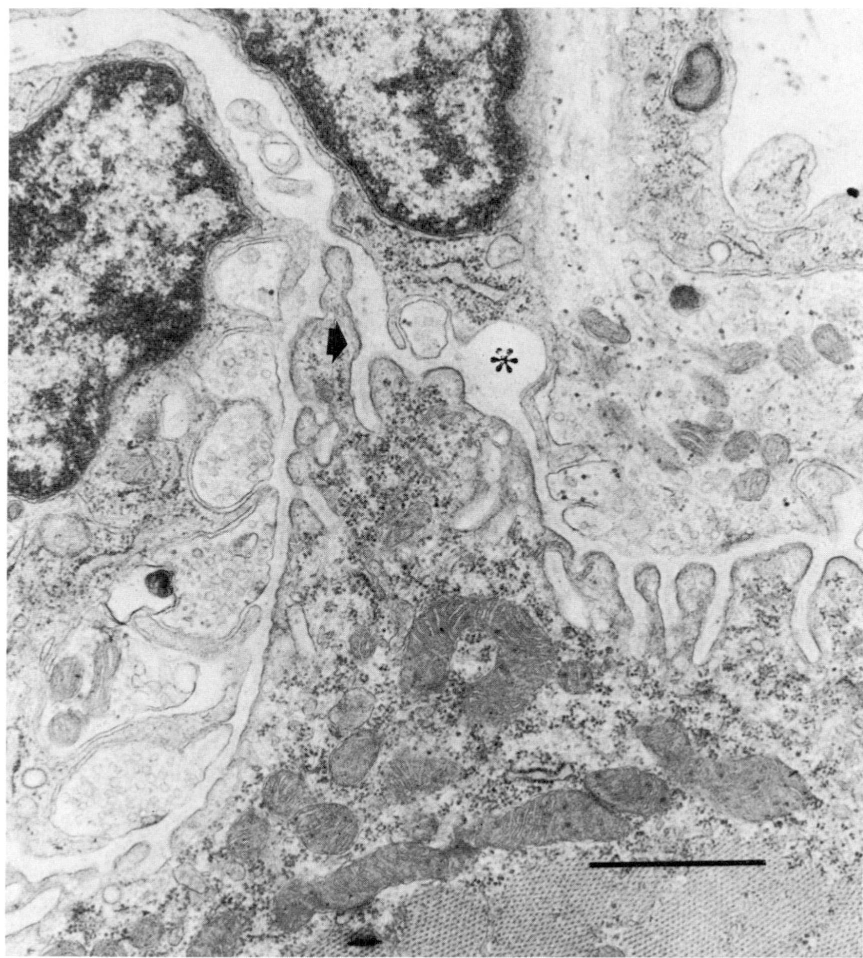

Figure 5. Electron micrograph of a neuromuscular junction from the diaphragm of a 1.5-day-old rabbit. Some junctional folds are apposed either by vacant spaces (asterisk) or by Schwann cell profiles (arrow). Scale, 1μm. (From Bixby.[38])

responsible, especially since a higher incidence of such profiles is seen during the synaptic retraction that occurs after axotomy.[38]

In other end-plates, misalignments of the opposite type are sometimes seen in which axonal profiles extend beyond the postsynaptic specializations (Fig. 6). As before, the misalignment might be attributed either to a presynaptic event—sprouting—or to a postsynaptic one—regression of junctional folds from regions they previously occupied. Again, it seems likely that presynaptic changes are at least partly re-

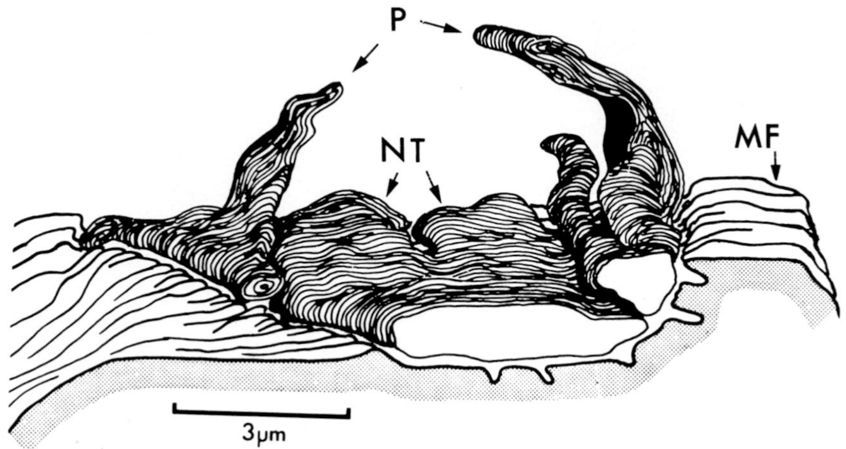

Figure 6. A partial reconstruction of the three-dimensional configuration of a nerve terminal (NT) from a neonatal rabbit diaphragm. The reconstruction was made by tracing the outlines of neuronal and muscle profiles from evenly-spaced sections through the central portion of the terminal, spacing successive contours so that the final drawing is to scale. Several protrusions (P) can be seen to rise above the muscle fiber (MF), in one case ending blindly several microns above the surface. (From Bixby.[38])

sponsible, especially since some of the profiles are directed well away from the surface of the muscle fiber. The incidence of vacant junctional folds and of terminal sprouts is difficult to quantify, but both seem to be relatively common in immature muscle, even in fibers which have become singly innervated.[38] This suggests that immature synapses are in a dynamic state, with any net changes in configuration depending on the balance of ongoing sprouting and regression of processes.

The available evidence suggests that nerve terminals are in a more quiescent state in adult mammalian muscle than during immature stages, but that they are not altogether static. The suggestion that continuous synaptic remodeling occurs at the neuromuscular junction is an old one,[47] and several recent studies have strengthened the evidence for this notion. Fine terminal sprouts can be seen at the light-microscopic level in a small but significant percentage of the terminals of normal adult muscles,[48–50] and the gradual increase in synaptic size and complexity that continues through adulthood implies that substantial new growth must have occurred. Signs of retraction and/or degeneration of terminal processes have also been observed for adult mammalian muscle.[48,49] The evidence for sprouting and regression is even stronger in adult amphibian muscle: sprouts are found overlying regions lacking end-plate cholinesterase, and cholinesterase-positive regions are found which lack innervation.[51–53] Interestingly, the ratio of sprouting to regression evidently shows seasonal variations.[52] Thus, the picture for adult neuromuscular synapses is similar to that described for sensory axons by Speidel,[54] in which sprouting and retraction are normal events *in vivo*. However, the frequency and extent of these events appear to be less than in immature muscles.

3.3. *Cellular Interactions Related to Synapse Elimination*

Questions of what mechanisms underly the process of synapse elimination can be asked at several levels. The evidence that synapses are removed by a process of retraction rather than degeneration has already been discussed. It is appropriate to turn next to the question of which cells are involved in the interaction. Does synapse elimination directly involve all of the synaptic terminals coexisting on any particular fiber, and do muscle fibers and/or Schwann cells play a role? That muscle fibers as well as synaptic terminals are involved at least as a passive substrate can be inferred from the observation that each fiber consistently retains one and only one synaptic input, so that the probability of any given synapse surviving depends on whether other synapses are made on the same fiber. Hence, mechanisms which involve retraction of synapses without regard to the presence or absence of other inputs to each muscle fiber are unlikely (see section 3.4).

Evidence that muscle fibers can play an active role in synapse elimination has been obtained in experiments involving cross-innervation at multiple ectopic sites on a fiber. In both immature[7] and adult[32] soleus muscles cross-innervated by a foreign nerve, synapses can be formed at multiple sites distributed more or less randomly on each fiber. Over a period of weeks most of the closely spaced polyneuronal inputs disappear, indicating that selective elimination can occur even when synapses are not in direct contact with one another. Similar interactions between spatially separate inputs occur during normal development of amphibian muscle.[16] The distance over which this interaction can take place is difficult to ascertain precisely but appears to be somewhere between 1 and a few millimeters.[7,32] Since a synapse on one fiber does not obviously affect the survival of synapses within this radius on adjacent muscle fibers, it follows that the interactions occurring on individual fibers cannot be attributed simply to some diffusible substance spreading between synapses. Rather, the muscle fiber itself must be involved in initiation or mediation of the signals that lead to synapse elimination.

The third cell type which might be involved in synapse elimination is the Schwann cell. Early in development individual Schwann cells often enwrap more than one axon, so it is conceivable that a single Schwann cell could be responsible for the selection of which preterminal axon is to be the surviving input to any given end-plate. Obviously, a simple mechanism of this type would not account for the aforementioned observation that interactions leading to synapse elimination can occur over considerable distances. Nonetheless, Schwann cells might confer a competitive advantage to particular synapses, perhaps by myelinating their axons, so that a role for Schwann cells in long-distance synaptic interactions would still be a possibility.

To obtain further evidence on this issue, Bixby[38] examined the relationship of Schwann cells to motor axons in the neonatal rabbit diaphragm. The most important observation was that myelination of intramuscular nerve branches occurs sufficiently late in development that it is unlikely to have a major influence on synapse elimination. Although a substantial degree of myelination has occurred in large intramuscular nerve branches at the time of birth, no myelinated axons were found in fiber branches that were within 200 μm of the synaptic region. Moreover, motor axons were shown to branch frequently close to the synaptic region. Thus, during the period of maximal synapse elimination, myelination has not begun on the axonal branches supplying individual end-plates. It remains possible that Schwann cells influence synapse elimination in some way that is either unrelated to myelination altogether or in which myelination is delayed following the commitment to myelinate.

3.4. *Competitive Synapse Elimination and the Rules Governing It*

One of the intriguing issues pertaining to synapse elimination concerns the selection of which particular synapses are to survive and which to be removed. Experiments on normal and partially denervated muscle have implicated two distinct influences on the survival of synapses. One of the key observations is that motor units from partially denervated rat soleus muscles, in which all but one or a few motor axons are severed at birth, end up significantly smaller than their starting size but significantly larger than they would be in a normal adult muscle.[7,23] The fact that the motor units are smaller than at birth indicates that motor neurons have an intrinsic tendency to withdraw a large percentage of their initial complement of terminals, even at the expense of leaving some fibers completely denervated. Interestingly, though, this tendency for intrinsic withdrawal is not evident in the lumbrical muscle of the rat, inasmuch as motor units in partially denervated muscles remain as large as at birth.[55] Thus, even in the same species, the rules governing synapse elimination are not the same for all muscles.

The observation that motor units end up larger than normal after neonatal partial denervation, both in the soleus and the lumbrical muscle, suggests that competitive interactions between synapses play a role in synapse elimination. What is meant by competition in this context is that the probability of survival of any given synapse depends on the presence or absence of other synapses *on the same muscle fiber*. Strictly speaking, the partial denervation experiments do not provide unequivocal evidence for such competition. It could be argued that the survival of a greater than normal number of synapses arises indirectly, say, as a result of sprout-inducing factors released from neighboring denervated fibers and not as a result of interactions localized to individual fibers. It is thus important to look at other evidence bearing on the issue of competition. The failure to detect any transiently denervated fibers at any stage of normal maturation[7] is significant in this regard, as it suggests that the last synapse on a fiber is sure to survive and therefore that the probability of survival indeed depends on the presence or absence of other inputs to a fiber. An alternative explanation, though, is that some fibers do become denervated but are then reinnervated so rapidly that the transient denervation is not readily detectable. The impaired abilities of neonatal motor axons to sprout[7,23] or to regenerate new connections[56] (even though both are possible to some extent[7,57,58]) argue against this, but do not rule it out altogether.

Taken together, these observations provide strong but not compelling evidence that peripheral competitive interactions occur during synapse elimination. If competition does occur, the question then becomes one of whether some synapses might actually have an advantage over others. This need not be the case: one could imagine all synapses on a fiber having exactly the same probability of surviving, yet the situation would nonetheless be competitive if all but one eventually were eliminated. Obviously, a variety of factors might alter the probability of survival of any given synapse relative to its neighbors, and several of these possibilities have been investigated experimentally. One is that the size of a motor neuron's peripheral field might affect the likelihood that its synapses will be eliminated. Another is that its rostrocaudal position in the spinal cord might be important. A third is that synaptic activity might affect the probability of survival.

3.4.1. Interactions Related to Motor Unit Size. In a number of systems it has been found that a regenerating nerve can compete effectively with inputs from a different nerve which has sprouted into denervated territory.[35,59,60] Such interactions can even occur in situations where the regenerating nerve is not intrinsically better matched to the target than the sprouted nerve (see also Bixby and Van Essen[36] and section 2.4). A feature common to all these situations is that the regenerating nerve, which initially has no peripheral connections, is competing with neurons that either are overextended or at least have normal peripheral fields. Under these circumstances it is evident that regenerating axons have a strong tendency to form synapses; however, it is difficult to determine whether these synapses, once formed, are more likely to persist than the preexisting inputs because they belong to neurons with a relatively small total number of connections to maintain. It is possible to address this question more directly in neonatal muscle by looking for changes in the distributions of motor unit sizes as an index of whether the loss of synapses differs for large vs. small motor units. Figure 7 shows the distribution of motor unit sizes, as estimated from the tension generated by stimulating individual motor units, for rat soleus muscles of various ages. An important feature of this pattern is that the scatter in motor unit tensions is generally higher in the muscles examined before day 10, when polyneuronal innervation is extensive, than in the one muscle examined at age 6 weeks. We therefore suggested that over the long run large motor units may be at a competitive disadvantage compared to smaller motor units.[7] However, it is noteworthy that there is as much if not more relative scatter in motor unit sizes at days 15 and 17, when nearly all fibers have become singly innervated, than at earlier stages. This suggests that any competitive advantage of smaller motor units may not be expressed until the synapse elimination process is largely over. Moreover, there are several additional complicating factors to be considered. One problem is the limited sample size for the data shown in Fig. 7. A similar range of motor unit tensions in neonatal animals was reported by Thompson and Jansen,[23] but they found a larger scatter in adult motor unit tensions than that shown in Fig. 7 and in the study by Close.[61] Also, there is considerable heterogeneity in muscle fiber size, especially in neonatal muscles, which could significantly affect the relationship between the tension generated by a motor unit and the number of muscle fibers it contains. In particular, some of the scatter seen in immature muscles might arise if there were systematic differences in the average size of muscle fibers innervated by different motor axons. Thus, the question of whether there are significant changes in the scatter of motor unit sizes during postnatal development clearly deserves further attention.

To clarify this issue we have recently begun a series of experiments similar to those just described, but on the rabbit soleus instead of the rat's. The advantages of using the rabbit soleus include its larger size, larger number of motor units, greater homogeneity of muscle fiber di-

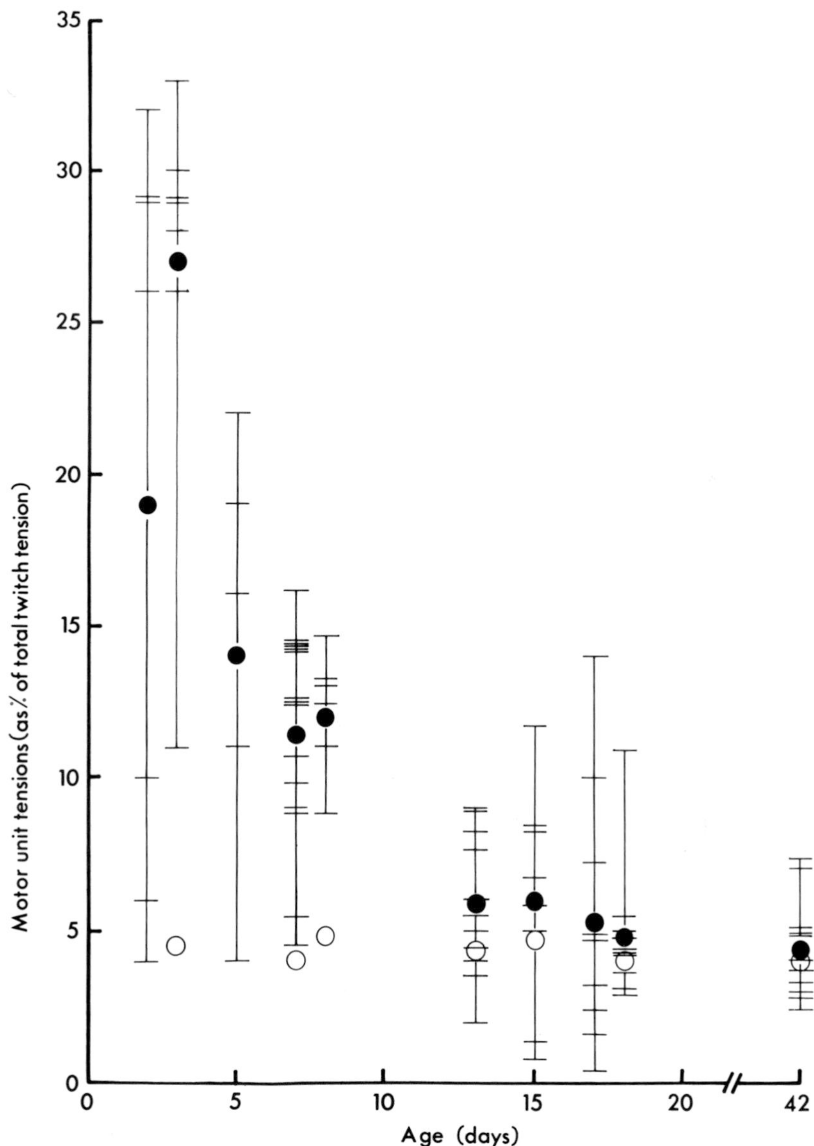

Figure 7. Motor unit sizes at different postnatal ages in the rat soleus muscle. Each vertical line represents results from one experiment. The ordinate shows the size of individual motor units expressed as a percentage of the maximal tension elicited by direct stimulation of the muscle. Filled circles give the mean size of motor units in each muscle; horizontal lines indicate the values for the lowest-threshold motor unit in each ventral root filament. Open circles show the average motor unit size that would be expected in the absence of polyneuronal innervation, based on the total number of motor units supplying the muscle. (From Brown *et al.*[7])

ameters, and lack of postnatal increases in muscle fiber number. In order to make accurate comparisons of the distribution of motor unit sizes at various developmental ages, it is necessary to have a quantitative measure of the degree of scatter in motor unit size for any given muscle. We have used the standard deviation of the individual motor unit tensions scaled to their mean value. This measure, which we term the "intrinsic diversity," should remain constant if all motor neurons were to lose a fixed percentage of their terminals. Our principal finding to date is that the intrinsic diversity in motor unit sizes actually increases significantly during the first two postnatal weeks, when the bulk of synapse elimination takes place.[28] During the 1st postnatal week the intrinsic diversity has an average value of 0.48 (seven muscles); this corresponds to about two-thirds of the motor units spanning a threefold range in size, and already at this stage some motor units are as small as the average size in the adult. The intrinsic diversity increases substantially during the 2nd week, reaching an average value of 0.93 in the five muscles examined between days 12 and 18. This corresponds to two-thirds of the motor units extending over a more than fivefold range. During this early postnatal period, when there is a threefold decrease in average motor unit size, a few motor units remain as large as the largest neonatal motor units (innervating 10% or more of the muscle). Other motor units undergo a steep decline in size, reaching a stage at which they innervate less than 0.1% of the muscle. This diversification in motor unit size is unlikely to be attributable to changes in the spectrum of muscle fiber diameters, since rabbit soleus muscle fibers become more, not less, uniform in size during maturation; moreover, we have observed that fibers are relatively homogeneous in size from postnatal day 8 onwards.

It seems reasonable to conclude that in the rabbit soleus small motor units are not at a competitive advantage during the period when most synapse elimination takes place. Indeed, it may be that small motor units are at a disadvantage and large motor units at an advantage. However, some diversification in motor unit size would be expected even if the loss of synapses were completely random with respect to motor unit size; we are currently exploring whether our data could be fit by simple models of this type. Another question being addressed is whether the extreme diversity in motor unit sizes found at days 12–18 persists into adulthood. If the final distribution is significantly more homogenous, it would imply an important additional stage of synaptic reorganization.

Recently, Miyata and Yoshioka[62] suggested that synapse elimination in rat soleus muscle occurs only for those motor units which originate in spinal root L4, and not for those originating from L5. The reported difference is remarkably large, with a fourfold reduction in the number of inputs from L4 and no change in the number from L5. It is important to consider alternative interpretations of their observations, however, as several technical difficulties might seriously bias the data. Foremost among these is the fact that the relative inputs from L4 and L5 to the soleus muscle vary considerably among individuals. Without some independent measure of the total number of motor axons from each spinal root in the experimental muscles, individual variations in the innervation pattern could affect their results to a much greater degree than might seem likely from the confidence limits they assigned to their estimates. This point is all the more worrisome because systematic differences in innervation patterns in different litters, which we have found to occur in the rabbit soleus (H. Gordon and D.V.E., unpublished), might bias the results if different litters had been examined at early and late developmental stages. Also, the inputs from L4 and L5 might be concentrated in different parts of the soleus muscle, as has been shown for other mammalian muscles,[63] and this could lead to serious sampling errors if the same region were not sampled in each experiment.

In order to see whether there are differences in synapse elimination for the spinal roots innervating the rabbit soleus, we have determined the average tension of S1 and S2 motor units at various postnatal ages. Shortly after birth (days 0–5), motor unit tensions, expressed as a percentage of maximal direct tension, average 5.5% for S1 and 5.0% for S2. These values decline to 1.8% for S1 and 1.9% for S2 in muscles examined between days 10 and 18. Clearly, there is a substantial decrease in motor unit tensions for both S1 and S2, and we conclude that synapse elimination occurs for motor units of both roots, contrary to the claim for the rat soleus. The decrease in motor unit tension is slightly greater for S1 than for S2, but further experiments are necessary to determine whether the difference is significant. In any event, the conclusion seems warranted that rostro-caudal differences in synapse elimination occur to at most a small degree in the rabbit soleus and have not been convincingly shown to occur in the rat.

3.4.2. The Role of Activity. The possibility that activity could play a role in the formation, growth, and/or stabilization of synaptic connections has long been considered an attractive basis for explaining some of the ways in which experience plays a crucial role in the orderly maturation of the nervous system (cf. Harris[64]). One of the advantages of the neuromuscular junction as a model system is the feasibility of examining the effects on synapse formation and elimination of altered nerve activity produced by either paralysis or chronic stimulation. It is now well established that nerve activity is unnecessary for synapse formation, given that blockage of nerve conduction or synaptic transmission does not impair the formation of connections *in vivo* or *in vitro*.[64,65] In contrast, several previous reports have suggested that activity may play a prominent role in synapse elimination, as polyneuronal innervation persists longer than normal in immature muscles whose nerve supply has been paralyzed with tetrodotoxin (TTX)[66] or whose activity has been reduced by tenotomy[67] or spinal transection.[62] Similar results have been obtained after paralysis of regenerating motor nerves to adult muscle.[68] Finally, an enhanced rate of synapse elimination in immature muscle has been reported after chronic muscle stimulation.[26] However, in none of these studies is it certain that the results reflect a direct effect of activity on synapse elimination. For example, with all of the experiments involving paralysis or reduced activity it seems possible that the residual polyneuronal innervation reflects the initiation of nerve sprouting rather than a reduction in synapse elimination (cf. Brown *et al.*[57]). This is not a problem with the chronic stimulation experiments reported by O'Brien *et al.*,[26] but there are two other difficulties with these experiments. First, the reduced level of polyneuronal innervation detected physiologically in the stimulated muscles was not found using anatomical techniques. This could mean that activity increased the percentage of intact but genuinely nonfunctional synapses. Alternatively, scar formation or irritation associated with the implantation and stimulation procedure might have rendered neuromuscular junctions more susceptible to transmission block during the final experiment. This objection is not a trivial one since even for the control muscles the incidence of polyneuronal innervation was somewhat lower than reported elsewhere.[7,25] The second point of concern is that in muscles contralateral to the stimulated side there were indications of an increased rate of synapse elimination. This was attributed to increased activity via the crossed-extensor reflex. However, these observations also raise the possibility that systemic effects, perhaps related to stress rather than activity, might provoke a general increase in the rate of synapse elimination. While either mechanism would be of interest, evidence is not as yet available for distinguishing among these and other possibilities.

Another general point about the studies mentioned above is that they all involve inactivation or activation of the entire population of inputs to the experimental muscle. Hence, they do not bear directly on the issue of whether differential activity levels affect the probability of elimination of inactive vs. active inputs. In order to address this issue we have examined the consequences of paralyzing only one of the spinal roots supplying the rabbit soleus (H. Gordon and D.V.E., unpublished). By inserting a small, silastic-coated plug containing TTX into spinal nerve S2 it is possible to obtain a fully reversible block lasting 4 days or more. S2 generally contains only a small fraction of the total population of soleus motor axons, and tension overlap measurements indicate that, at the time of the TTX implant (postnatal days 3–5), nearly all soleus muscle fibers innervated through S2 are also innervated through S1. Therefore, few fibers were rendered completely inactive by the partial paralysis, and the possibility of inactivity-induced sprouting should not complicate the interpretation of the results.

In control experiments in which S2 had been implanted with a silastic plug lacking TTX we found that the median size of S2 motor units was on average 1.3 times the size of S1 motor units (nine experiments). After 4 or 5 days of TTX block S2 motor units were 1.0 times the size of S1 motor units (five experiments). It is clear, on the one hand, that several days of paralysis did not put S2 motor units at a major disadvantage; they ended up nearly as large as they would have been in the absence of paralysis. On the other hand, the small difference between control and experimental groups may reflect a genuine effect of paralysis. Further experiments are necessary to resolve this latter issue; what can be concluded at present is that synapses belonging to inactive motor neurons are at most at a rather modest disadvantage when in competition with normally active ones. It is somewhat surprising that a larger effect of differential activity levels on synapse elimination was not seen in view of the aforementioned reports suggesting a major role of activity. It may be that longer periods of differential activity than 3–6 days are necessary for a more pronounced effect to be established, and methods to extend this period are currently being explored.

4. MODELS AND POSSIBLE MOLECULAR MECHANISMS

4.1. *Positive vs. Negative Feedback*

Although it seems clear that the controlled elimination of synapses during development requires some type of intercellular communication, most likely a direct signal between muscle and nerve, the questions pertaining to the molecular nature of the signal are largely unresolved. In general terms it has been pointed out that synapse elimination might involve either positive- or negative-feedback mechanisms.[27,69,70] Positive feedback might involve competition for one or more trophic factors or growth-promoting substances. Negative feedback might involve interactions with one or more substances which inhibit growth or promote retraction.

A specific suggestion for a negative-feedback interaction has been made by O'Brien *et al.*, who have obtained evidence that acetylcholine promotes the release of proteases from immature muscle[26] and that these proteases can lead to degradation of presynaptic terminals *in vitro.*[71] Accordingly, they propose that proteases released during normal muscle activity tend to degrade all of the existing synapses on a fiber, but that some inputs are more resistant to this degradative influence than others owing to differences in the degree to which they are supplied with the materials necessary for terminal replenishment or regrowth. This hypothesis has the advantage of being specific and invoking known intercellular signals, acetylcholine and a protease, whose levels can be experimentally manipulated. On the other hand, the available evidence is by no means compelling. It is not surprising that protease levels exist which can damage presynaptic terminals. However, to establish a clear role of proteases in the normal process of synapse elimination it is necessary to show effects at levels which occur normally and which involve retraction of terminals without severe disruption of intracellular morphology. A more critical test would be to determine whether the normal occurrence of synapse elimination is halted by blocking protease activity *in vivo*. Also, it should be noted that the protease hypothesis in its present form cannot account for the competitive interactions of synapses separated by up to 1 mm. O'Brien *et al.*[26] suggest that extracellular diffusion of protease could lead to interactions over the necessary distances, but this fails to explain why the competition occurs only between synapses coexisting on a single fiber and not between closely spaced synapses on adjoining fibers.

A positive-feedback mechanism for synaptic interactions might involve a specific trophic factor released by muscle, taken up by nerve terminals, and essential for their survival or growth. An obvious analogy, as has been pointed out by others,[69] is the effect of nerve growth factor (NGF) on sympathetic and sensory neurons. NGF is taken up and retrogradely transported by neurons, and can have general effects on neuronal survival and growth (cf. Greene and Shooter[72]) as well as local stimulatory effects on individual neurites[73,74] (see also Chapters 6 and 9). Evidence for a trophic factor secreted by muscle has been obtained in *in vitro* experiments.[75,76] On the other hand, a positive-feedback mechanism need not involve the uptake of any specific factors into the nerve terminal. Direct contact with an end-plate seems to be important in terminal survival and growth, and it has been suggested that the interactions leading to synapse elimination are contact-mediated events.[27,70] One specific suggestion is that the competition is for access to the same marker or markers in the basal lamina that serve as a scaffold for the induction and maintenance of connections.[70] It would be particularly attractive if both polyneuronal innervation and its subsequent elimination could be explained in terms of interactions already known to be operative during the formation of synapses. This notion is explored in detail in the following section.

4.2. *A Model for Synapse Formation, Polyneuronal Innervation, and Synapse Elimination*

4.2.1. *Relevant Developmental Interactions.* The formation of neuromuscular connections is a complex, multifaceted phenomenon whose underlying mechanisms are only partially understood.[3,33,70] It is convenient to distinguish three major aspects of synaptogenesis which together provide the basis for a model capable of accounting for polyneuronal innervation and synapse elimination. They will be reviewed only briefly, since much of the relevant experimental evidence has already been discussed here (section 3.2) and elsewhere.[3,33,70]

a. Sprouting and Retraction. One of the important properties of motor neurons is a tendency for continuous sprouting and retraction of terminal processes. As argued above, the degree of "spontaneous" sprouting (i.e., that occurring in the absence of experimental perturbation) apparently changes as neuromuscular connections mature, but both tendencies persist, at least to some degree, in normal adult muscle. The balance between sprouting and retraction can be altered dramatically by procedures such as partial denervation or muscle paralysis.[77] It is very likely that muscle inactivity leads to release or exposure of a "sprouting factor" responsible for the increased incidence and extent of newly sprouted terminal processes occurring under such circumstances. It should be noted, though, that the direct effect of the sprouting factor could be either to increase the tendency for terminals to extend new processes or to decrease the probability of such processes being retracted.

It is not firmly established whether the stimulus for sprouting is a diffusible factor, as suggested by some experiments,[78] or a contact-mediated interaction, as suggested by others.[79] An interesting possibility is that both mechanisms are operative to varying degrees in different experimental situations. A single sprouting factor could even serve both roles, according to whether it was free to diffuse or was bound to cell membranes or an extracellular matrix.

Unfortunately, little is known about the mechanisms whereby terminal processes are extended and retracted, except that they presumably involve the polymerization, depolymerization, or reorganization of actin and/or other cytoskeletal elements.[80] Even less is known about how these events are controlled by external stimuli, such as sprouting factor, or by internal influences emanating from the cell body. What is most important to recognize in the present context is that, by analogy with hormonal interactions, regulation might occur in a variety of ways, and in particular that regulation by external stimuli need not involve the uptake of any specific factors into the nerve terminal. Sprouting factor might work, for example, by affecting ion fluxes into the terminal, by altering the levels of intracellular regulatory molecules (e.g., second messengers), or by changing membrane-to-substrate adhesivity (see Chapter 6).

b. Innervation Factor. Synapse formation can occur anywhere on an uninnervated muscle fiber, apparently at random.[3,9,33] This must involve a specific recognition between nerve and muscle, since connections are not made with other cell types (e.g., fibroblasts, Schwann cells) with which a growing nerve comes into contact. It is possible that the "innervation factor" which initiates synaptogenesis is the same as the factor which promotes contact-mediated sprouting, but they could equally well be separate factors.[70] Once synaptogenesis begins at any particular site, the receptivity of the extrasynaptic region is quickly suppressed. It is simplest to assume that this involves loss or redistribution of the aforementioned innervation factor, but the possibility of an increased level of an extrajunctional factor inhibiting synapse formation cannot be ruled out.

c. Scaffolds and Stabilization. Over a period of hours or days, nerve contact induces a stable synaptic scaffold in the basal lamina. The simplest hypothesis is that the nerve induces the aggregation or selective incorporation of the same innervation factor that is initially distributed over the entire myotube,[70] but it might instead be one or more other factors. Although the role of the nerve in inducing the scaffold is clear, it is not yet known whether the nerve or the muscle is responsible for its synthesis. It is useful to note, though, that there does exist a clear example of a basal lamina constituent induced by nerve but synthesized by muscle. Lømo and Slater[81] showed that transient contact by a foreign nerve could lead to the deposition of acetylcholinesterase by active muscle fibers at sites of nerve contact, but occurring subsequent to nerve removal. This implies a signal from nerve to muscle which might be released by the nerve terminal or might instead be contact mediated. The synaptic scaffold must have several diverse effects on the induction of pre- and postsynaptic specializations. Most important for the present discussion is that it must somehow stabilize the terminal. As mentioned already for the sprouting factor, this could occur by decreasing the tendency for spontaneous regression and/or by increasing the tendency for local sprouting, since stability would be enhanced as long as the ratio of sprouting to regression were increased. Also, as with sprouting factor, these effects need not involve the actual uptake of scaffolding or other synaptic markers.

In brief, the discussion has been focussed on two spontaneously occurring phenomena, sprouting and regression, and their modulation by several neuromuscular interactions involving a sprouting factor, an innervation factor, and a synaptic scaffolding. All three factors conceivably might be the same substance acting somewhat differently according to its physical state (bound vs. free) and concentration. Regardless of their molecular identity, though, none of the interactions they mediate presupposes that muscle fibers should receive multiple inputs at one stage and remove all but one at another. Taken together, however, they provide an adequate framework for explaining the occurrence and nature of polyneuronal innervation, as well as the way in which excess inputs are removed, as will be detailed in the following section. The essential features of the model are that (1) during stages in which there is a bias for sprouting over regression, polyneuronal innervation tends to occur, and (2) during stages in which this bias is reduced or reversed, synapse elimination occurs among terminals competing for access to the stabilizing influence of the synaptic scaffold.

4.2.2. Development and Application of the Model. For any model to maintain serious consideration it must be able to account for a variety of features concerning the maturation of neuromuscular connections as it occurs normally and after various experimental perturbations. At the same time, one does not want the model to become more specific or arbitrary than is warranted by the available experimental evidence. With these considerations in mind a general model for neuromuscular maturation will be developed, drawing on the interactions outlined in the preceding section, and invoking them in whatever fashion proves necessary to explain important developmental phenomena.

a. The Occurrence of Focal Polyneuronal Innervation. The first question is why, since synapse formation can so quickly render the extrasynaptic region of a muscle fiber refractory to innervation, are additional inputs so readily accepted at the initial end-plate region. Although puzzling at first, this outcome can be readily explained by consideration of the dynamic events of synaptogenesis. At early stages of neuromuscular innervation motor axons sprout profusely within the muscle, presumably because there is a high intrinsic tendency to sprout at this stage of development, coupled with a strong sprouting stimulus provided by muscle cells which have not yet been innervated. Consequently, many sprouts would come into contact with innervated fibers at both synaptic and extrasynaptic sites. Such contacts might occur entirely by chance, but the probability of contacting preexisting end-plates would be enhanced by any tendency of growing motor axons to fasciculate with each other, as commonly occurs during nerve outgrowth elsewhere *in vivo*[82,83] as well as *in vitro*[84] (see Chapters 6, 7, and 8). Sprouts which reach extrasynaptic regions of an innervated muscle fiber would fail to form synapses, presumably because of the rapid disappearance or blockage of innervation factor, perhaps by the initial synapse. (For nonmammalian muscles which have distributed innervation, the depletion of innervation factor may occur only within a limited region around each synapse.) Those sprouts which reach the immediate vicinity of a preexisting end-plate would, in contrast to the others, have a significant chance of forming a stable connection. This is because the synaptic scaffold, always receptive to innervation, would generally be partially exposed as a result of the spontaneous retraction of terminal processes going on at all times. Although these naked sites would often be covered up by reexpansion of existing inputs, it seems likely that sprouts from nearby axons would occasionally arrive at the right moment, make contact, and immediately be stabilized. They would then have the opportunity to expand their foothold by competing for access to a larger portion of the existing scaffold as well as helping induce new scaffolding. Thus, the establishment of focal polyneuronal innervation seems like a natural, perhaps inevitable, consequence of a situation in which there is a high incidence of sprouting and retraction of axonal processes embedded in a closely packed matrix of muscle cells. Just why sprouting and retraction should be so extensive at this stage of development is not so easy to answer. It may simply reflect the dynamic state typical of immature neurons in general. Alternatively, it may reflect the specific interactions necessary to ensure the prompt innervation and even induction[55] of appropriate numbers of muscle cells.

b. Competitive Elimination of Synapses. Given a dynamic situation in which multiple terminals on a single end-plate are simultaneously sprouting and retracting processes, there are several ways in which single innervation could come about.

1. One way in which synapses might be lost is if the size of a synaptic terminal affects its tendencies to sprout and/or regress. A larger terminal might have a higher probability of sprouting or a lower probability of retracting processes per unit area of synaptic contact. This would confer a competitive advantage to the larger terminal and lead ultimately to the complete elimination of smaller terminals. Exactly why these probabilities would be size dependent cannot be specified because

of our ignorance about the mechanisms of sprouting and regression. Presumably, though, the control of these processes involves specific membrane receptors (perhaps a receptor to mediate the scaffolding's stabilizing influence) as well as intracellular regulatory substances. Unless the density of receptors and the levels of regulatory substances are *completely* independent of terminal size, it would seem likely that terminals of a particular size or range of sizes would have a competitive advantage over terminals of other sizes. If the relationships were such that smaller terminals were at an advantage over larger ones, then not only the establishment, but the indefinite persistence, of polyneuronal innervation would be favored. If, on the other hand, larger terminals were at an advantage (either from the outset or as a result of a developmental change), then smaller terminals would tend to recede and eventually disappear. The important points are first, that the entire process of synapse elimination is one which can operate by differential biasing of sprouting vs. retraction tendencies of terminals competing for access to the synaptic scaffold. The winning terminal succeeds because of its likelihood of taking over regions of scaffold left naked by partial retraction of losing terminal(s) and because of its likelihood of maintaining this expanded territory. Second, only a slight competitive edge, if held for several days, would be needed to achieve this outcome.

2. Another possibility is that synapse elimination is simply a consequence of stochastic fluctuations in terminal extent, without any consistent advantage associated with larger terminals. Suppose, for example, that at the microscopic level both regression and sprouting of processes are probabilistic events and that there is a finite probability that any given synapse will suddenly retract all of its processes, thereby losing its foothold on the synaptic scaffold. Once contact is broken, the axon might suddenly become more likely to regress altogether, because it has lost whatever stabilizing, regression-inhibiting, or sprout-inducing influence is provided by the scaffold, and also because the newly vacated part of the end-plate would tend to be taken over by other terminals.

Once a fiber becomes singly innervated, though, its terminal would tend to occupy the entire end-plate; the spontaneous fluctuations in terminal size would occur around a larger mean than in the multiply innervated state. Hence, there would be a much lower probability of complete terminal regression, which is consistent with the evidence against the occurrence of transiently denervated fibers.

3. A third basis for the removal of synapses concerns the role of the motor neuron cell body in providing its terminals with the constituents necessary for survival. That the periphery is critically dependent on the cell body is suggested by the rapid withdrawal and degeneration

produced by axotomy and by the intrinsic tendency for motor neurons to withdraw peripheral synapses during early postnatal development. In terms of how central influences manifest themselves at the periphery, it is again easy to imagine a variety of plausible interactions. For example, motor neurons might differ in the degree to which they are able to supply their terminals with any of a variety of substances involved in regulation of sprouting or retraction (e.g., constituents needed to recognize or respond to factors in the synaptic scaffold). These differences might be related to motor unit size, activity levels, or other intrinsic features of motor neurons. Whatever their nature, their occurrence would lead to the elimination of disadvantaged inputs by differential biasing of sprouting vs. retraction, as already discussed.

c. Synaptic Withdrawal after Partial Denervation. The observation that wholesale synapse elimination occurs even in partially denervated soleus muscles containing only one or a few motor units points to an intrinsic tendency of motor neurons (in some muscles) to withdraw most of their synapses at a particular stage of development. It might seem that this result could be fully explained simply by invoking an enhancement of the normal tendency for spontaneous retraction of processes. However, the situation is not so straightforward. In particular, it is necessary to consider why the outcome is not an across-the-board reduction in the size of all terminals (or just a uniform failure to grow), rather than one in which some terminals grow larger and others disappear altogether despite the absence of direct competition with other terminals. In essence, it seems that there must be a competitive advantage of some terminals, presumably the larger ones, over other terminals, presumably the smaller ones, belonging to the *same* motor neuron. The basis of this competition is unknown, but it is plausible to suppose that it involves a nonlinear relationship between the size of a terminal and the supply of substances needed for growth, maintenance, or survival (e.g., ones which regulate sprouting and retraction). If larger terminals were able to claim a disproportionate share of the materials transported down the axon (or if they were more efficient in divesting themselves of harmful waste products), then a positive-feedback mechanism would exist that would tend to increase the disparity between large and small terminals. In the partial denervation situation this mechanism alone would be sufficient to lead to complete withdrawal of synapses, while during normal maturation it could play a major role in biasing the outcome of competitions between synapses belonging to different motor neurons. In the extreme case one might anticipate that such a mechanism would favor the establishment of one or a few "giant" synapses by each motor neuron. The fact that this does not occur indicates that the optimal terminal size is not the largest possible, either because of the nature of the nonlinearities relating terminal size to trophic supplies or because other interactions (relating, say, to a limited supply of scaffolding by muscle fibers) become progressively more important as terminal size increases.

d. Maintenance of Single Innervation in the Adult. Two major changes occur during maturation which together can account for the absence of a significant degree of polyneuronal innervation in normal adult mammalian muscle. Even though sprouting and regression of processes evidently persist in the adult, they appear to be quantitatively less extensive than in the neonate. Coupled with this is the greater size of muscle fibers and hence greater average separation between neighboring end-plates. Thus there would be little chance that a process sprouting from a terminal or preterminal axon would reach another end-plate and even less chance that it would encounter a vacant site on that end-plate where it could establish a foothold.

e. Distributed Synapses after Cross-innervation. The fact that synapses are readily formed at multiple sites along a single muscle fiber in cross-innervation experiments contrasts sharply with the absence of distributed innervation during normal mammalian development, but is reminiscent of the pattern in lower vertebrates. Presumably, the difference is one of timing and/or spatial interactions, in that the suppression of susceptibility to innervation outside a newly formed synapse either takes place more slowly or spreads more slowly in adult and early postnatal muscles than in embryonic ones.

f. Elimination of Distributed Inputs. The mechanism proposed above for the elimination of focal polyneuronal innervation involves multiple synapses competing for access to the same synaptic scaffold. Obviously, this cannot account for competitive interactions between spatially separate synapses, so it is necessary to consider alternative possibilities. This can still be done within the framework of the interactions already associated with synapse formation. For example, suppose that the synaptic scaffolding is synthesized by the muscle, turns over at a finite rate once it is incorporated into the basal lamina, and is replenished from a limited supply per unit length of muscle fiber. If nearby nerve terminals on the same fiber differ in their effectiveness at inducing the incorporation of this factor into their respective end-plates, then a feedback loop could be established in which a synapse initially at a small disadvantage would be less effective at inducing the replenishment of its scaffolding and would therefore tend to sprout less and regress more. This would put it at an even greater disadvantage at replenishing its scaffolding and could ultimately lead to its complete withdrawal.

The fact that different mechanisms are invoked to explain the elimination of distributed vs. focal polyneuronal innervation might seem to be a drawback to the general model described here. On the other hand, there are several reasons for not regarding this as a serious problem. First, the observation that synapse elimination is markedly prolonged in time course when it involves competition at a distance[7] indicates that some aspects of the interactions indeed are not identical in the two situations. Second, the proposed mechanisms are not as different as they might seem at first glance. They both involve similar signals at the end-plate. In the case of focal innervation the key assumption is that contact with the scaffolding directly affects the tendency of a terminal to sprout and/or regress. It is also necessary to assume that the nerve has induced the scaffolding in the first place, but the particular nature of this induction is not critical. In the case of more distant interactions, the first assumption about feedback effects of the scaffolding on the nerve is maintained, and in addition it is necessary to specify that both nerve and muscle must be directly involved in the regulation of the scaffolding. The third point is that there already exists evidence from cross-innervation experiments that the susceptibility of a denervated end-plate to reinnervation is gradually suppressed when a synapse exists elsewhere on the same fiber.[7,31]

If it is true that the key to spatial interactions is a competition for the incorporation of synaptic scaffolding, then the same interactions might also occur in individual polyneuronally innervated end-plates: some terminals would be more effective than others at inducing the replenishment of scaffolding. Whether this would play a significant role in the competition for survival would depend on two factors. The first concerns whether an individual terminal affects the replenishment of scaffolding throughout the end-plate or only in that portion which it occupies. The second concerns the degree to which terminals tend to intermix and exchange places on an end-plate as a result of the dynamics of sprouting and regression. No detailed evidence bearing on either of these issues is available, however.

g. Survival of Synapses from the Same Neuron. The observation that closely spaced terminals belonging to the same motor neuron are occasionally encountered in cross-innervated muscles[32] suggests that their common origin confers some resistance to the interactions that lead to synapse elimination. As Kuffler *et al.*[32] point out, it hardly seems likely that this survival is related to unique chemical markers on each terminal. They suggest instead that the muscle fiber produces a trophic factor at a rate inversely related to its activity level. Dually innervated fibers driven by the same motor neuron would tend to have lower activity than polyneuronally innervated fibers and hence would produce more trophic substance and enhance the survival probabilities of both synapses. This suggestion can be incorporated into the present model by supposing that it is the production of synaptic scaffolding which is inversely related to activity. Moreover, the tendency for synapse elimination would also be reduced because there is no possibility of one synapse having an advantage over the other by virtue of its parentage. Yet another possibility is that whatever feedback a neuron obtains from its association with an end-plate spreads to other nearby terminals of the same neuron. This might involve the widespread distribution of a trophic factor itself or of some intracellular regulatory substance. It will not be easy to distinguish among these possibilities and others, such as a protection from degradation conferred by synchrony of pre- and postsynaptic activity.[85] One point which will be important to determine is whether common parentage of synapses coexisting on a fiber is sufficient to guarantee their mutual survival or merely makes it more likely.

4.2.3. *Recapitulation and Testing of the Model.* The model for neuromuscular maturation can be summarized as follows. Motor nerve terminals are continually sprouting and retracting, but the balance between the two processes as well as their overall extent are subject to various external and internal influences. The major external influences are contact with a sprouting factor whose production is inhibited by muscle activity, and with a synaptic scaffolding whose production or aggregation is induced by the nerve (but with varying degrees of effectiveness for different terminals) and is replenished by the muscle fiber from a supply of limited amount per unit length of fiber (and perhaps of variable amount according to muscle activity levels). The major internal influences involve the supply of materials which directly or indirectly affect sprouting and retraction; the distribution of these materials probably depends nonlinearly on terminal size and may also depend on other features such as motor unit size and activity levels.

Many aspects of this model are similar to, and have drawn heavily from, general models of synapse elimination that have been suggested by others.[27,69,70] The major differences are that the present model (1) accounts for the occurrence of polyneuronal innervation as well as synapse elimination; (2) attributes synapse elimination to the competition for synaptic scaffolding, a factor whose existence is already strongly suspected, without invoking the actual uptake of this factor; and (3) suggests a specific way in which the competition is expressed, namely, by alterations or fluctuations in sprouting vs. retraction tendencies, rather than the more general notion of acquisition of a factor necessary for growth or survival. In a sense, this model is a specific formulation of the idea of competition for "synaptic space" proposed for both neuromuscular[86] and CNS[87] reinnervation, in that it spells out what is distinctive about synaptic vs. extrasynaptic space and suggests how the competition could occur.

Given our fragmentary understanding of the molecular basis of neuromuscular interactions, it should be clear that the evidence favoring the various aspects of the present model is indirect and in no way compelling. The ultimate worth of the model may lie mainly in its usefulness as a guide to further lines of experimentation, and in this respect several comments are worth making. Perhaps the most important is to emphasize the need for a better understanding of the mechanisms of sprouting and retraction. These are surely very complex phenomena subject to regulation in a variety of ways. It is of great interest to know what molecular interactions are responsible for changes in the configuration of a terminal and over what extent these interactions can take place (e.g., what portion of a terminal is affected by a local sprouting stimulus). Such questions are particularly amenable to analysis *in vitro*, and it seems reasonable to anticipate substantial progress from the structural and biochemical approaches currently underway in many laboratories (see Chapter 6).

A second approach that shows considerable promise is the effort to identify specific basal lamina constituents, hopefully including the scaffolding itself, i.e., the factor(s) responsible for terminal stabilization. Success has already been achieved in obtaining synapse-specific antibodies,[88] and there seem to be no insurmountable obstacles to finding antibodies to constituents demonstrably involved in developmental interactions (see also Chapter 3). Once the scaffolding is identified, it may become possible to assess its role in synapse elimination more directly by blocking it with antibodies or otherwise changing its effective distribution.

Lastly, it should be pointed out that the focus of the present model on the synaptic scaffold is not meant to deny the plausibility of additional substances, "trophic" or otherwise, playing important roles in synapse elimination. There is no compelling need as yet to invoke such substances to explain the interactions that are known, but neither is there any strong basis for suspecting that they do not exist. Obviously, the search for additional synapse-specific factors should continue, and at such time as they are found their possible role in synapse elimination should receive careful scrutiny.

5. OVERVIEW AND CONCLUSION

5.1. *Synapse Elimination Elsewhere in the Nervous System*

A detailed discussion of synapse elimination in other parts of the nervous system besides the neuromuscular junction is outside the scope of this article. Nonetheless it is useful to comment briefly on the relevance that neuromuscular synapse elimination has to the understanding of general principles of neural development. The most important point in this respect is that synapse elimination evidently plays a major role in the normal development of many different parts of the nervous system. Evidence for synapse elimination during maturation has been obtained in vertebrate sympathetic and parasympathetic ganglia,[89–91] in the spinal cord,[92,93] cerebellum,[94] and cerebral cortex,[95,96] and in invertebrate muscles.[97] There is also indirect evidence for a major shifting of connections within the vertebrate retina[98] and between retina and tectum[99,100] owing to differential growth of topographically organized sheets of cells. Even in the CNS of adult mammals there may be a significant degree of synaptic remodeling,[101,102] although the occurrence of degenerating debris raises the possibility that the changes are largely due to cell death.

The mechanism of synapse elimination is not well understood in any of these systems, but several interesting insights have emerged concerning its functional significance. In sympathetic ganglia the loss of synapses is correlated with changes in dendritic organization, and there is a correlation between the complexity of dendritic arborization and the number of synaptic inputs retained in the adult.[69,90,91] Thus, a major aspect of synapse elimination in the autonomic system may be related to the segregation of synaptic inputs onto specific dendritic domains.

In the visual system there is strong evidence that synapse elimination plays a major role in the maturation of ocular dominance columns in the visual cortex. In both cats and monkeys geniculocortical inputs subserving each eye are distributed uniformly in horizontal extent through layer IV early in development, whereas in adults the inputs are segregated into well-defined ocular dominance columns.[30,103,104] Since electrophysiological recordings from layer IV show a high degree of binocular activation in neonates but not adults, it seems likely that connections which are present and functional at birth disappear during maturation. The critical role which binocular competition plays in the reorganization of visual cortical connections has been examined by a variety of approaches (see Chapter 11). Of particular interest is the recent evidence that chronic binocular inactivity produced by intraocular TTX injections[105] and perhaps also dark-rearing[106] (but see Stryker[105]) prevent the normal segregation of geniculocortical afferents in kittens. This striking effect of altered impulse activity contrasts with the difficulty in establishing any direct and unambiguous effect of TTX paralysis on neuromuscular synapse elimination (see Section 3.4.2). It remains to be determined whether this reflects an inherent difference between the systems or is instead related to a shorter duration of the block in the neuromuscular experiments.

5.2. *Concluding Remarks*

It might seem wasteful that the majority of synaptic connections established in the neuromuscular system, and perhaps throughout the nervous system, should be summarily removed not long after they are formed. However, the inefficiency may be less than it seems at first glance, as the materials obtained from a retracting synapse are presumably available for redistribution to other terminals of the same neuron. By contrast, the phenomenon of neuronal cell death, well documented in many parts of the nervous system (see Chapter 9), is more extravagant insofar as it involves complete cellular degeneration and degradation. These considerations aside, the intriguing feature of synapse elimination is that it adds a further dimension to the issue of specificity and plasticity of the nervous system. Proper maturation of the nervous system requires not only that a particular set of connections be formed, but that an appropriate subset of these be taken away. It is probably not a matter of redundant mechanisms, but rather of complementary ones which yield a final product more refined than that attainable by either operating alone.

Obviously there is a high degree of specificity in the initial establishment of connections. In the neuromuscular system there are few outright errors in early development[10,107,108]; nor does there appear to be any marked change in the location or overall extent of muscle fibers belonging to individual motor units.[10] If there is a major functional role of synapse elimination in this system, it is probably related to some form of numerical matching, such as the attainment of an appropriate distribution of motor unit sizes. In the visual cortex the degree of specificity demanded in the adult is enormously greater, but this specificity is only partially achieved during prenatal development. At birth or shortly thereafter, the connections are sufficiently precise that cortical cells have well-defined receptive fields and specific functional properties such as orientation selectivity; however, ocular dominance columns are not fully established, and many cells have immature properties, particularly with respect to binocular interactions.[109] Evidently, the attainment of mature properties necessitates a stage of fine tuning in which visual experience plays a major role. It seems likely, on the basis of evidence discussed above, that the elimination of synapses during this stage involves the weeding out of connections which turn out to be inappropriate, and not just the adjustment of their overall number.

One of the major goals in the analysis of synapse elimination anywhere in the nervous system is to elucidate the molecular nature of the intercellular and intracellular interactions involved in the process. There is good reason to believe that neuromuscular synapse elimination must involve bidirectional signals between nerve and muscle, but the identity of these signals remains unknown. The argument was presented above that it is possible to account for known aspects of synapse elimination in terms of competition for access to synaptic markers in the basal lamina and differential capacities to induce these markers and respond to them. Thus the transition from polyneuronal to single innervation may come about by the operation of the same mechanisms involved in establishing polyneuronal innervation in the first place, with the changed outcome resulting from quantitative mechanistic differences. Alternatively, there may well be specific trophic factors and/or inhibitory factors. Distinguishing among these and perhaps other possibilities will be a challenging task for the future.

ACKNOWLEDGMENTS

I am indebted to H. Gordon and J. L. Bixby for insightful discussions and valuable criticisms of the manuscript, and to P. Brown and C. Katz for typing the manuscript. Work from my laboratory was supported by the Alfred P. Sloan Foundation, by the Pew Memorial Trust, and by BRSG Grant RR07003 awarded by the Division of Research Resources, NIH.

6. REFERENCES

1. Cowan, W. M., 1978, Aspects of neural development, *Int. Rev. Physiol.* **17**:149.
2. Jacobson, M., 1978, *Developmental Neurobiology*, 2nd ed., Plenum Press, New York.
3. Dennis, M. J., 1981, Development of the neuromuscular junction: Inductive interactions between cells, *Ann. Rev. Neurosci.* **4**:43.
4. Tello, J. F., 1917, Genesis de las terminaciones nerviosas motrices y sensitivas, *Trab. Lab. Invest. Biol. Madrid* **15**:101.

5. Cuajunco, F., 1942, Development of the human motor end-plate, *Carnegie Inst. Contr. Embryol.* **30:**129.
6. Redfern, P. A., 1970, Neuromuscular transmission in new-born rats, *J. Physiol.* **209:**701.
7. Brown, M. C., Jansen, J. K. S., and Van Essen, D., 1976, Polyneuronal innervation of skeletal muscle in new-born rats and its elimination during maturation, *J. Physiol.* **261:**387.
8. Bagust, J., Lewis, D. M., and Westerman, R. A., 1973, Polyneuronal innervation of kitten skeletal muscle, *J. Physiol.* **229:**241.
9. Bennett, M. R., and Pettigrew, A. G., 1974, The formation of synapses in striated muscle during development, *J. Physiol.* **241:**515.
10. Dennis, M. J., Ziskind-Conhaim, L., and Harris, A. J., 1981, Development of neuromuscular junctions in rat embryos, *Dev. Biol.* **81:**266.
11. Ontell, M., and Dunn, R. F., 1978, Neonatal muscle growth: A quantitative study, *Am. J. Anat.* **152:**539.
12. Betz, W. J., Caldwell, J. H., and Ribchester, R. R., 1979, The size of motor units during post-natal development of rat lumbrical muscle, *J. Physiol.* **297:**463.
13. Lubinska, L., and Zelená, J., 1966, Formation of new sites of acetylcholinesterase activity in denervated muscle of young rats, *Nature* (*London*) **210:**39.
14. Riley, D. A., 1976, Multiple axon branches innervating single endplates of kitten soleus myofibers, *Brain Res.* **110:**158.
15. Bixby, J. L., and Van Essen, D. C., 1979, Regional differences in the timing of synapse elimination in skeletal muscles of the neonatal rabbit, *Brain Res.* **169:**275.
16. Bennett, M. R., and Pettigrew, A. G., 1975, The formation of synapses in amphibian striated muscle during development, *J. Physiol.* **252:**203.
17. Rosenthal, J. L., and Taraskevitch, P. S., 1977, Reduction of multiaxonal innervation at the neuromuscular junction of the rat during development, *J. Physiol.* **270:**299.
18. Harris-Flanagan, A. E., 1969, Differentiation and degeneration in the motor horn of the foetal mouse, *J. Morphol.* **129:**281.
19. Chiakulas, J. J., and Pauly, J. E., 1965, A study of postnatal growth of skeletal muscle in the rat, *Anat. Rec.* **152:**55.
20. Rayne, J., and Crawford, G. N. C., 1975, Increase in fibre numbers of the rat pterygoid muscles during postnatal growth, *J. Anat.* **119:**347.
21. Rowe, R. W. D., and Goldspink, G., 1969, Muscle fibre growth in five different muscles in both sexes of mice. I. Normal mice, *J. Anat.* **104:**519.
22. Enesco, M., and Puddy, D., 1964, Increase in the number of nuclei and weight in skeletal muscle of rats of various ages, *Am. J. Anat.* **114:**235.
23. Thompson, W., and Jansen, J. K. S., 1977, The extent of sprouting of remaining motor units in partly denervated immature and adult rat soleus muscle, *Neuroscience* **2:**523.
24. Westerman, R. A., Lewis, D. M., Bagust, J., Edjtehadi, G. D., and Pallot, D., 1973, Communication between nerves and muscles: Postnatal development in kitten hindlimb fast and slow twitch muscle, in: *Memory and Transfer of Information*, (H. P. Zippel, ed.), pp. 255–291, Plenum Press, New York.
25. Riley, D. A., 1977, Spontaneous elimination of nerve terminals from the endplates of developing skeletal myofibers, *Brain Res.* **134:**279.
26. O'Brien, R. A. D., Östberg, A. J. C.,and Vrbová, G., 1978, Observations on the elimination of polyneuronal innervation in developing mammalian skeletal muscle, *J. Physiol.* **282:**571.
27. Brown, M. C., Holland, R. L., and Hopkins, W. G., 1981, Excess neuronal inputs

during development, in: *Development in the Nervous System,* (D. R. Garrod and J. D. Feldman, eds.), Cambridge University Press, Cambridge, in press.
28. Gordon, H., and Van Essen, D. C., 1981, Motor units diversify in size as synapse elimination proceeds in the neonatal rabbit soleus muscle, *Soc. Neurosci. Abstr.,* **7**:179.
29. Hubel, D. H., and Wiesel, T. N., 1970, The period of susceptibility to the physiological effects of unilateral eye closure in kittens, *J. Physiol.* **206**:419.
30. LeVay, S., Wiesel, T. N., and Hubel, D. H., 1980, The development of ocular dominance columns in normal and visually deprived monkeys, *J. Comp. Neurol.* **191**:1.
31. Frank, E., Jansen, J. K. S., Lømo, T., and Westgaard, R. H., 1975, The interaction between foreign and original motor nerves innervating the soleus muscle of rats, *J. Physiol.* **247**:725.
32. Kuffler, D. P., Thompson, W., and Jansen, J. K. S., 1980, The fate of foreign endplates in cross-innervated rat soleus muscle. *Proc. R. Soc. London Ser. B* **208**:189.
33. Lømo, T., 1980, What controls the development of neuromuscular junctions? *Trends Neurosci.* **3**:126.
34. McArdle, J. J., 1975, Complex end-plate potentials at the regenerating neuromuscular junction of the rat, *Exp. Neurol.* **49**:629.
35. Brown, M. C., and Ironton, R., 1978, Sprouting and regression of neuromuscular synapses in partially denervated mammalian muscles, *J. Physiol.* **278**:325.
36. Bixby, J. L., and Van Essen, D. C., 1979, Competition between foreign and original nerves in adult mammalian skeletal muscle, *Nature* (*London*) **282**:726.
37. Korneliussen, H., and Jansen, J. K. S., 1976, Morphological aspects of the elimination of polyneuronal innervation of skeletal muscle fibres in newborn rats, *J. Neurocytol.* **5**:591.
38. Bixby, J. L., 1981, Ultrastructural observations on synapse elimination in neonatal rabbit skeletal muscle, *J. Neurocytol.* **10**:81.
39. Riley, D. A., 1981, Ultrastructural evidence of axon retraction during the spontaneous elimination of polyneuronal innervation of the rat soleus muscle, *J. Neurocytol.* **10**:425.
40. Guth, L., and Zalewski, A. A., 1963, Disposition of cholinesterase following implantation of nerve into innervated and denervated muscle, *Exp. Neurol.* **7**:316.
41. Guth, L., Zalewski, A. A., and Brown, W. C., 1966, Quantitative changes in cholinesterase activity of denervated sole plates following implantation of nerve into muscle, *Exp. Neurol.* **16**:136.
42. Gutmann, E., and Hanzlíková, V., 1967, Effects of accessory nerve supply to muscle achieved by implantation into muscle during regeneration of its nerve, *Physiol. Bohemoslov.* **16**:244.
43. Frank, E., Gautvik, K., and Sommerschild, H., 1975, Cholinergic receptors at denervated mammalian motor end-plates, *Acta Physiol. Scand.* **95**:66.
44. Marshall, L. M., Sanes, J. R., and McMahan, U. J., 1977, Reinnervation of original synaptic sites on muscle fiber basement membrane after disruption of the muscle cells, *Proc. Natl. Acad. Sci. U.S.A.* **74**:3073.
45. Sanes, J. R., Marshall, L. M., and McMahan, U. J., 1978, Reinnervation of muscle fiber basal lamina after removal of myofibers. Differentiation of regenerating axons at original synaptic sites, *J. Cell Biol.* **78**:176.
46. Burden, S. J., Sargent, P. B., and McMahan, U. J., 1979, Acetylcholine receptors in regenerating muscle accumulate at original synaptic sites in the absence of the nerve, *J. Cell Biol.* **82**:412.

47. Young, J. Z., 1952, Growth and plasticity in the nervous system, *Proc. R. Soc. London Ser. B* **139**:18.
48. Barker, D., and Ip, M. C., 1966, Sprouting and degeneration of mammalian motor axons in normal and de-afferentated skeletal muscle, *Proc. R. Soc. London Ser. B* **163**:538.
49. Tuffery, A. R., 1971, Growth and degeneration of motor end-plates in normal cat hind limb muscles, *J. Anat.* **110**:221.
50. Brown, M. C., and Ironton, R., 1977, Motor neurone sprouting induced by prolonged tetrodotoxin block of nerve action potentials, *Nature (London)* **265**:459.
51. Letinsky, M. S., Fischbeck, K. H., and McMahan, U. J., 1976, Precision of reinnervation of original postsynaptic sites in frog muscle after a nerve crush, *J. Neurocytol.* **5**:691.
52. Wernig, A., Pécot-Dechavassine, M., and Stöver, H., 1980, Sprouting and regression of the nerve at the frog neuromuscular junction in normal conditions and after prolonged paralysis with curare, *J. Neurocytol.* **9**:277.
53. Haimann, C., Mallart, A., Tomás i Ferré, J., and Zilber-Gachelin, N. F., 1981, Patterns of motor innervation in the pectoral muscle of adult *Xenopus laevis*: Evidence for possible synaptic remodeling, *J. Physiol.* **310**:241.
54. Speidel, C. C., 1942, Studies of living nerves. VII. Growth adjustments of cutaneous terminal arborizations, *J. Comp. Neurol.* **76**:57.
55. Betz, W. J., Caldwell, J. H., and Ribchester, R. R., 1980, The effects of partial denervation at birth on the development of muscle fibres and motor units in rat lumbrical muscle, *J. Physiol.* **303**:265.
56. Dennis, M. J., and Harris, A. J., 1980, Transient inability of neonatal rat motoneurons to reinnervate muscle, *Dev. Biol.* **74**:173.
57. Brown, M. C., Holland, R. L., and Hopkins, W. G., 1980, Some effects of botulinum toxin on the motor innervation of neonatal rat muscles, *J. Physiol.* **307**:17p.
58. Bennett, M. R., and Pettigrew, A. G., 1974, The formation of synapses in reinnervated and cross-reinnervated striated muscle during development, *J. Physiol.* **241**:547.
59. Mark, R. F., 1980, Synaptic repression at neuromuscular junctions, *Physiol. Rev.* **60**:355.
60. Proctor, W., Frenk, S., Taylor, B., and Roper, S., 1979, "Hybrid" synapses formed by foreign innervation of parasympathetic neurons: A model for selectivity during competitive reinnervation, *Proc. Natl. Acad. Sci. U.S.A.* **76**:4695.
61. Close, R., 1967, Properties of motor units in fast and slow skeletal muscles of the rat, *J. Physiol.* **193**:45.
62. Miyata, Y., and Yoshioka, K., 1980, Selective elimination of motor nerve terminals in the rat soleus muscle during development, *J. Physiol.* **309**:631.
63. Swett, J. E., Eldred, E., and Buchwald, J. S., 1970, Somatotopic cord-to-muscle relations in efferent innervation of cat gatrocnemius, *Am. J. Physiol.* **219**:762.
64. Harris, W. A., 1981, Neural activity and development, *Ann. Rev. Physiol.* **43**:689.
65. Cangiano, A., Lømo, T., Lutzemberger, L., and Sveen, O., 1980, Effects of chronic nerve conduction block on formation of neuromuscular junctions and junctional AChE in the rat, *Acta Physiol. Scand.* **109**:283.
66. Thompson, W., Kuffler, D. P., and Jansen, J. K. S., 1979, The effect of prolonged, reversible block of nerve impulses on the elimination of polyneuronal innervation of new-born rat skeletal muscle fibers, *Neuroscience* **4**:271.
67. Benoit, P., and Changeux, J.-P., 1975, Consequences of tenotomy on the evolution of multiinnervation in developing rat soleus muscle, *Brain Res.* **99**:354.
68. Benoit, P., and Changeux, J.-P., 1978, Consequences of blocking the nerve with a

local anaesthetic on the evolution of multiinnervation at the regenerating neuromuscular junction of the rat, *Brain Res.* **149:**89.
69. Purves, D., and Lichtman, J. W., 1980, Elimination of synapses in the developing nervous system, *Science* **210:**153.
70. Jansen, J. K. S., Thompson, W., and Kuffler, D. P., 1978, The formation and maintenance of synaptic connections as illustrated by studies of the neuromuscular junction, *Progr. Brain Res.* **48:**3.
71. O'Brien, R. A. D., Östberg, A. J., and Vrbová, G., 1980, The effect of acetylcholine on the function and structure of the developing mammalian neuromuscular junction, *Neuroscience* **5:**1367.
72. Greene, L. A., and Shooter, E. M., 1980, The nerve growth factor: Biochemistry, synthesis, and mechanism of action., *Ann. Rev. Neurosci.* **3:**353.
73. Gundersen, R. W., and Barrett, J. N., 1979, Neuronal chemotaxis: Chick dorsal-root axons turn toward high concentrations of nerve growth factor, *Science* **206:**1079.
74. Campenot, R. B., 1977, Local control of neurite development by nerve growth factor, *Proc. Natl. Acad. Sci. U.S.A.* **74:**4516.
75. Bennett, M. R., and Nurcombe, V., 1979, The survival and development of cholinergic neurons in skeletal muscle conditioned media, *Brain Res.* **173:**543.
76. Obata, K., and Tanaka, H., 1980, Conditioned medium promotes neurite growth from both central and peripheral neurons, *Neurosci. Lett.* **16:**27.
77. Brown, M. C., Holland, R. L., and Hopkins, W. G., 1981, Motor nerve sprouting, *Ann. Rev. Neurosci.* **4:**17.
78. Betz, W. J., Caldwell, J. H., and Ribchester, R. R., 1980, Sprouting of active nerve terminals in partially inactive muscles of the rat, *J. Physiol.* **303:**281.
79. Brown, M. C., Holland, R. L., Hopkins, W. G., and Keynes, R. J., 1981, An assessment of the spread of the signal for terminal sprouting within and between muscles, *Brain Res.* **210:**145.
80. Bray, D., and Gilbert, D., 1981, Cytoskeletal elements in neurons, *Ann. Rev. Neurosci.* **4:**505.
81. Lømo, T., and Slater, C. R., 1980, Control of junctional acetylcholinesterase by neural and muscular influences in the rat, *J. Physiol.* **303:**191.
82. Bate, C. M., 1976, Pioneer neurons in an insect embryo, *Nature (London)* **260:**54.
83. Grant, P., and Rubin, E., 1980, Ontogeny of the retina and optic nerve in *Xenopus laevis*. II. Ontogeny of the optic fiber pattern in the retina, *J. Comp. Neurol.* **189:**671.
84. Rutishauser, U., Gall, W. E., and Edelman, G. M., 1978, Adhesion among neural cells of the chick embryo. IV. Role of the cell surface molecule CAM in the formation of neurite bundles in cultures of spinal ganglia, *J. Cell Biol.* **79:**382.
85. Stent, G. S., 1973, A physiological mechanism for Hebb's postulate of learning, *Proc. Natl. Acad. Sci. U.S.A.* **70:**997.
86. Slack, J. R., 1978, Interaction between foreign and regenerating axons in axolotl muscle. *Brain Res.* **146:**172.
87. Meyer, R. L., 1979, "Extra" optic fibers exclude normal fibers from tectal regions in goldfish, *J. Comp. Neurol.* **183:**883.
88. Sanes, J. R., and Hall, Z. W., 1979, Antibodies that bind specifically to synaptic sites on muscle fiber basal lamina, *J. Cell Biol.* **83:**357.
89. Lichtman, J. W., 1977, The reorganization of synaptic connexions in the rat submandibular ganglion during postnatal development, *J. Physiol.* **273:**155.
90. Lichtman, J. W., and Purves, D., 1980, The elimination of redundant preganglionic innervation to hamster sympathetic ganglion cells in early post-natal life, *J. Physiol.* **301:**213.

91. Purves, D., and Hume, R. I., 1981, The relation of postsynaptic geometry to the number of presynaptic axons that innervate autonomic ganglion cells, *J. Neurosci.* **1:**441.
92. Ronnevi, L. O., 1977, Spontaneous phagocytosis of boutons on spinal motoneurons during early postnatal development: An electron microscopical study in the cat, *J. Neurocytol.* **6:**487.
93. Knyihar, E., Csillik, B., and Rakic, P., 1978, Transient synapses in the embryonic primate spinal cord, *Science* **202:**1206.
94. Crepel, F., Mariani, J. and Delhaye-Bouchad, N., 1976, Evidence for a multiple innervation of Purkinje cells by climbing fibers in the immature rat cerebellum, *J. Neurobiol.* **7:**567.
95. Boothe, R. G., Greenough, W. T., Lund, J. S., and Wrege, K., 1979, A quantitative investigation of spine and dendrite development of neurons in visual cortex (area 17) of *Macaca nemestrina* monkeys, *J. Comp. Neurol.* **186:**473.
96. Innocenti, G. M., 1981, Growth and reshaping of axons in the establishment of visual callosal connections, *Science* **212:**824.
97. Stephens, P. J., and Govind, C. K., 1981, Peripheral innervation fields of single lobster motoneurons defined by synapse elimination during development, *Brain Res.* **212:**476.
98. Hollyfield, J. G., 1971, Differential growth of the neural retina in *Xenopus laevis* larvae, *Dev. Biol.* **24:**264.
99. Meyer, R. L., 1978, Evidence from thymidine labeling for continuing growth of retina and tectum in juvenile goldfish, *Exp. Neurol.* **59:**99.
100. Gaze, R. M., Keating, M. J., Östberg, A., and Chung, S.-H., 1979, The relationship between retinal and tectal growth in larval *Xenopus*: Implications for the development of the retino-tectal projection, *J. Embryol. Exp. Morphol.* **53:**103.
101. Sotelo, C., and Palay, S. L., 1971, Altered axons and axon terminals in the lateral vestibular nucleus of the rat, *Lab. Invest.* **25:**653.
102. Chan-Palay, V., 1973, Neuronal plasticity in the cerebellar cortex and lateral nucleus, *Z. Anat. Entwicklungsgesch.* **142:**23.
103. Rakic, P., 1976, Prenatal genesis of connections subserving ocular dominance in the rhesus monkey, *Nature (London)* **261:**467.
104. LeVay, S., Stryker, M. P., and Shatz, C. J., 1978, Ocular dominance columns and their development in layer IV of the cat's visual cortex: A quantitative study, *J. Comp. Neurol.* **179:**223.
105. Stryker, M. P., 1981, Late segregation of geniculate afferents to the cat's visual cortex after recovery from binocular impulse blockade, *Soc. Neurosci. Abstr.* **7:**842.
106. Swindale, N. V., 1981, Absence of ocular dominance patches in dark-reared cats, *Nature* (*London*) **290:**332.
107. Dennis, M. J., and Harris, A. J., 1979, Elimination of inappropriate nerve-muscle connections during development of rat embryos, *Progr. Brain Res.* **49:**359.
108. Landmesser, L. T., 1980, The generation of neuromuscular specificity, *Ann. Rev. Neurosci.* **3:**279.
109. Pettigrew, J. D., 1974, The effect of visual experience on the development of stimulus specificity by kitten cortical neurones, *J. Physiol.* **237:**49.

11

Regeneration and Regulation in the Developing Central Nervous System

with Special Reference to the Reconstitution of the Optic Tectum of the Chick Following Removal of the Mesencephalic Alar Plate

W. MAXWELL COWAN and THOMAS E. FINGER

1. INTRODUCTION

Since the publication in 1958 of Liu and Chamber's[1] seminal study on the reorganization of connections in the adult cat spinal cord after the selective elimination of certain of its afferent inputs, there has been a veritable flood of papers dealing with various aspects of the phenomenon which has come to be known as "neuromorphological plasticity." Since much of this work has been reviewed in a number of recent publications,[2–5] we need not consider it at length here, except to point out that there is now a substantial body of evidence for essentially three

W. MAXWELL COWAN · The Salk Institute for Biological Studies, San Diego, CA 92138. THOMAS E. FINGER · Department of Anatomy, University of Colorado Medical Center, Denver, CO 80262.

This work was supported in part by the Clayton Foundation for Research, of which W. M. C. is a Senior Investigator, and by grant EY-03653 (formerly EY-1255) from the National Eye Institute.

different types of response to partial denervation in many regions of the brain and spinal cord. The first and perhaps most common response is *axonal sprouting*, which, at least in some systems, may lead to virtually a complete reinnervation of the deafferented region by collaterals from adjoining intact axons. Second, in other situations, and especially in the developing nervous system, partial deafferentation may lead either to *the misrouting of axons* into regions that they would not normally ennervate or, alternatively, to *the persistence of fibers* that normally degenerate or are withdrawn. And third, certain neuronal systems, such as the central aminergic pathways, appear to be capable of *true regeneration* following surgical interruption.

Interest in these various reactions has been so great that to a considerable extent it has obscured the fact that for close to three-quarters of a century it has been known that at early stages in development the vertebrate nervous system may display considerable regeneration, not just of selected fiber systems but of entire segments of the brain and spinal cord. Since this work appears to be largely unknown (or, at least, to have been generally neglected), before presenting some of our own findings on the capacity of the chick optic tectum to regenerate after early lesions of the mesencephalic alar plate, we shall briefly review a number of the more critical studies that have been published on regeneration in the developing brain.

2. REVIEW OF PREVIOUS STUDIES OF REGENERATION IN THE DEVELOPING CENTRAL NERVOUS SYSTEM

The first indication that central neural tissue (like most other embryonic tissues) has the capacity for regulation, came from Lewis's[6] observation that after small lesions of the neural plate in the amphibian *Rana palustris*, the ablated tissue is rapidly reconstituted by the proliferation of cells in the neighboring, undamaged parts of the neural plate, and their subsequent migration into the ablated region. At about the same time, Bell[7,8] showed, in embryos at a somewhat later stage in development, that after unilateral excision of the forebrain rudiment the damaged region is replaced by a thin sheet of tissue that contains both nerve cells and neuronal processes. Essentially the same observation was made about five years later by Spemann,[9] who found that after removing much of the rostral half of the neural plate, the forebrain was replaced by an epithelial sheet that contained many identifiable nerve cells.

In 1916, in what was at one time a widely quoted study, Burr[10] suggested that the ingrowth of extrinsic afferents was essential for the reconstitution of the amphibian forebrain, because when the nasal pit (from which the olfactory epithelium is derived) was removed together with the presumptive forebrain, regeneration never proceeded beyond the "epithelial-sheet stage." According to Burr, if the nasal pit was left intact the reconstitution of the forebrain was often complete. This interpretation was subsequently called in question by Spirito,[11–13] who, in a series of less frequently cited papers, demonstrated quite clearly that regeneration of the forebrain could often occur in the absence of its olfactory input, and most later work has tended to support his view that neither extrinsic nor central afferents are necessary for the regeneration of the embryonic central nervous system.*

The most extensive series of studies on early central nervous system regeneration is that of Detwiler, who between 1944 and 1947 reported the results of four separate groups of experiments on the reconstitution of the medulla,[14] of the forebrain,[15] of the midbrain,[16] and of the brachial region of the spinal cord[17] in the salamander *Ambystoma punctatum.* The principal finding was essentially the same in all four studies, namely, that after excising one half of the presumptive brain regions or a few segments of the spinal cord, at early embryonic stages, the ablated part could be completely replaced by tissue derived from the corresponding region on the opposite side of the brain or cord (but, significantly, *not* from tissue rostral or caudal to the ablated part). We shall not consider each study separately, but because of its relevance for our own findings on the regeneration of the tectum, we should cite his observations on the reconstitution of the amphibian midbrain. In a series of some 60 salamanders, the right half of the developing midbrain was excised at embryonic stages 20 or 21, and the animals were sacrificed between stage 30 and mid-larval life (stage 46). By stage 30 (i.e., four days after the initial operation) a single layer of epithelial cells, derived from the contralateral side, had bridged the interval between the dorsal and ventral margins of the midbrain, and enclosed a newly constituted mesencephalic ventricle. By stage 37, the regenerated lateral wall of the midbrain was thickened considerably, apparently as the result of accelerated mitotic activity along its ventricular margin. By the 44th postoperative day (stage 46) the regenerated side was essentially indistinguishable from the unoperated half of the midbrain. From counts of the numbers of mitotic figures in the ventricular zone at the level of the midbrain ablation, and at levels rostral and caudal to this, Detwiler

* Of course, at later stages in development, the ingrowth of afferents is as important for the growth and maintenance of the neurons in the regenerated nervous system as it is during normal neural development (Cowan[52] and Kelly and Cowan[67]).

confirmed that the reconstituted tissue is derived entirely from the unoperated half of the midbrain and that the intact brain rostral or caudal to this makes no contribution to the regenerative process.

If Detwiler's was the most extensive series of studies of regeneration in the amphibian central nervous system, undoubtedly the most careful and complete analysis was that of Harrison[18] on the reconstitution of the hindbrain following unilateral extirpation of the relevant part of the neural plate in *Ambystoma.* In this important paper Harrison resolved more clearly than any of his predecessors a number of important issues, and at the same time made a number of significant new observations. First, he established beyond doubt that regeneration occurred exclusively from the contralateral, unoperated side; this was done both negatively, by demonstrating that the hindbrain could not be reconstituted if the initial lesion was bilateral, and also positively, by the use of the supravital dye Nile blue sulphate applied to the unoperated half of the hindbrain primordium. Second, he provided the first good quantitative data on the extent of the regeneration by volumetric measurements of the reconstituted half of the hindbrain: in his best cases the regenerated region achieved a volume about 70% of that of the normal hindbrain (in animals at the same stage in development). Third, from careful analyses of mitotic activity he was able to show that initially cell proliferation in the regenerating tissue lags behind that on the unoperated side and in control animals at comparable stages, but since mitosis continues in the operated region long after it has ceased in the unoperated side, the early lag period is largely compensated for. Fourth, he adduced some evidence to suggest that the underlying mesoderm may play some part in the regenerative response, because when it was ablated together with the presumptive hindbrain, neural reconstitution was never as complete as in those cases in which the mesoderm had been undisturbed. Finally, he suggested that early injury to the neural plate may have widespread effects on cell proliferation throughout the brain, since mitotic activity (as judged by the number of mitotic figures) appeared to be enhanced even in regions quite far removed from the injured area. Clearly, this does not imply that such remote regions contribute to the regenerative response, only that mitosis is widely affected in some way—possibly as the result of a nonspecific prolongation of the cell cycle.

Harrison was well aware that a major limitation in his work (and in that of his predecessors) was that the assessment of the regeneration was at relatively gross (almost macroscopic) level, and that in the absence of more detailed neuroanatomical observations, no sweeping generalizations could be drawn about the degree to which individual neuronal populations, let alone specific neural pathways, had been reformed. To date this important issue has only been addressed in the amphibian nervous system by Holtzer,[19] who for the first time used a reliable neurofibrillar stain (Bodian's protargol method) for the analysis of his material on the reconstitution of the urodele spinal cord following the unilateral removal of three spinal segments. This method enabled him to identify a number of distinctive cell groups in the reconstituted tissue, and to relate the extent to which they could regenerate to the developmental stage at which the operation was performed. In the youngest embryos—operated upon between stages 18 and 24—regeneration was essentially complete, whereas in animals operated upon between stages 33 and 42 only the dorsal internuncial cells appeared on the operated side. He also traced the course taken by the axons of motoneurons and of some of the more dorsally placed spinal interneurons. The progressive restriction in the regenerative capacity of the cord led Holtzer to suggest that the developing spinal cord undergoes a form of mosaic differentiation (see also Chapter 2), and that although each component retains the capacity for regenerative hyperplasia at least for some period, it can only give rise, in the regenerated region, to cells of its own type. In other words, each neuronal population differentiates autonomously and does not seem to be influenced to any significant extent by the condition of the neighboring groups of cells.

At the time these later studies on regeneration in the amphibian nervous system were published it was widely believed that the regenerative capacity of the amphibian neural plate (and its various derivatives) was similar, at least in principle, to the capacity of certain central pathways to regenerate in amphibians and fish after surgical interruption, a phenomenon known to occur since the mid-1920s.[20] The regeneration of the optic nerves and tract in teleosts and amphibians had been effectively exploited by Sperry and his associates in a series of now classical experiments,[21–24] but since no comparable axonal regeneration could be demonstrated in the amniote brain, it was generally assumed that there was little point in looking for the restitution of brain parts in the central nervous systems of amniotes. This view seemed to gain credence when Wenger[25] published the results of her study on the effects of various ablations of the brachial segments of the developing chick spinal cord. In none of her experiments (which included hemiablations and quadrantic extirpations, carried out between the 15 and 25 somite stages) was there the slightest indication of regeneration of the spinal cord. Her conclusion that "by the end of the second day [of incubation] there exists in the neural epithelium . . . a mosaic pattern, with each component being independent of the others, *incapable of regulation or regeneration,* and capable of producing only a limited number and certain types of cells," was generally taken to mean that the developing chick spinal cord (and, by extension, the entire avian central nervous system) had no regenerative capacity.

A number of incidental observations from the earlier literature on the development of the avian nervous system[26,27] were consonant with this interpretation, but as Watterson and Fowler[28] were soon to point out, two critical factors had been neglected in the interpretation of Wenger's findings (and of the observations in the other studies cited); these were (1) the developmental stage at which the experiments were carried out; and (2) the nature of the experimental manipulation. Instead of surgically ablating different parts of the chick spinal cord, Watterson and Fowler divided the roof plate region at various levels along the midsagittal plane, at the 12- to 28-somite stage, and inserted small strips of mesodermal tissue (including somites and adjacent nephrotome) between the separated lateral halves of the cord at various levels. In several of these experiments each lateral half of the cord developed more or less normally, but in a significant proportion (11 out of 17 cases) one or both of the separated lateral halves of the cord reconstituted its own medial wall and, in time, gave rise to more than simply a half cord. In no case was the reconstitution of the cord complete. In fact, the regeneration was essentially limited to the alar plate derivatives, including the dorsal horn, the dorsal and lateral columns, and occasionally some of the interneuronal cell groups near the base of the dorsal horn; motoneurons and other basal plate derivatives were never seen in the reconstituted parts of the cord, although occasionally displaced motoneurons were found in the region adjoining the regenerated tissue.

The finding that the alar plate region of the chick spinal cord retains a considerable capacity for regeneration paved the way for a number of similar studies on other regions of the avian nervous system. Of these only two are sufficiently well documented to warrant consideration here. The first was a study by Birge and Hillman[29] of regeneration in the chick hindbrain. For this several different types of ablation were made in the presumptive hindbrain of chicks between 30 and 38 hr of incubation (corresponding approximately to the 7- and 12-somite stages, or stages 9 and 10 of the Hamburger and Hamilton[30] series). As Harrison[18] had earlier found in *Ambystoma,* no regeneration occurred after bilateral ablations of the metencephalic alar and basal plate regions, and in most cases with more restricted lesions the surviving tissues appeared to develop autonomously along their own lines. However, in many cases in which only the alar plate region of one side was ablated, a secondary hyperplasia occurred, and in some brains this hyperplasia was of such magnitude that by the 10th day of incubation the region which Birge and Hillman identified as the "anterior cerebellar lobe" of the unoperated side had almost doubled its normal volume, and the so-called "middle cerebellar lobe" was approximately one and one-half times its normal size. Most of these volumetric increases were maintained through the later stages in development, but in several cases they subsequently declined, by about 20–30% at day 18. Interestingly, what they termed the "posterior cerebellar lobe" showed no comparable hyperplasia at any stage.

These findings stimulated Birge to carry out an even more extensive series of experiments on the development of the chick midbrain.[31] Using the same electrocauterization technique adapted for his previous work, five different types of experiment were performed: unilateral alar plate extirpations, unilateral alar and basal plate ablations, bilateral reductions in the prospective alar plates, bilateral basal plate ablations, and complete removal of the midbrain. All the operations were done early on the 2nd day of incubation, between 28 and 38 hr of incubation (i.e., at Hamburger and Hamilton stages 9 and 10), and the embryos were killed at intervals between the 2nd and 20th days of incubation. Since in none of the experiments in which the basal plate was ablated was there any indication of regulation, and as this region did not appear to contribute to the regeneration of the alar plate, these cases will not be considered further, except to say that they provide additional evidence for the very early determination of all basal plate derivatives, and they confirm that the development of the alar plate is largely independent of the fate or presence of the basal plate.

The most interesting of Birge's cases were those in which the mesencaphalic alar plate was removed on one side. Within just a few hours of the operation, the neuroepithelium lining the tectal ventricle on the *unoperated* side had begun to expand and to bend towards the exposed basal plate of the opposite side. Although the ventricle (or mesocoele) remained open to the exterior, the overlying mesodermal tissues showed no tendency to encroach onto the basal plate (possibly because of the continuing secretion of fluid by the neuroepithelial cells as Weiss[32] and Holtzer[19] had earlier suggested). From mitotic counts it was evident that even at this early stage cell proliferation in the intact neuroepithelium was accelerated (by about 30–35% compared to control embryos at the same stage in development). Interestingly, there was no increase in the number of mitotic figures in the region along the cut edge of the alar plate; rather the accelerated cell division appeared to involve only the more lateral portions of the ventricular zone. By the following day, the volume of the intact alar plate was increased by about 15% and more than half the original tissue defect was closed by the flexure of the hyperplastic tissue. By the 5th day of incubation the hyperplasia was even more marked, the numbers of mitoses being increased by about 30% and the volume of the surviving tectum being about 40% larger than that of an intact "half tectum" in a normal animal. By the 7th day the original tissue defect was completely bridged, and from this stage onwards, it is reasonable to speak of the "regeneration of the ablated tectal lobe." By the 9th day, the "regenerated" and "intact" optic lobes were rather similar in appearance, and the entire alar plate region closely resembled the tectum of normal chicks at the corresponding developmental age, except in one important respect. Instead of there being two distinct optic lobes* separated by a relatively cell free tectal roof plate region, the newly constituted tectum had the appearance of a single, dome-shaped structure, bridging across the midline. From the 12th day of incubation (when cell proliferation in the ventricular zone has essentially ceased[33,34]) to just before hatching, the two halves of the tectum continued to expand uniformly, and in Birge's best cases their combined volumes were found to be equal to (and in some instances to actually exceed) the combined volumes of the two optic lobes in normal animals. Moreover, the general appearance of the regenerated tectum was essentially normal, although no detailed analyses of its cytoarchitecture seem to have been carried out. Because no comparable hyperplasia or regeneration occurred after *bilateral* alar plate ablations, Birge concluded that neither the diencephalon nor the hindbrain could contribute to the replacement of the tectum and, as we have mentioned above, the mesencephalic basal plate was similarly incapable of giving rise to tectal tissue. The fate of the roof plate region was less obvious. Since the roof plate was consistently absent after regeneration of the tectum Birge was of the opinion that it was the least determined region within the midbrain and that it actively participated in the regeneration of the tectum. If this is so, it would appear to be the only structure within the developing brain that is capable of giving rise to a tissue of quite different type.

We have described Birge's findings in some detail not only because

* As the terminology that has been used for the optic tectum is rather confused, it is worth mentioning here that we shall use the term *optic tectum* to refer to the entire tectal region, and the descriptive term *optic lobes* for the lateral halves of the tectum. Each optic lobe normally receives its retinal input from the contralateral eye, and is separated from its fellow of the opposite side by the relatively cell-free *tectal roof plate*—see Fig. 1A). For convenience we shall speak of the *two halves of the tectum* when we refer to the expanded, dome-shaped tectum that is usually formed after unilateral alar plate ablations. Each half of the tectum in these cases corresponds morphologically (if not in size) to one optic lobe in an intact animal.

they served as the starting point for our own work, but also because they provided the first really convincing evidence that during embryonic development an entire brain region can be reconstituted, *with an apparently normal internal morphology*. In this respect, his findings are of inherently greater interest than the occurrence of what has come to be known as "tectal overgrowth," although the latter seems to have attracted considerably more interest in the last two decades.[35–39] Tectal overgrowth has many of the features of a neoplastic transformation. It can occur after almost any direct injury to the chick tectum during the first 4 or 5 days of incubation, and indeed it is known to occur fairly consistently after removal of the rostral part of the notochord on the 3rd day of incubation.[39] The occurrence of tectal overgrowth is marked by an uncontrolled proliferation within the ventricular zone and the formation of tumorlike masses of tectal tissue. Within the overgrown tissue, zones of relatively normal cytoarchitecture are found; however, interspersed between these are regions in which the tectal architecture is totally disrupted and others in which there are islands containing curious rosettelike clusters of epithelial cells. It is not known what causes this anomalous tectal growth, nor apparently has any attempt been made to determine whether the overgrown tissue receives a retinal input or is capable of forming connections with other parts of the brain.

3. RECENT OBSERVATIONS ON THE REGENERATION OF THE CHICK OPTIC TECTUM

Since the publication of Birge's[31] important study, a great deal has been learned about the normal development and morphology of the avian optic tectum, and a number of new methods have been introduced which have made possible the experimental analysis of the patterns of connections formed during development. We have taken advantage of some of these recent technical advances to reexamine the whole problem of regeneration in the chick optic tectum and to explore a number of issues that Birge was unable to answer with the techniques available to him. In particular, we have paid rather more attention to the cytoarchitectonic organization of the regenerated tectum and to the sequence in which the neurons in the various tectal laminae are generated. We have also examined the capacity of the regenerated tectum to form an orderly retino-topic map, and the extent to which the retinal projection to the regenerated tectum can be modified by the early removal of one eye. Before presenting the results of these recent studies, however, a brief account of the normal morphology and development of the chick optic tectum is required, because it is only against this background that the pattern of embryonic regeneration can be critically evaluated.

3.1. *The Normal Morphology of the Chick Optic Tectum*

The morphology of the avian optic tectum has been described by a number of workers over the past 80 years.[40–45] As a result of these studies there is now general agreement about the overall organization and the pattern of lamination within the mature tectum, but unfortunately a good deal of confusion has been introduced in the literature through the use of differing terminologies. Ramón y Cajal's[41] system of numbering the various cellular and fiber layers consecutively from the surface to the tectal ventricle has the merit of simplicity (at least for the adult tectum) and has been widely adopted, but the terminology most commonly used in the United States and Great Britain is that first suggested by Huber and Crosby[42] and subsequently modified by Jungherr[43] and by Cowan *et al.*[45]. This recognizes 6 major layers that have been named from without inwards:

1. The *stratum opticum* (SO).
2. The *stratum griseum et fibrosum superficiale* (SGFS).
3. The *stratum griseum centrale* (SGC).
4. The *stratum album centrale* (SAC).
5. The *stratum griseum periventriculare* (SGP).
6. The *stratum fibrosum periventriculare* (SFP).

The arrangement of these various layers is shown in Fig. 1, from which it is also evident that the SGFS is subdivisible into at least 10 layers; these have been designated by the letters a–j by Cowan *et al.*[45] The arrangement and relative thickness of the layers varies somewhat in different regions of the tectum, but for our purposes the simplified description given above may be accepted as adequately covering the greater part of the tectum.

In normal animals there is a precisely ordered projection of the retina upon the contralateral optic lobe with the superior and inferior quadrants of the retina projecting to the ventral and dorsal halves of the tectum respectively, and the nasal and temporal quadrants, respectively, projecting upon the caudal and rostral halves of the tectum.[46,47] From Golgi, axonal degeneration, and autoradiographic studies, it is now known that retinal afferents terminate within the outer six laminae of the SGFS, the majority ending superficially in laminae a and b, and at a deeper level in laminae d and e.[41,45,48] The major efferent projections of the tectum arise from the large neurons within the SGC and are

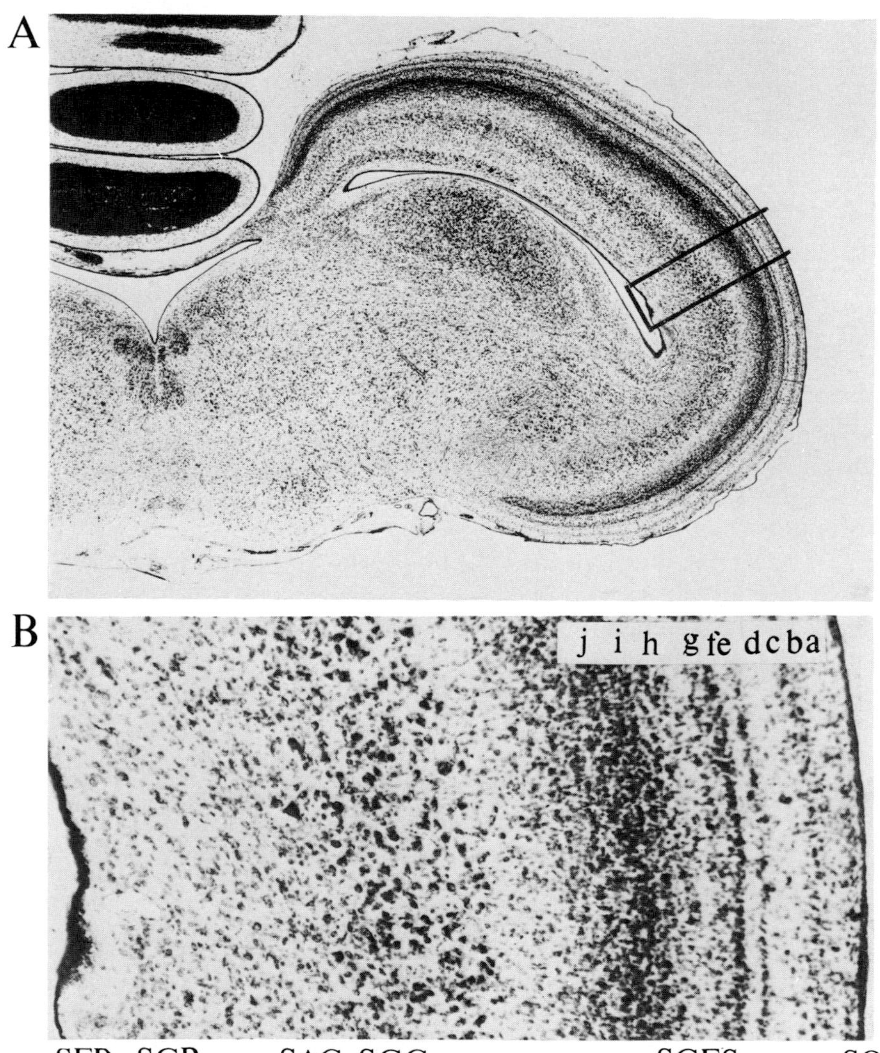

Figure 1. (A) A low-power photomicrograph of a section through the caudal third of the optic tectum in a normal 19-day-old chick embryo to show the general organization and topographic relationships of the tectum. (B) This enlarged view of the region contained within the rectangular area marked in (A) illustrates the arrangement of the various sublayers within the *stratum griseum et fibrosum superficiale*.

distributed to a number of structures within the diencephalon and brainstem,[49–51] but most of the retino-topically ordered projections arise within the deeper layers of the SGFS. Among the latter the projections to the isthmic nuclei (including the *nuclei isthmi parvocellularis* and *magnocellularis* and the nucleus of origin of centrifugal fibers to the retina—the *isthmo-optic nucleus*[52,53]) are of particular relevance to the present study; they have been shown to arise principally from the fusiform cells in laminae *h* and *i*.[51,54,55] The other connections of the tectum need not be reviewed here, except to point out that there is a reciprocal projection to the SGFS from the *nucleus isthmi parvocellularis,* the axons of the relevant isthmic neurons ending mainly in laminae d and e of the SGFS.

3.2. *The Normal Development of the Chick Optic Tectum*

A number of studies of the development of the optic tectum have appeared in the past 15 years, and although several details have yet to be elucidated, we can now give a fairly complete account, at least at a descriptive level, of the major events in its histogenesis and of its sequential invasion by optic nerve fibers.

The tectum develops from the mesencephalic alar plate. At an early stage (around the 2nd day of incubation—stages 8 or 9 of the Hamburger and Hamilton series) the alar plate is only poorly delimited from the adjoining diencephalon and hindbrain, and from the basal plate structures that give rise to the midbrain tegmentum. At this time there is no clear indication of the future roof plate region in the midline, and the alar plate as a whole consists only of a ventricular zone, comprising the neuroepithelial lining of the mesencephalic ventricle, and a narrow marginal zone beneath the developing leptomeninges. Over a period of 10 days an increasing number of cellular layers appear, and by the 14th–16th days of incubation the central region of the tectum has acquired its mature appearance.[56]

All tectal cell proliferation occurs within the ventricular zone, and from both mitotic counts[33] and [^{3}H]thymidine autoradiography[34] it is evident that a distinct temporo-spatial gradient of cell proliferation extends from the rostro-lateral part of the tectum toward its caudo-medial pole, such that from the 3rd day of incubation onward the rostral and lateral parts of the tectum are more advanced than the caudo-medial region by the equivalent of about 2 days of development. The peak period of cell proliferation occurs between the 4th and 6th days of incubation, and cell division is essentially complete by about day 12. Using a variant of the cumulative [^{3}H]thymidine labeling procedure, Fujita[56] and LaVail and Cowan[57] have shown that the cellular layers of the tectum are generated in an unusual sequence. The deepest layers (extending from the SGP to the SGC) are the first to be generated—with the cells in these layers withdrawing from the mitotic cycle at intervals between the 3rd and 6th days of incubation. This group of layers is followed by the generation of the cells in the outer part of the SGFS including laminae a–g; collectively, the cells in these layers are formed between the 5th and 8th days of incubation. Finally, the deeper cells of the SGFS, comprising laminae h, i, and j, are generated between the 6th and 9th days. While there is obviously some overlap in the duration of these waves of cell division and outward neuronal migration, when the tectum as a whole is considered they are as sufficiently clear-cut as the generation of the various layers in the mammalian neocortex. Moreover, within each of the three zones that can be defined on the basis of the time of origin of their neurons, secondary inside-out and outside-in gradients (with respect to the ventricular zone) can be recognized (see Fig. 2).

These events can be summarized briefly by stating that the development of the tectum is marked by three successive and partly over-

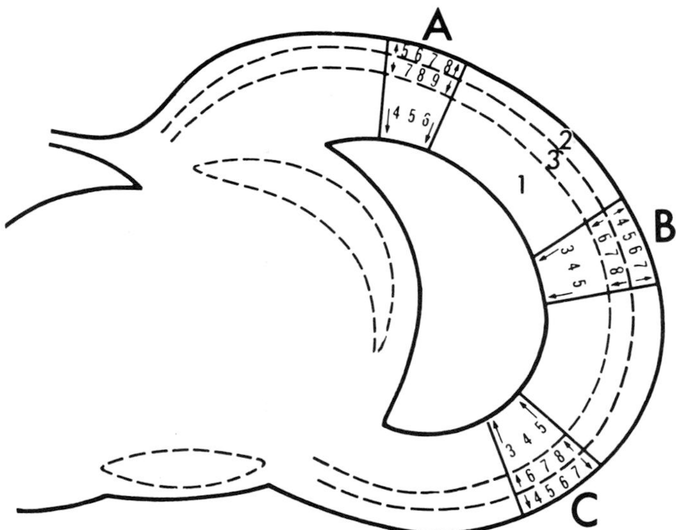

Figure 2. The cells in the various layers of the optic tectum are generated in three distinct groups; these are designated in this figure according to their relative time of origin by the numbers 1, 2, and 3. Within each of these developmental zones secondary inside-out or outside-in gradients occur; these are indicated by the small arrows; and the general ventrolateral to dorso-medial gradient is shown by the times of origin of the cells (in days) in the three sectors marked A, B, and C. (Modified, with permission, from LaVail and Cowan.[34])

lapping phases: (1) A phase that extends from the end of the 2nd day to about the 8th day of incubation that is characterized principally by cell proliferation. (2) A phase of neuronal deployment during which the cells migrate away from the ventricular zone and come to occupy the various layers that make up the tectum; this phase extends from about the 4th to the 12th days of incubation and is marked by the assembly of first the deeper tectal layers, then the outer seven layers of the SGFS (laminae a–g) and finally the three deeper layers of the SGFS (laminae h, i, and j). (3) A phase of neuronal growth and maturation during which the volume of the tectum increases considerably; this expansion is due mainly to the growth of the cells, the elaboration of their processes,[58,59] and the invasion of the tectum by its various afferent inputs.

To date the only afferent fiber system whose development has been analyzed in any detail is that from the contralateral retina. The optic nerve fibers first reach the rostro-lateral pole of the tectum on the 6th day of incubation.[60–62] By the 9th day they have extended across the surface of most of the rostral half of the tectum, and they finally reach its caudo-medial pole around day 12. For the most part the fibers remain with the SO until about the 8th or 9th day, when they begin to invade the outer layers of the SGFS. There is some uncertainty as to where this first occurs. McGraw and McLaughlin[63] believe that it begins at the point where the optic tract first contacts the tectum, but Crossland *et al.*[62] and Rager[64] have evidence (from autoradiographs and Golgi preparations, respectively) that the first significant penetration of the SGFS by optic nerve fibers occurs close to the center of the tectum, at or near the site of representation of the central retina. Subsequently, according to these authors, a progressive expansion of the invaded region occurs more or less concentrically, so that the SGFS at the peripheral margin of the tectum is not fully innervated by optic nerve fibers until about the 16th or 18th day of incubation. As Crossland *et al.*[62] have pointed out, if this pattern accurately reflects the sequence of synapse formation by optic nerve fibers, retinal synaptogenesis in the tectum would closely parallel the sequence of retinal ganglion cell generation. The first retinal ganglion cells to be formed are located near the upper end of the choroid fissure around day 4, and over the next 8 days there is a broad wave of ganglion cell genesis that extends more or less radially from the region of the future area centralis to the retinal periphery.[65] The importance of this is that if we could be sure that the radial sequence of ganglion cell formation is matched by a corresponding radial sequence in the invasion of the optic tectum, it would be unnecessary to postulate a continuous restructuring of the retino-tectal projection, despite the markedly different sequence of tectal cell genesis (which, as we have pointed out, proceeds in a curvilinear fashion from the rostro-lateral to the caudo-medial pole of the tectum).

Only one further point about the development of the retino-tectal projection requires comment here: if part of the optic cup is removed, prior to the outgrowth of optic nerve fibers, the axons of the surviving retinal ganglion cells consistently grow back to those regions of the tectum that they would normally occupy.[66] Under these circumstances the tectal region corresponding to the ablated part of the retina always remains free of optic nerve fibers and, in time, shows the same type of secondary (or transneuronal) degenerative changes that are seen throughout the tectum after complete removal of the contralateral eye.[67]

3.3. *A Reexamination of Tectal Regeneration in the Chick*

Since it appeared that Birge's[31] study had not been repeated, it seemed appropriate to reexamine the whole problem of tectal regeneration in the chick, and in particular to take advantage of some of the experimental techniques now available for determining the time of origin of the cells in the regenerated region and to map certain of the connections that it is capable of forming. If Birge is correct in thinking that the regenerated part of the tectum is derived from the alar plate of the *contralateral side,* it is a matter of some interest to establish whether the connections formed by the regenerated tissue are appropriate for the side it comes to occupy, or if they simply represent an extension of the connections of the side from which its cells are ultimately derived. In addition, because of the absence of a roof plate region between the two halves of the reconstituted tectum, we were interested to know how this would affect the distribution of optic nerve fibers in the SO when both eyes were present, and when one eye was removed early in development. In the sections that follow we shall briefly summarize some of our findings on these and certain related problems, based on an analysis of approximately 80 out of a total of over 400 chick embryos in which different parts of the mesencephalic alar plate were removed during the latter part of the second day of incubation (between Hamburger and Hamilton stages 9 and 11, i.e., after 38–45 hours of incubation).

3.3.1. The Experimental Procedure. In the majority of the embryos we have analyzed, one half of the mesencephalic alar plate was surgically ablated as shown in Fig. 3A. Although we cannot be sure in any given case that the entire region had been removed, every effort was made to resect the tissue right up to the midline, and as far laterally as was possible without seriously damaging the underlying basal plate

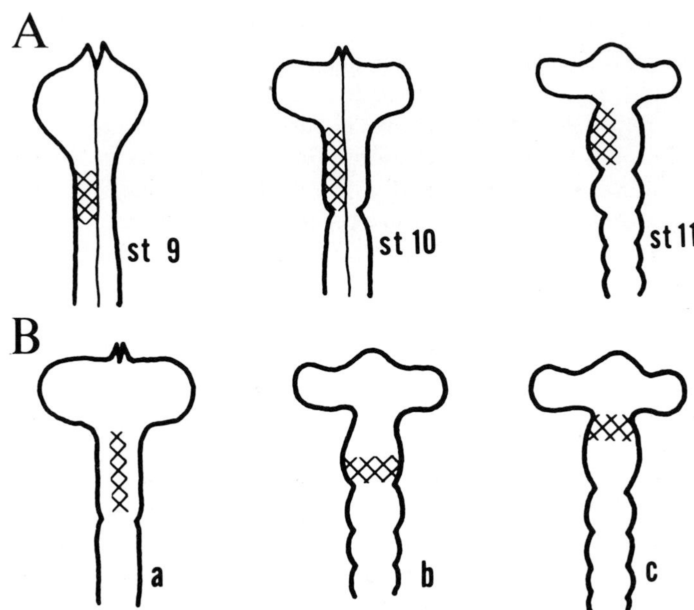

Figure 3. (A) The cross-hatched areas show the extent of the unilateral mesencephalic alar plate extirpations of the kind carried out in the majority of our experiments, at stages 9, 10, and 11 of the Hamburger and Hamilton[30] series. (B) In addition to the standard operation illustrated in (A), we have carried out three types of experimental control: removal of a parasagittal strip of mesencephalic alar plate tissue (a), and bilateral removals of either the caudal (b) or rostral (c) halves of the alar plate.

region. Since even at stage 10 the boundaries of the mesencephalon are not clearly defined, one can never be certain about the full extent of the alar plate lesion; but with this reservation, we shall refer hereafter to experiments of this kind as *unilateral alar plate ablations.* In a small number of cases various alternative types of alar plate lesion were made (see Fig. 3B). These included: (1) bilateral ablations of either the rostral or the caudal half of the mesencephalic alar plate, (2) bilateral removals of a narrow parasagittal strip of alar mesencephalic plate tissue, and (3) unilateral alar plate removals at stages 8 or 12. All the operations were performed aseptically through a small opening in the shell, with the aid of a Zeiss operating microscope and fine glass needles, after supravital staining of the embryos with neutral red.

To determine the time of origin of the cells and the pattern of neuronal migration in the regenerating tectum, in one series of embryos with unilateral alar plate ablations tritiated [^{3}H]thymidine (10 μCi in 10 μl, Spec. Act. 20 Ci/mM) was injected onto the vitelline membrane, either on a single day, or on 2 or 3 successive days, at appropriate intervals after the lesion. Most of the injected embryos were allowed to survive until the 10th or 12th day of incubation (stages 34–38), but some were sacrificed within 30 min of the administration of the isotope and others were kept alive until just before hatching (day 20—stage 45). The brains were processed for histological examination and autoradiography following the protocol described by Cowan *et al.*[68]

To determine the distribution of the retinal projection onto the regenerated tectum, two types of experiments were carried out. In the first, [^{3}H]proline (L-2,3,^{3}H-(N), Spec. Act. 35 Ci/mM) was injected into the vitreous of one eye (either that on the side contralateral to the earlier alar plate ablation or that on the side contralateral to the "control" half of the tectum) at a predetermined time (usually around stage 42). These animals were killed 6 hr after the [^{3}H]proline injection, which, as we have previously shown, is adequate to allow for rapid axonal transport along the axons of the retinal ganglion cells to the tectum.[48] In the second series of experiments one optic cup was removed at the same time, or shortly after, the ablation of the mesencephalic alar plate. In about half of these cases the eye on the same side as the alar plate ablation was removed; in the remainder the contralateral eye was resected. Two or 3 days before hatching [^{3}H]proline was injected into the remaining eye, 6 hr before the animals were killed and their brains prepared for autoradiography.

3.3.2. Observations on the Reconstitution of Tectal Cytoarchitecture. From the series of animals sacrificed at various intervals after unilateral removal of the mesencephalic alar plate we have been able to reconstruct the series of events that in time leads to the reconstitution of the optic tectum with a more or less normal cytoarchitecture. However, before presenting our observations on the sequential development of the regenerated tissue, it may be appropriate to begin this section with a description of the final appearance of the reconstituted tectum, and then to describe how this comes to be formed.

Figure 4A shows the appearance of a section through the central part of the tectum in a chick that was sacrificed on the 18th day of incubation, 16 days after what was judged to be a complete unilateral ablation of the mesencephalic alar plate. For comparison, a comparable section through the tectum of a normal chick at the same age is shown in Fig. 4B. The immediate and most striking difference between the two structures is the absence in the experimental brain of the roof plate region which normally separates the two optic lobes. A second difference is that the area occupied by the optic tectum in the experimental animal is reduced, if one compares it with the combined cross-sectional

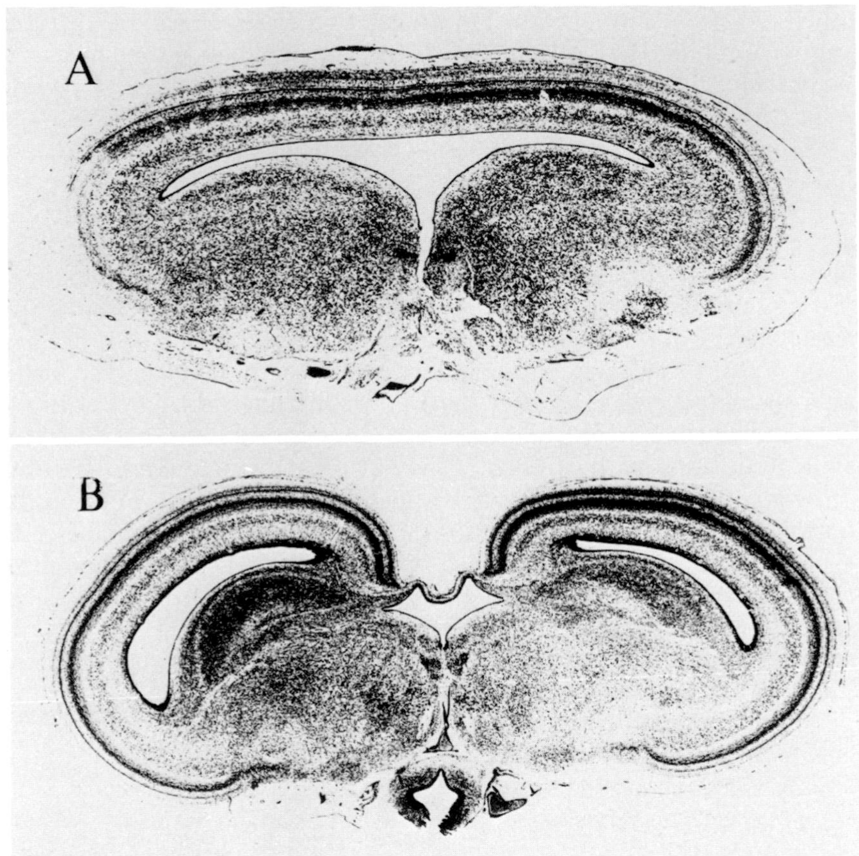

Figure 4. (A) Low-power photomicrograph of a section through the tectum of an 18-day-old chick in which the mesencephalic alar plate on the left side had been ablated on the 2nd day of incubation. Observe how the regenerated tectum forms a broad, dome-shaped structure spanning the midline, and note the absence of the roof plate region that normally separates the optic lobes of the two sides, as shown in (B), which is a comparable micrograph from a control embryo at the same age.

areas of the two optic lobes in the control animal. Measurements of the total volume of the tectum in this and similar cases confirm that the reconstituted tectum is nearly always smaller than that of two normal optic lobes. In the case illustrated in Fig. 4A the volume of the operated tectum amounted to just over 70% of that of a normal 18-day-old chick. The actual reduction in volume varied from case to case; in five brains analyzed quantitatively in this way the volume of the reconstituted tectum ranged from 65 to 76% of the normal value. Although this is significantly less than the amount of regeneration that Birge reported in his best preparations, it is clear from the illustrations in his paper that in every other respect our findings are similar to his. In particular, it is clear that the reduction in volume that we have found is not due to the selective loss of certain parts of the tectum or to the absence of particular tectal laminae: each of the layers that can be recognized in the normal tectum is present in the regenerated material, and each appears to contain the same types of cell (or at least those types that can be recognized in Nissl preparations) in the same proportions, and with the same density (Fig. 5). In the case of the SGC (for which it is possible to obtain reasonably accurate estimates of cell number[67]) we have found that the relative numbers of cells in the regenerated tectum closely parallel the volume of the tectum as a whole; in three specimens in which the volume and neuronal packing density in the SGC were measured it was found that the volume of the layer was about 70% of that in the two optic lobes of a control animal, and that the cell density was unchanged.

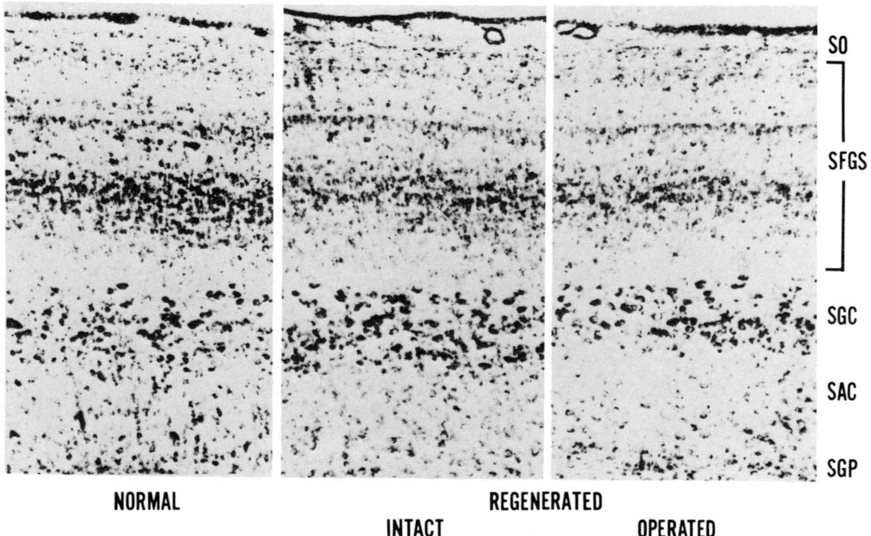

Figure 5. These three photomicrographs from comparable regions in the tectum of a normal control animal, and from the unoperated (intact) and operated sides of a chick with a prior mesencephalic alar plate ablation, make it clear that all the layers that one can normally see in the tectum are present in the regenerated tissue, and that the reduction in total volume that we have commonly found in our experimental animals is due to a general reduction in the size of the regenerated tectum rather than to the selective loss of specific classes of neurons in particular layers.

In a smaller number of cases, the general appearance of the regenerated tectal tissue was the same, but instead of spanning the midline the tectum was clearly divided into two lobes by a more or less normal-appearing roof plate region. At present it is not clear why a tectal roof plate developed in these brains: the embryos were operated upon at the same ages (stages 9– to 10+), the same operative procedure was used, and the animals were reared under the same conditions and were maintained for the same postoperative period. The most likely explanation is that in these cases a smaller amount of alar plate tissue had been resected, even though every effort was made to remove the tissue up to the midline. As we have pointed out, in the absence of definable landmarks it is difficult to be certain, in any given case, exactly how much tissue was removed, and it is probable that in some experiments a narrow strip of alar plate tissue to the side of the midline was left intact. If this were the case, we assume that most of the regeneration would occur from the surviving presumptive tectal tissue on the side of the lesion (rather than from the contralateral side) and for this reason, it is perhaps not surprising that the presumptive roof plate region did not undergo regulation. It is of interest that in one of these brains the regenerated optic lobe was as large as that in a normal chick of the same age, but in all the others the volume of the optic lobe on the unoperated side was only about 80% of that in normal chicks, and the regenerated lobe was always somewhat smaller than this (the actual volumes ranging between 60 and 76% of the normal value). It is difficult to account for the reduction in the size of the lobe on the unoperated side in these brains unless perhaps the tissue on the unoperated side contributed to the regenerative response; however, at this time we cannot rule out that the control optic lobes were small because the operative procedure had some nonspecific retarding effect on tectal growth. In this context it is noteworthy that in the one case in which the intact optic lobe was of normal size, the regenerated lobe was among the largest we have seen. Whatever the explanation for the failure of the roof plate to develop in the majority of our mesencephalic alar plate ablations may prove to be, the fact that a normal-appearing roof plate was found in a few cases makes it clear that regulation of the presumptive roof plate region is not an obligatory requirement for tectal regeneration, as Birge[31] has suggested.

The normal development of the roof plate region is poorly understood. According to Wilson[39] its presence is first recognizable on the 4th day of incubation; prior to this the alar plate tissue along the midline is indistinguishable from that on either side. On the 4th day the tissue along the midline becomes progressively thinner and shows a diminished number of cells. By the 6th day it is much reduced in thickness, and apart from a few of the larger cells of the mesencephalic nucleus of the trigeminal nerve that have invaded the region from the neural crest[69,70] it is essentially free of neurons. It is not known to what extent the normal disappearance of cells from the roof plate region is due to their degeneration or to their lateral migration. Our material does not bear directly on this issue, but it does indicate that the tissue in the midline is the most subject to regulation, and as we shall see, the absence of a roof plate permits certain unusual patterns of connectivity.

3.3.3. The Temporal Pattern of Tectal Regeneration. The earliest indication that the tectum will be reconstituted is the appearance of a thin epithelial sheet along the medial, cut edge of the alar plate. Although it is not clear just when this epithelial sheet begins to be generated, within 3 days of the lesion it has usually bridged the interval between the unoperated side of the tectum and the cut edge of the basal plate. By the 6th day of incubation (stage 27) the medial one-half to two-thirds of this epithelial sheet has become somewhat thicker, and although it is still appreciably thinner than the tectal issue on the unoperated side of the tectum, it has all the features of an established neuroepithelium, and has already given rise to many postmitotic neurons. At this stage the lateral third or so of the bridging neuroepithelium is still rather thin, and in fact, measurements of the relative thickness of the neuroepithelium on the two sides indicate that the regenerated tissue as a whole is only about half the thickness of the wall of the developing tectum on the intact side. And whereas on the intact side blood vessels have already invaded the tissue, there is no indication of vascularization on the reconstituted side. From a comparison of the appearance of the regenerating tissue with the structure of the normally developing tectum at the 6-day stage,[57] it is evident that the development of the regenerated tissue is retarded by the equivalent of about 48 hr; even when compared with the tissue on the unoperated side, it is retarded by at least 24 hr.

By day 8 (stage 30) it is evident that there has been a considerable acceleration in the development of the regenerated tectum, and at this stage the tectal tissue on the two sides appears rather similar. However, from measurements of the thickness of the first layer of differentiated neurons (corresponding to layer ii in LaVail and Cowan's[57] description) it is evident that the regenerated half of the tectum is still somewhat retarded, but the degree of retardation now corresponds to something less than 24 hr. On the intact side this layer varies in thickness from about 65 μm laterally to about 6 μm near the midline (at a level corresponding to the junction of the middle and caudal thirds of the tectum), while on the reconstituted side it is just under 40 μm thick in its lateral part and, again, about 6 μm near the midline (Fig. 6). Even more in-

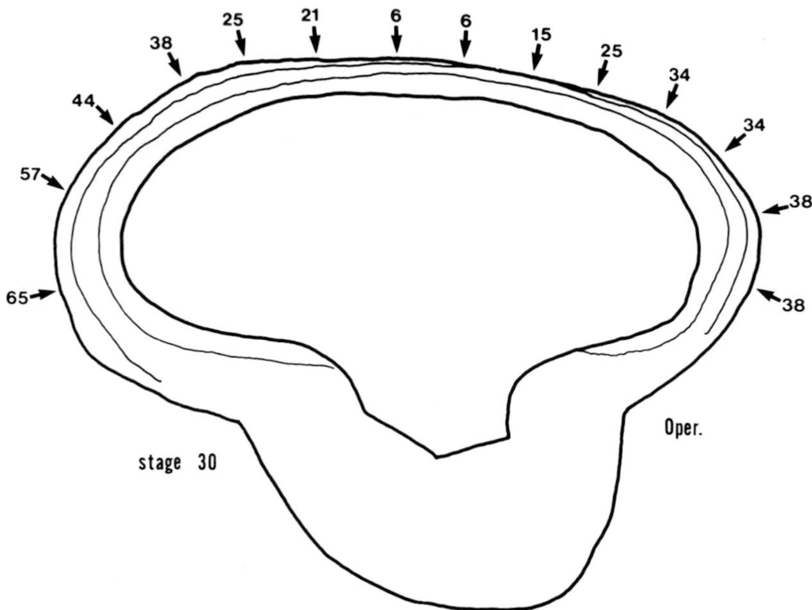

Figure 6. This drawing of the tectum of an embryo at stage 30 illustrates the common finding that the lateral to medial gradient in cell proliferation and cytoarchitectonic differentiation is reestablished within the regenerated tectum, even though development on the regenerated side lags behind that on the unoperated side. The numbers indicate the relative thickness of LaVail and Cowan's[57] developmental layer ii, at each of several points across the perimeter of the unoperated and operated (oper) sides.

teresting at this stage is the finding that the rostro-caudal and latero-medial gradients in cytoarchitectonic deafferentation, which are such a striking feature in the normal development of the tectum, are both clearly recognizable on the regenerated side. That the rostro-caudal gradient should be reestablished is perhaps not unexpected since it is clearly evident on the unoperated side from which the regeneration proceeds, but the existence of a relatively normal gradient along the lateral to medial dimension of the regenerated tectum is surprising, since it is the mirror image of the corresponding gradient on the unoperated side. This suggests that once the reconstituted neuroepithelium bridges the gap in the alar plate, it comes under the influence of the morphogenetic gradient-determining mechanisms that normally operate across the lateral to medial dimension of the developing brain. The effect of this is that even though the regenerated tissue is derived from the medial part of the alar plate of the opposite side, the lateral to medial gradient determining mechanism acting on that side is no longer effective; instead the corresponding gradient on the reconstituted side takes over and becomes the primary determinant of development on this side. In this respect the regenerating tectum appears to behave in a manner analogous to that seen when the entire midbrain is reversed 180° around its longitudinal axis at stage 10. After such rotations Cowan and Wenger found that the normally retarded caudal part of the tectum appears to accelerate its rate of growth so that by the 9th or 10th day of incubation this region was appreciably further advanced in its cytoarchitectonic differentiation than the original rostral part of the tectum.[71]

In a smaller number of cases the more or less uniform lateral to medial gradient usually seen across the extent of the regenerated tectum was not present. In these cases both the lateral and medial parts of the regenerated tissue were more advanced in their development than the central region. One such case is illustrated in Fig. 7, from which it can be seen that the central portion of the regenerated tectum is only about 60–70% of the thickness of the tissue along either its medial or its lateral borders. Since, as we have remarked above, measurements of the thickness of the tectal wall provide a good indication of its relative development, it appears that the central portion of the regenerated tectum was retarded in these brains by the equivalent of about 24–36 hr. At present we cannot resolve whether this appearance was brought about by some disturbance in the normal operation of the lateral to medial gradient determining mechanism, or if it is attributable to some other

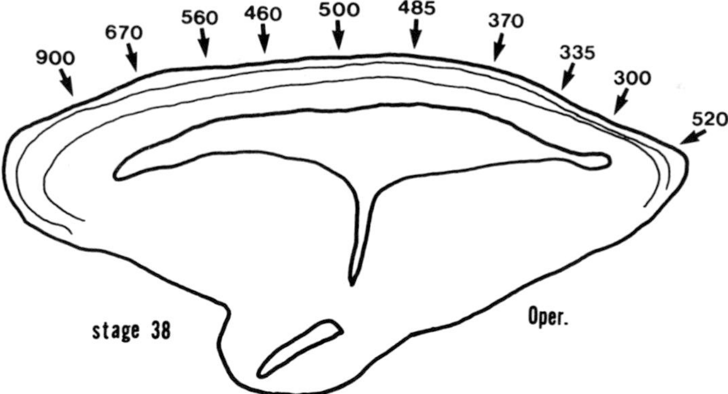

Figure 7. This drawing of a section through the middle of the tectum in a stage 38 embryo, illustrates that in some cases the central part of the regenerated tectal tissue is appreciably thinner than at either edge. This is most easily accounted for on the assumption that in these cases regeneration has occurred both from the contralateral side and from the side of the original alar plate lesion, possibly from residual presumptive tectal tissue along the lateral margin of the mesencephalic alar plate.

factor. An alternative explanation is that in these cases the regeneration of the tectum was initiated from both the medial and lateral cut edges of the alar plate. It is worth repeating that although every effort was made to ablate the entire half of the alar plate it is likely that in some cases a small lateral fragment of tissue was left intact along the junction between the alar and basal plates. If this happened, it seems not unlikely that the surviving lateral alar plate tissue might contribute to the neuroepithelium that bridges the gap in the roof of the mesencephalon, and that regeneration would then proceed from both the lateral and medial sides. A similar pattern of development was seen in some of the embryos that were sacrificed at earlier stages. In these the regenerated tectum was often thrown into accordionlike folds (see Fig. 8), and from measurements of the thickness of the regenerated tissue at several points along its medio-lateral extent, it is evident that the central region is appreciably retarded in its development, compared to the more lateral and medial parts (Fig. 8). Indeed in the thinnest region of the brain shown in Fig. 8, few differentiated neurons were to be seen in the region corresponding to LaVail and Cowan's[57] layer ii, even as late as stage 34.

That regeneration does not occur from either the rostral or caudal cut edges of the alar plate has been clearly demonstrated in a separate series of experiments in which partial bilateral alar plate ablations were made. One example from this group of experiments will serve to make the point. In this case the caudal half of the mesencephalic alar plate

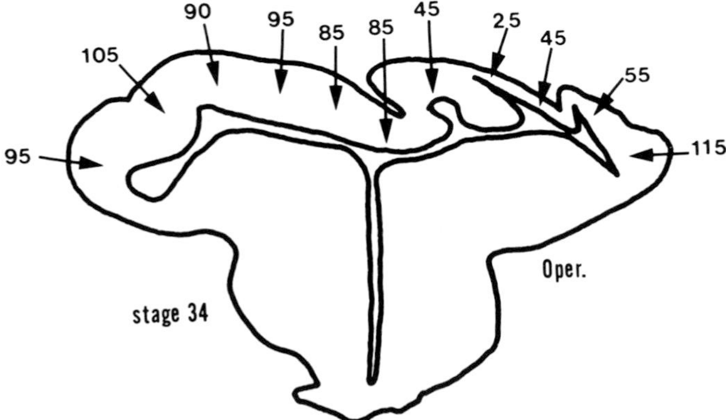

Figure 8. Occasionally the wall of the regenerating tectum is thrown into accordionlike folds, but even when this occurs it is possible to see differences in the rate of growth of the tectum. In the case from which this drawing was made, the development of the central part of the regenerated side lagged behind that along either its medial or lateral margins, at stage 34.

was removed bilaterally at stage 10. When the animal was killed on the 18th day of incubation, the tectum was found to have the same dome-shaped appearance seen in our other experiments in which the roof plate was missing. However, when the volume of the entire tectum was measured it was found to be only 48% of that of the combined optic lobes in a normal chick, and since no more than half the alar plate had been removed, it is evident that no tectal regeneration had occurred. As the total amount of tissue removed in this and the other cases in this series was essentially the same as in our other experiments, and since the same operative procedure was used, it seems reasonable to conclude with Birge[31] that tectal regeneration can only occur from alar plate tissue *at the same rostro-caudal level,* and that in this respect the reconstitution of the chick optic tectum obeys the same general rules as have been observed for other parts of the neuraxis and for other species (see review above).

3.3.4. *The Time of Origin of Neurons in the Regenerated Tectum.* From experiments in which [^{3}H]thymidine was administered at different times after the initial alar plate ablation, we have been able to confirm that the normal *sequence* in the generation of the various tectal layers is maintained in the regenerating tissue, even though the *absolute* time at which the different classes of neurons are formed is delayed by as much as 24–48 hr.* Thus the same three developmental zones recognized by LaVail and Cowan[34] are evident in the regenerated tissue, and within each of these zones the same inside-out and outside-in radial gradients are apparent. Again it will suffice to illustrate this point by reference to a single case. In this animal, half of the alar plate was resected at stage 10; [^{3}H]thymidine was injected on the 8th and 9th days of incubation, and the brain was fixed on day 10 (stage 36). In normal chicks cell proliferation is at a relatively low level by day 10[33,34] and most of the neurons generated at this time are destined for the deeper laminae of the SGFS (especially, layers i and j—corresponding to LaVail and Cowan's developmental layer vi). In the experimental brain heavily labeled neurons were seen on both the operated and unoperated sides only in the deeper part of this developmental layer; at rostral levels the labeled cells were limited to a narrow zone close to the midline, but toward the caudal pole of the tectum they were found throughout the layer except along the lateral margin of the tectum. However, the two sides are clearly different: at each rostrocaudal level the mediolateral

* The actual delay varies from layer to layer and from region to region. The earliest formed layers at the rostral pole of the tectum show the greatest delay; those whose cells are generated rather late in tectal development may be delayed by no more than 6 hr.

extent of the zone containing labeled neurons is appreciably greater on the operated than on the unoperated side. We have illustrated this for one representative level in Fig. 9. At this level labeled cells were confined to a region 0.8 mm along the medial edge of the unoperated side, but extended laterally for almost twice this distance on the regenerated side. From the data presented in LaVail and Cowan's[34] study we have calculated that at the 8-day stage, the rostrolateral to dorsomedial wave of cell proliferation proceeds at the rate of about 3 mm of tectal surface per day. If no allowance is made for slowing in the experimental animals, we estimate that the difference in the mediolateral extent of cell labeling on the two sides in this brain would correspond to a relative delay in cell genesis on the regenerated side of about 6–7 hr.

In summary, following the reconstitution of the neuroepithelium, cell proliferation in the regenerating tectum shows the same general

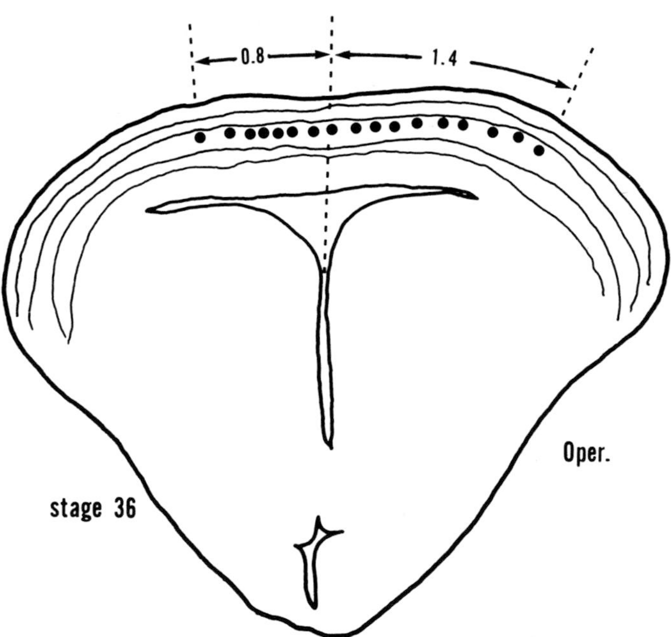

Figure 9. It is clear from [^{3}H]thymidine labeling experiments that cell proliferation on the regenerating side of the tectum lags behind that on the unoperated side. In this embryo [^{3}H]thymidine was administered on the 8th and 9th day of incubation, and on day 10, when the brain was fixed for autoradiography, labeled neurons in the deeper layers of the SGFS (layers i and j) were found over a distance of 0.8 mm from the midline on the unoperated side, and up to 1.4 mm on the regenerating side. The large dots indicate the relative positions of the labeled cells on the two sides; the differences in their distribution correspond to a retardation of about 6–7 hr in the genesis of the cells on the operated side.

pattern as in the normal tectum in that it proceeds along the same rostral to caudal and lateral to medial gradients, and the cells destined for the various laminae are generated in the same distinctive sequence. The only significant difference in cell generation appears to be due to the initial delay occasioned by the reconstitution of the neuroepithelium. From this we conclude that whereas the *absolute time* at which any given neuronal population is formed is not critical, in a complex, multilayered region such as the tectum the *relative sequence* in which neurons of different phenotypes are generated is rigidly maintained. Our observations further suggest that the newly constituted neuroepithelium not only contains stem cells for each class of tectal neuron, but also that the precursor cells are present in the appropriate relative numbers. Unfortunately, at present we have no useful markers to distinguish neurons of different lineages or to identify neural stem cells within the developing nervous system (see chapters 1, 2, and 3), and the factors that regulate their proliferation are wholly unknown.

3.4. *Experiments on the Organization and Plasticity of the Retinal Projection upon the Regenerated Optic Tectum*

Since with the exception of Holtzer's[19] study of regeneration in the amphibian spinal cord no attempt seems to have been made to examine the connections formed by reconstituted regions of the brain or spinal cord, we have taken advantage of one of the newer methods for tracing connections in the developing nervous system to examine the projection of the retina upon the regenerated chick optic tectum. This was of interest, first because we had found that the regenerated tectal tissue is usually derived entirely from the contralateral side, and we wished to know whether the reconstituted part of the tectum receives a projection from the contralateral eye and, if so, is the projection retinotopically organized as in normal animals or in some altered manner? Second, we wished to determine whether in the absence of the roof plate the retinal fibers from the two eyes would remain confined to their respective sides of the tectum, and if they did so when both eyes were present, would they still respect the midline if one eye were removed at some stage before the normal outgrowth of retinal ganglion cell axons? And third, when it became clear that the reconstituted side of the optic tectum was often appreciably reduced in size, we were interested to see if the size disparity which this created had any effect on the other known projections of the retina to the diencephalon and midbrain.

3.4.1. The Distribution of Retinal Fibers to the Regenerated Tectum. In the first group of experiments of this kind we attempted to label all the ganglion cells in one eye (usually on the side contralateral to the earlier alar plate ablation, but sometimes on the same side) by a relatively large (10 μl) intraocular injection of [^{3}H]proline, and subsequently mapped the resulting axonal transport to the tectum autoradiographically. In each of these brains the retinal projection from the injected eye was found to be distributed exclusively to the contralateral side of the brain. And, as in normal animals, fibers were given off to a number of di- and mesencephalic visual relay centers including the so-called ventral lateral geniculate nucleus, the dorsolateral and lateral anterior thalamic nuclei, the ectomammillary nucleus, the mesencephalic lentiform nucleus, and the pretectal region.[45,72] The labeled fibers entered the optic tectum by way of the marginal optic tract and were distributed through the SO to the outer laminae of the SGFS. Here the distribution of grain densities was essentially the same as that seen in normal posthatched chicks,[48] the highest grain densities being found in layers b and d, and there was a somewhat smaller peak in layers e and f; deep to layer f the grain density fell abruptly to the background level. What was particularly interesting was the abrupt way in which the labeling in both the SO and the SGFS terminated near the midpoint of the dome-shaped tectum (Fig. 10).

Measurements of the extent of the tectal surface covered by the labeled fibers in different cases indicates that in some brains the projection from the retina on the side contralateral to the alar plate lesion occupied slightly more than half the tectal surface; in other cases it was slightly less than half. But in every case the boundary between the

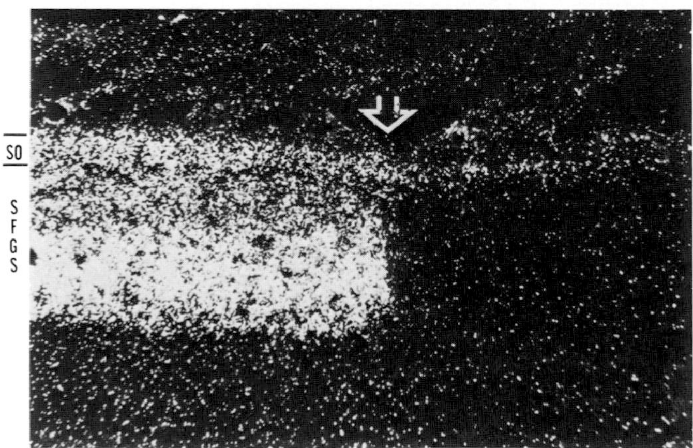

Figure 10. When both eyes are intact, the retinal projection to the regenerated tectum is distributed only to the contralateral side, and as this dark-field photomicrograph indicates, after an injection of [^{3}H]proline into the eye the labeled axons in the SO and in the SGFS stop abruptly at the midline (arrow).

labeled and unlabeled regions was very sharp. Although we have not directly examined the projection of the two retinae in the same animal (using a double-labeling procedure), from the study of different cases in which the projection from the retina either ipsilateral or contralateral to the alar plate removal was mapped, it seems fairly clear that at least by day 18 the two projections together cover the entire tectal surface and that the territories they occupy are mutually exclusive. We have not examined animals prepared in this way at earlier stages in development, so at present we do not know if there is a degree of overlap between the projections from the two retinae when the fibers first invade the tectum; if there is, it is evident that by the 17th or 18th day of incubation the overlapping fibers must have been eliminated.

Qualitatively the projections to different regions of the tectum are similar on the two sides, but it is difficult to determine whether they are quantitatively the same. We have found no difference in the relative thickness of layers a–g of the SGFS on the two sides, although in some cases that zone is slightly thinner on either side of the midline than further laterally. Grain density measurements of the labeled retinal projections indicate that in this parasagittal zone the numbers of silver grains are about 20–25% lower than those in the adjoining regions, but it is not clear if this is due to an actual reduction in the relative number of axons and axon terminals adjoining the midline region, or if it is due to some heterogeneity in the labeling of the retina by the injected isotope.

In a separate series of experiments, small injections of [^{3}H]proline were made directly into the retina so as to label (in different animals) the projections from each retinal quadrant. Although no attempt was made to systematically map the projection of each part of the retina upon the regenerated tectum, the size and location of the various isotope injections differed sufficiently in the various cases to permit us to state that at least in its general arrangement, the retino-topic organization of the projection upon the regenerated optic tectum is essentially normal. In separate experiments we have evidence that the nasal and temporal halves of the retina project to the caudal and rostral parts of the regenerated tectum, respectively, and that the superior and inferior quadrants respectively project upon the lateral and medial halves of the reconstituted tissue. It remains to be determined if the receptive fields and other physiological properties of the neurons in the regenerated tectum are also normal; this will require rearing the operated chicks through hatching, a procedure that usually carries a rather high mortality.[66]

3.4.2. The Retinal Projection to the Regenerated Tectum in Monocular Chicks. When it became evident that the retinal projections from the two eyes remain segregated within the appropriate halves of the reconstituted tectum, we performed another series of experiments to see what would happen when one eye was removed shortly after the alar plate ablation. In particular we were interested to know if the fibers from the remaining retina would remain confined to the contralateral half of the regenerated tectum or if, in the absence of a roof plate, they would spread across the midline into the ipsilateral half tectum. At present the number of cases of this kind that we have examined is rather small, but the findings are sufficiently clear cut to warrant their being placed on record.

In these animals some 24–36 hr after the resection of one half of the mesencephalic alar plate, the optic cup on the opposite side (or in some animals the eye on the same side) was surgically removed between stages 14 and 17. When the animals had reached stages 43 or 44, the heads were reexposed and a relatively large injection (10–20 μl) of [^{3}H] proline was made into the surviving eye. Six hours later the animals were killed and their brains prepared for autoradiography.

Regardless of which eye had been removed the relevant findings in every successful case were the same: the retinal projection to the tectum from the surviving eye spread across the midline for a considerable distance within the SO, and contributed fibers not only to the SGFS of the contralateral side but also to the appropriate laminae over the greater part of the tectum on the *ipsilateral* side. One example of this type of expanded retinal projection is illustrated in Fig. 11. This figure is representative of the findings in all the experiments of this kind and shows quite clearly that the density of the projection to the SGFS is by no means uniform across its extent; on the side contralateral to the injected eye it appears qualitatively to be essentially the same as in the animals that had both eyes intact, but beyond the midline the density of the projection (both within the SO and in the SGFS) falls off progressively as one proceeds laterally from the midline. Approximately two-thirds of the way around the perimeter of the tectum the labeling of the retinal fibers is at, or close to, the background level. As we have not yet analyzed these brains quantitatively, the exact point at which the projection to the ipsilateral tectum ends is unknown, and it is possible that in some cases a small number of retinal fibers may even reach the extreme lateral edge of the ipsilateral half tectum. However, it is clear that the general extent of the projection is the same regardless of whether the projection was from the eye on the same or the opposite side as the alar plate ablation (i.e., irrespective of whether the fibers entered the tectum from the regenerated or the unoperated side).

It is not clear from the material we have available whether the altered retinal projection that occurs under these circumstances is to be

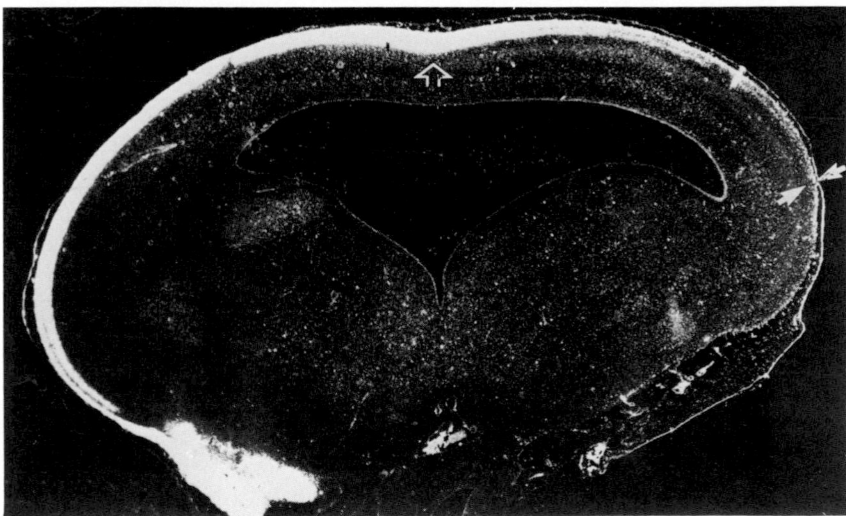

Figure 11. If one eye is removed together with half of the mesencephalic alar plate (on the same or the opposite side), the optic nerve fibers from the surviving retina are not prevented from spreading across the midline by a cell-free roof plate. In this low-power dark-field photomicrograph the labeled retinal fibers continue, in the SO and the SGFS, across the midline (marked by the open arrowhead) into the opposite half of the tectum, where they continue at least as far as the point marked by the double arrowheads.

regarded as simply a generalized expansion of the projection from the surviving retina, or if there is a duplication of the projection to the two halves of the dome-shaped tectum. To clarify this we are currently repeating these experiments with localized intraretinal injections of [^{3}H] proline. If these result in a "mirror image" distribution of label on the two sides, they would strongly suggest that the projection to each of the two halves of the tectum is retino-topically ordered. On the other hand, if each injection results in a single, localized region of labeling within the dome-shaped tectum, it would appear that the projection has simply expanded to occupy most of the territory available for retinal afferents.

The outcome of these experiments will have important implications for the whole question of plasticity in the avian retino-tectal projection. Our previous work on this system has pointed to its being rather rigidly determined from an early stage in development. For example, after early partial lesions of the optic cup, the remaining retinal tissue in the operated eye has always been found to project to a localized region within the contralateral optic tectum. And, as judged from the pattern of the concomitant cell loss seen in the isthmo-optic nucleus, the axons of the surviving retinal ganglion cells always seemed to terminate within the appropriate sector of the tectum.[48] Within the limits of the methods available for the analysis of the retinal projection in such experiments there was no indication that it had expanded to any significant degree; indeed in every case in which the retinal lesion had been placed after stage 12 a clearly defined region in the contralateral tectum was free of retinal fibers and showed the characteristic atrophic changes that occur after complete deafferentation.[67] The finding of an expanded (or duplicated) retinal projection in monocular chicks which have undergone tectal regeneration is the first indication that this system may be capable of the same type of plasticity that has been observed in other vertebrates (see, for example, Yoon,[73] Sharma,[74] Schmidt *et al.*,[75] and Gaze.[76])

These findings also suggest that the roof plate region normally presents a significant barrier to the spread of retinal fibers from one optic lobe to the other. We have examined the brains of a large number of chicks in which one eye had been removed (without manipulating the alar plate or tectum); in none of those animals in which the roof plate had developed normally have we observed optic nerve fibers crossing the midline in the tectum to reach the optic lobe of the opposite side. Although an ipsilateral retino-tectal projection is frequently found in such monocular chicks (especially if the eye removal is carried out relatively early in development, specifically before stage 12[77]), invariably the fibers to the ipsilateral tectum follow a quite different route than that seen in our experiments with alar plate and optic cup removals.*

The fact that in the reconstituted tectum retinal fibers from one eye can extend into the territory normally occupied by the fibers from the opposite eye also suggests that when both eyes are present the fibers normally compete with each other near the midline, and that the sharp boundary which is seen between the two retinal projections reflects this competitive interaction. Competition of this kind is known to occur in several other neural systems (see Chapter 10), and has been particularly well documented during the development of the eye dominance columns found in area 17 in the monkey.[78,79]

3.4.3. *The Retinal Projection in Animals with Partial Tectal Regeneration.* We have observed a quite different type of plasticity in the chicks in which the tectum showed only partial regeneration. While these animals were of only limited interest for the analysis of tectal regeneration *per se,* in the few cases in which [^{3}H]proline had been injected into

* In a small number of monocular chicks the development of the roof plate region seems (for some unknown reason) to be impaired. In these brains there is usually a narrow zone in which the tectal tissue of the two optic lobes is continuous; wherever this occurred we have found evidence for a crossed retinotectal projection similar to that described above.

the eye contralateral to the partially regenerated tectum we have been able to examine the effects of a fortuitously induced size disparity on the retinal projection. In the majority of the brains of this type that we have examined, the volume of the regenerated part of the tectum was less than 50% of that of a normal optic lobe, so the size disparity was substantial. Interestingly, in these cases the retinal projection from the eye contralateral to the alar plate lesion did not occupy half the dome-shaped tectal surface, but rather remained confined to the relatively small regenerated sector, and stopped abruptly along a line that morphologically would appear to correspond to the original midline. As we did not independently label the projections from the other retinae in these cases, we do not have direct evidence for their distribution, but there seems no reason to doubt that they occupied the rest of the tectum, in a more or less normal fashion. We should add that as we have not attempted to map the retino-topic organization of the projections to the partially regenerated tecta, we do not know if the connections formed were derived from all parts of the retina or if only certain retinal regions were represented. It will be important to establish this point, because it should help to clarify the interpretation of the findings of the nontectal central projections in these brains.

The latter show a number of interesting features. First, it is our impression that many of the projections to such visual relay nuclei as the ventral lateral geniculate nucleus, the dorsolateral and lateral anterior thalamic nuclei, the mesencephalic lentiform nucleus, and the pretectal area, are rather heavier than normal (as judged by the distribution and density of the silver grains seen over the nuclei in our autoradiographs). Since quantitative estimates of the magnitude of projections are difficult to make in autoradiographs (unless there is an appropriate built-in control in the preparation—see Cowan and Cuenod[80]), we cannot state with certainty that there are more retinal fibers and synapses in these nuclei than would normally be found, but it seems likely that this will prove to be the case. Second, in all cases of this type that we have examined there have been a number of labeled projections to the ipsilateral visual thalamic and pretectal nuclei, which follow a wholly aberrant course. As in normal chicks, the retinal fibers from the eye contralateral to the partially regenerated tectum decussate completely at the optic chiasm. However, on reaching the pretectal region some of the fibers again cross the midline in what appears to be a "pretectal commissure," that is quite distinct from the normal posterior commissure. After crossing the midline, some of the aberrant fibers terminate in the pretectal area, but others continue rostrally to end in the ipsilateral dorsolateral anterior thalamic nucleus, and in some cases also in the lateral anterior thalamic nucleus. Interestingly, none of the aberrant fibers entered the other visual relay nuclei on this side, and in particular, none extended into the nucleus rotundus of either side. The absence of a projection to the nucleus rotundus is noteworthy because this nucleus is known to receive a substantial visual input from the optic tectum.[49,50,81]

In many respects these experiments in which there is a marked disparity between the magnitude of the retinal input and the size of the available target area in the tectum are comparable to the experiments of Schneider and his colleagues[82,83] in which early postnatal lesions were placed in the superior colliculus of hamsters. In both instances aberrant connections were formed and the "normal" retinal recipient structures appeared to receive an abnormally heavy retinal input. Schneider has referred to this phenomenon as a "pruning response" and has suggested that it represents an attempt by the neurons that were deprived of their normal target to form and maintain a normal or near-normal total number of synaptic connections. It is interesting that in our experiments the aberrant projections formed in the presence of an unusually small tectum were not distributed to all the available visual relay centers on the ipsilateral side of the brain, but only to a distinct subset of these centers. Just what determines which nuclei receive aberrant projections and which are to be excluded from receiving such inputs is unknown. Conceivably it may be simply the proximity of the nucleus to the recrossed retinal projection, but it is possible that a hierarchy of affinities within the visual system limits the patterns of connections that can be formed (cf. the analogous situation described by Hollyday *et al.*[84] in chicks with supernumerary limbs). Until we know more about the normal central distribution of the axons of different classes of retinal ganglion cells in the avian brain, it will be difficult to resolve this issue.

We should also like to know what percentage of the retinal ganglion cells survive in brains with partially regenerated tecta. Hughes and LaVelle[85] have shown that if a substantial part of the tectum is ablated on the 4th or 5th day of incubation, a majority of the cells in the associated parts of the retina undergo a secondary degeneration (see Chapter 9 for discussion of the role of targets in neuronal survival). As they did not examine the nontectal projections of the affected retinae, it is uncertain if the types of pruning reaction we have observed also occurred in their material; this point bears further investigation, and it will be especially important to determine whether the age of the animal at the time of the tectal lesion is critical for the establishment of aberrant, or unusually heavy, retinal projections to other visual centers.

3.4.4. Retinal Projections to Regions of Abnormal Tectal Regeneration. In some of the brains we have examined, parts of the regenerated tectum showed areas of distinctly abnormal lamination. Most commonly the affected areas appeared as relatively small regions (~100 μm in diameter) in which the normal tectal lamination was missing. In these cases, the labeled optic nerve fibers simply passed over the surface of the dyslaminate sector, in a band that was continuous with the SO, but none of the fibers extended inwards into the disorganized tissue itself. In a small number of cases the reverse situation pertained: there were several small islands with relatively normal lamination embedded in a mass of disorganized tissue. Although this disorganized tissue appeared to contain many neurons, the labeled retinal fibers simply passed over, or through, the affected areas, seemingly without terminating in them. But whenever the fibers reached an island of normal-appearing tissue, there was always evidence of labeled axons (and presumably axon terminals) in the appropriate outer layers of the SGFS. We have not analyzed these cases in detail, but the basic observation is noteworthy because it suggests rather strongly that ingrowing optic nerve fibers are capable of "recognizing" regions of normal tectal architecture, and that they only invade and form synapses in those zones in which the relevant cell types are present and in their normal topographic arrangement. It is premature to infer from this that the axons respond to cues that are present only on the surfaces of cells in the outer tectal layers, and that the relevant cues are missing in the dyslaminate zones (however, see Chapters 6 and 10 for discussions of this possibility). An alternative explanation might be that the mechanism responsible for the normal pattern of tectal lamination is also critically implicated in the target-locus recognition process. A more systematic examination of the structure of the dyslaminate tissue might throw some light on this issue, but for the present it is worth emphasizing that a normal cytoarchitecture does not appear to be an essential prerequisite for the establishment of an ordered system of connections in other neural tissues. For example in the cerebral and cerebellar cortices of homozygous reeler mice, in which the normal cytoarchitectonic organization is grossly disrupted, it has been shown that the relevant afferent fibers are able to identify their appropriate neuronal targets and to establish connections that appear to be functionally quite normal.[86–88]

Acknowledgments

This work was supported in part by the Clayton Foundation for Research, of which W. M. C. is a Senior Investigator, and by grant EY-03653 (formerly EY-1255) from the National Eye Institute.

4. REFERENCES

1. Liu, C., and Chambers, W. W., 1958, Intraspinal sprouting of dorsal root axons, *Arch. Neurol. Psychiatr.* **79:**46.
2. Cotman, C. W. (ed.), 1978, *Neuronal Plasticity,* Raven Press, New York.
3. Lund, R. D., 1978, *Development and Plasticity of the Brain,* Oxford University Press, New York.
4. Bjorklund, A., and Stenevi, U., 1979, Regeneration of monoaminergic and cholinergic neurons in the mammalian central nervous system, *Physiol. Rev.* **59:**62.
5. Tsukahara, N., 1981, Synaptic plasticity in the mammalian central nervous system, *Ann Rev. Neurosci.* **4:**351.
6. Lewis, W. H., 1906, Experiments on the regeneration and differentiation of the central nervous system in amphibian embryos, *Am. J. Anat.* **5:**XI.
7. Bell, E. T., 1906, Experimental studies on the development of the eye and the nasal cavities in frog embryos, *Anat. Anz.* **29:**185.
8. Bell, E. T., 1907, Some experiments on the development and regeneration of the eye and the nasal organ in frog embryos, *Wilhelm Roux Arch. Entwicklungsmech. Org.* **23:**457.
9. Spemann, H., 1912, Zur Entwicklung des Wirbeltieranges, *Zool. Jahr.* **32:**1.
10. Burr, H. S., 1916, Regeneration in the brain of *Amblystoma, J. Comp. Neurol.* **26:**203.
11. Spirito, A., 1928, Processi regolativi della regione encefalica degli embrioni di Anuri, *Rend. R. Accad. Naz. Lincei Naples* **8:**429.
12. Spirito, A., 1929, Processi di rigenerazione e di regolazione nella regione encefalica degli embrioni di Urodeli, *Rend. R. Accad. Naz. Lincei Naples* **10:**215.
13. Spirito, A., 1930, Rigenerazioni e regolazioni nell' encefalo degli Amfibi, *Wilhelm Roux Arch. Entwicklungsmech. Org.* **122:**152.
14. Detwiler, S. R., 1944, Restitution of the medulla following unilateral excision in the embryo, *J. Exp. Zool.* **96:**129.
15. Detwiler, S. R., 1945, The results of unilateral and bilateral extirpation of the forebrain of *Amblystoma, J. Exp. Zool.* **100:**103.
16. Detwiler, S. R., 1946, Midbrain regeneration in *Amblystoma, Anat. Rec.* **94:**229.
17. Detwiler, S. R., 1947, Restitution of the brachial region of the cord following unilateral excision in the embryo, *J. Exp. Zool.* **104:**53.
18. Harrison, R. G., 1947, Wound healing and reconstitution of the central nervous system of the amphibian embryo after removal of parts of the neural plate, *J. Exp. Zool.* **106:**27.
19. Holtzer, H., 1951, Reconstitution of the urodele spinal cord following unilateral ablation. Part I. Chronology of neuron regulation, *J. Exp. Zool.* **117:**523.
20. Matthey, R., 1925, Recuperation de la vue apres resection des nerfs optiques chez le triton, *C. R. Soc. Biol.* **93:**904.
21. Sperry, R. W., 1943, Effect of 180° rotation of the retinal field on visuotopic motor coordination, *J. Exp. Zool.* **92:**263.
22. Sperry, R. W., 1948, Patterning of central synapses in regeneration of the optic nerve in teleosts, *Physiol. Zool.* **21:**351.
23. Arora, H. L., and Sperry, R. W., 1962, Optic nerve regeneration after surgical cross-union of medial and lateral optic tracts, *Am. Zool.* **2:**389.
24. Attardi, D. G., and Sperry, R. W., 1963, Preferential selection of central pathways by regenerating optic fibers, *Exp. Neurol.* **7:**46.
25. Wenger, E., 1950, An experimental analysis of relations between parts of the brachial spinal cord of the embryonic chick, *J. Exp. Zool.* **114:**51.

26. Levi-Montalcini, R., 1945, Corrélations dans le développement des differentes parties du système nerveux. II. Corrélations entre le développement de l'encéphale et celui de la moelle épinière dans l'embryon de poulet, *Arch. Biol.* **56:**71.
27. Yntema, C. L., and Hammond, W. S., 1945, Depletions and abnormalities in the cervical sympathetic system of the chick following extirpations of the neural crest, *J. Exp. Zool.* **100:**237.
28. Watterson, R. L., and Fowler, I., 1953, Regulative development in lateral halves of chick neural tubes, *Anat. Rec.* **117:**773.
29. Birge, W. J., and Hilleman, H. H., 1953, Metencephalic development and differentiation following experimental lesions in the early chick embryo, *J. Exp. Zool.* **124:**545.
30. Hamburger, V., and Hamilton, H., 1951, A series of normal stages in the development of the chick embryo, *J. Morphol.* **88:**49.
31. Birge, W. J., 1959, An analysis of differentiation and regulation in the mesencephalon of the chick embryo, *Am. J. Anat.* **104:**431.
32. Weiss, P., 1934, Secretory activity of the inner layer of the embryonic midbrain of the chick as revealed by tissue culture, *Anat. Rec.* **58:**299.
33. Cowan, W. M., Martin, A. H., and Wenger, E., 1968, Mitotic patterns in the optic tectum of the chick during normal development and after early removal of the optic vesicle, *J. Exp. Zool.* **169:**71.
34. LaVail, J. H., and Cowan, W. M., 1971, The development of the chick optic tectum. II. Autoradiographic studies, *Brain Res.* **28:**421.
35. Bergquist, H., 1959, Experiments on the overgrowth phenomenon in the brains of chick embryos, *J. Embryol. Exp. Morphol.* **7:**122.
36. Källén, B., 1961, Studies on cell proliferation in the brain of chick embryos with special reference to the mesencephalon, *Z. Anat. Entwicklungsgesch.* **122:**388.
37. Källén, B., 1962, Overgrowth malformation and neoplasia in embryonic brain, *Confin. Neurol.* **22:**40.
38. Wilson, D. B., 1971, Distribution of thymidine-H^3 in the overgrown brain of the chick embryo, *J. Comp. Neurol.* **141:**37.
39. Wilson, D. B., 1972, Effects of embryonic overgrowth on the avian optic tectum, *Am. J. Anat.* **135:**549.
40. van Gehuchten, A., 1892, La structure des lobes optiques chez embryon de poulet, *Cellule* **8:**5.
41. Ramón y Cajal, S., 1911. *Histologie du Système Nerveux de l'Homme et des Vertébrés. II,* Maloine, Paris.
42. Huber, G. C., and Crosby, E. C., 1929, The nuclei and fiber paths of the avian diencephalon, with consideration of telencephalic and certain mesencephalic centers and connections, *J. Comp. Neurol.* **48:**1.
43. Jungherr, E., 1945, Certain nuclear groups of the avian mesencephalon, *J. Comp. Neurol.* **82:**55.
44. Cragg, B. G., Evans, D. H. L., and Hamlyn, L. H., 1954, The optic tectum of *Gallus domesticus*: A correlation of the electrical responses with the histological structure, *J. Anat.* **88:**292.
45. Cowan, W. M., Adamson, L., and Powell, T. P. S., 1961, An experimental study of the avian visual system, *J. Anat.* **95:**545.
46. Hamdi, J. A., and Whitteridge, D., 1954, The representation of the retina on the optic tectum of the pigeon, *Q. J. Exp. Physiol.* **39:**111.
47. McGill, J. I., Powell, T. P. S., and Cowan, W. M., 1966, The retinal representation upon the optic tectum and isthmo-optic nucleus in the pigeon, *J. Anat.* **100:**5.

48. Crossland, W. J., Cowan, W. M., and Kelly, J. P., 1973, Observations on the transport of radioactively labeled proteins in the visual system of the chick, *Brain Res.* **56**:77.
49. Hart, J. R., 1969, *Some Observations on the Development of the Avian Optic Tectum*, Ph.D. dissertation, University of Wisconsin, Madison, WI.
50. Karten, H. J., 1965, Projections of the optic tectum in the pigeon (*Columba livia*), *Anat. Rec.* **151**:369.
51. Hunt, S. P., and Kunzle, H., 1976, Observations on the projections and intrinsic organization of the pigeon optic tectum: An autoradiographic study based on anterograde and retrograde axonal and dendritic flow, *J. Comp. Neurol.* **170**:153.
52. Cowan, W. M., 1970, Centrifugal fibers to the avian retina, *Br. Med. Bull.* **26**:1.
53. Cowan, W. M., and Powell, T. P. S., 1963, Centrifugal fibers in the avian visual system, *Proc. R. Soc. London Ser. B* **158**:232.
54. Crossland, W. J., and Hughes, C. P., 1978, Observations on the afferent and efferent connections of the avian isthmo-optic nucleus, *Brain Res.* **145**:239.
55. Streit, P., Reubi, J. C., Wolfensberger, M., Henke, H., and Cuenod, M., 1979, Transmitter-specific retrograde tracing of pathways?, *Progr. Brain Res.* **51**:489.
56. Fujita, S., 1964, Analysis of neuron differentiation in the central nervous system by tritiated thymidine autoradiography, *J. Comp. Neurol.* **122**:311.
57. LaVail, J. H., and Cowan, W. M., 1971, The development of the chick optic tectum. I. Normal morphology and cytoarchitectonic development, *Brain Res.* **28**:391.
58. Domesick, V. B., and Morest, D. K., 1977*a*, Migration and differentation of ganglion cells in the optic tectum of the chick, *Neurosci.* **2**:459.
59. Domesick, V. B., and Morest, D. K., 1977*b*, Migration and differentiation of Shepherd's crook cells in the optic tectum of the chick, *Neurosci.* **2**:477.
60. De Long, G. R., and Coulombre, A. J., 1965, Development of the retinotectal topographic projection in the chick embryo, *Exp. Neurol.* **13**:351.
61. Goldberg, S., 1974, Studies on the mechanics of development of the visual pathways in the chick embryo, *Dev. Biol.* **36**:24.
62. Crossland, W. J., Cowan, W. M., and Rogers, L. A., 1975, Studies on the development of the chick optic tectum. IV. An autoradiographic study of the development of retino-tectal connections, *Brain Res.* **91**:1.
63. McGraw, C. F., and McLaughlin, B. J., 1980, Fine structural studies of synaptogenesis in the superficial layers of the chick optic tectum, *J. Neurocytol.* **9**:79.
64. Rager, G., 1976, Morphogenesis and physiogenesis of the retino-tectal connections in the chicken. II. The retino-tectal synapses, *Proc. R. Soc. London Ser. B* **192**:353.
65. Kahn, A. J., 1973, Ganglion cell formation in the chick neural retina, *Brain Res.* **63**:285.
66. Crossland, W. J., Cowan, W. M., Rogers, L. A., and Kelly, J. P., 1974, The specification of the retino-tectal projection in the chick, *J. Comp. Neurol.* **155**:127.
67. Kelly, J. P., and Cowan, W. M., 1972, Studies on the development of the chick optic tectum. III. Effects of early eye removal, *Brain Res.* **42**:263.
68. Cowan, W. M., Gottlieb, D. I., Hendrickson, A. E., Price, J. L., and Woolsey, T. A., 1972, The autoradiographic demonstration of axonal connections in the central nervous system, *Brain Res.* **37**:21.
69. Rogers, L. A., and Cowan, W. M., 1973, The development of the mesencephalic nucleus of the trigeminal nerve in the chick, *J. Comp. Neurol.* **147**:291.
70. Narayanan, C. H., and Narayanan, Y., 1978, Determination of the embryonic origin of the mesencephalic nucleus of the trigeminal nerve in birds, *J. Embryol. Exp. Morphol.* **43**:85.
71. Cowan, W. M., 1971, Studies on the development of the avian visual system, in: *Cellular Aspects of Neural Growth and Differentiation* (D. C. Pease, ed.), pp. 177–222, University of California Press, Berkeley and Los Angeles.

72. Reperant, J., 1973, Nouvelles données sur les projection visuelles chez le Pigeon (*Columba livia*), *J. Hirnforsch.* **14:**151.
73. Yoon, M., 1971, Reorganization of retinotectal projections following surgical operations on the optic tectum in goldfish, *Exp. Neurol.* **33:**395.
74. Sharma, S. C., 1972, Reformation of retinotectal projections after various tectal ablations in adult goldfish, *Exp. Neurol.* **34:**171.
75. Schmidt, J. T., Cicerone, C. M., and Easter, S. S., 1978, Expansion of the half retinal projection to the tectum in goldfish: An electrophysiological and anatomical study, *J. Comp. Neurol.* **177:**257.
76. Gaze, R. M., 1978, The problem of specificity in the formation of nerve connections, in: *Specificity of Embryological Interactions* (D. Garard, ed.), pp. 53–93, Chapman and Hall, London.
77. O'Leary, D. D. M., and Cowan, W. M., 1980, Observations on the effects of monocular and binocular eye removal on the development of the chick visual system, *Neurosci. Abstr.* **6:**297.
78. Hubel, D. H., Wiesel, T. N., and LeVay, S., 1977, Plasticity of ocular dominance columns in monkey striate cortex, *Philos. Trans. R. Soc. London Ser. B* **278:**377.
79. Rakic, P., 1977, Prenatal development of the visual system in the rhesus monkey, *Philos. Trans. Roy. Soc. London Ser. B* **278:**245.
80. Cowan, W. M., and Cuenod, M., 1975, The use of axonal transport for the study of neural connections: A retrospective survey, in: *The Use of Axonal Transport for Studies of Neuronal Connectivity* (W. M. Cowan and M. Cuenod, eds.), pp. 3–24, Elsevier, Amsterdam.
81. Karten, H. J., and Revzin, A. M., 1966, The afferent connections of the nucleus rotundus in the pigeon, *Brain Res.* **2:**368.
82. Schneider, G. E., 1973, Early lesions of superior colliculus: Factors affecting the formation of abnormal retinal projections, *Brain Behav. Evol.* **8:**73.
83. Schneider, G. E., and Jhaveri, S. R., 1974, Neuroanatomical correlates of spared or altered function after brain lesions in the newborn hamster, in: *Plasticity and Recovery of Function in the Central Nervous System* (D. G. Stein, J. J. Rosen, and N. Butters, eds.), pp. 65–109, Academic Press, New York.
84. Hollyday, M., Hamburger, V., and Farris, J. M. G., 1977, Localization of motor neuron pools supplying identified muscles in normal and supernumerary legs of chick embryo, *Proc. Natl. Acad. Sci. U.S.A.* **74:**3582.
85. Hughes, W. T., and LaVelle, A., 1975, The effects of early tectal lesions on development in the retinal ganglion cell layer of chick embryos, *J. Comp. Neurol.* **163:**265.
86. Drager, U. C., 1976, Reeler mutant mice: Physiology in primary visual cortex, *Exp. Brain Res. Suppl.* **1:**274.
87. Caviness, V. S., and Rakic, P., 1978, Mechanisms of cortical development: A view from mutations in mice, *Ann. Rev. Neurosci.* **1:**297.
88. Lemmon, V., and Pearlman, A. L., 1981, Does laminar position determine the receptive field properties of cortical neurons? a study of cortico-tectal cells in area 17 of the normal mouse and the reeler mutant, *J. Neurosci.* **1:**83.

Index